The H.I.S.S. of the A.S.P.

Understanding the Anomalously Sensitive Person

by

David Ritchey

The H.I.S.S. of the A.S.P.:
Understanding the
Anomalously Sensitive Person

By

David Ritchey

To order additional copies of this book or for book publishing information, or to contact the author:

Headline Books, Inc.
P.O. Box 52
Terra Alta, WV 26764
www.headlinebooks.com

Tel/Fax: 800-570-5951 or 304-789-5951
Email: ASPproject@headlinebooks.com
www.hissofasp.com

Cover Art by Glenn Lewis

ISBN 0929915291

Library of Congress Control Number: 2002116194

PRINTED IN THE UNITED STATES OF AMERICA

To my offspring
— Harper and Mac —
both of whom seemed to know,
either intuitively or experientially,
what it took me years of research
to figure out.

Acknowledgments

Most acknowledgments begin with a statement to the effect that the book could not have been written without the help of many other people. In the case of *The H.I.S.S. of the A.S.P.,* "many" means literally hundreds—and it would be impossible to acknowledge all of them by name.

Most of those who lent their assistance remain, by intention, anonymous. They are the 295 people in the HISS Reference Group who contributed about an hour of their time to complete the questionnaire.

Then there are the "old faithfuls," the eight original subjects each of whom answered almost 2000 questions in the early rounds of testing. These stalwart backers, without whom this project never would have gotten off the ground, have my profound gratitude. They are: Andrew Combe, Brian Ireland, Edward Kendall, Lea Kendall, Elizabeth Serkin, Carl Silver, Jessica Thomas and Lynda Vieytes.

Quite a few people helped to facilitate the distribution and collection of questionnaires. With apologies to those who have been overlooked, those remembered include: William Baldwin, Judith Baldwin, Ann Baruch, Deane Brown, Lyn Buchanan, Andrew Combe, Leni Erickson, Mary Jo Hackett, Bill Hays, Debbie Jarvis, Edward Kendall, Lea Kendall, Scott Mangham, Harley Pursglove, Mac Ritchey, Howard Schachter, Harper Schantz, Elizabeth Serkin, Michael Sutherland and Jenny Wade.

Several individuals helped me to organize my thinking long before development of the HISS ("Holistic Inventory of Stimulus Sensitivities") questionnaire even began. Numerous hours were spent in conversation with: Joan Borysenko, Myrin Borysenko, Kurt Ebert, Jim Hardt, David Hufford, Wayne London and Kenneth Ring. Ken's graciousness was especially striking—upon discovering that we were pursuing essentially the same idea, he shared with me his own research and suggested that I take it from there.

Those who read the first draft of this book and offered valuable feedback included: Laurence Austin, Andrew Combe, Lisa Hilty, Edward Kendall, Keven Murphy, Harley Pursglove, and Elizabeth Serkin.

The pathfinding work of other writers and researchers made my task considerably easier. Especially helpful were the efforts of: Elaine Aron, Albert Budden, Henry Corbin, Stanley Coren, Albert Galaburda, Howard Gardner, David Gelernter, Norman Geschwind, Ernest Hartmann, Ernest Hilgard, Julian Jaynes, Eve LaPlante, Joseph Chilton Pearce, Michael Persinger, Dean Radin, Kenneth Ring and Michael Talbot.

Development of the HISS was facilitated by my being able to draw upon ideas introduced in already extant questionnaires developed by, among others: Gilbert Atkinson, Marilyn Bates, Katherine Briggs, Eve Carlson, Bruce Greyson, Ernest Hartmann, Budd Hopkins, David Kiersey, Steven Lynn, Isabel Myers, Frank Putnam, Judith Rhue, Kenneth Ring and Auke Telegren.

Individuals who made unique contributions include: Susan Butler and Rob White (inspired drawings), Joanne Garland (tireless transcription), Michael Sutherland (statistical guidance), Lyn Buchanan, Donna Cashell, Harley Pursglove and Jenny Wade (all of whom took on aspects of this project as if it were their own) and B. J. "Bob" and Cathy Teets of Headline Books (who believed enough in the project to edit and publish this book).

Finally, there's my best friend, my most loyal supporter, my most ardent admirer, my black Labrador retriever, Raven, whose patience was boundless.

Contents

PART II: THE EVIDENCE

Foreword

BY KENNETH RING, PH.D.

Back in the late 1980s, when I was engaged in the research that eventually led to my book, *The Omega Project,* I found myself dealing with a conundrum that had previously stumped other researchers interested in the realm of extraordinary encounters such as near-death experiences and purported interaction with alien beings. The problem was this: why did only some people report such experiences while others who had either come close to death or had sighted apparent UFOs recounted nothing of the kind? In other words, what made certain individuals sensitive to these sometimes hard-to-credit "realities," which nevertheless seemed entirely real to them, whereas most people in comparable situations remained entirely oblivious? "'Twas a puzzlement." And not just to me. I remember asking one prominent researcher of near-death experiences how he accounted for such wild variability. His answer was as pithy as it was candid. "Ken," he said, "I haven't got a clue."

Well, after I had undertaken my own work, I thought I had found at least a few clues and, in a couple of initial articles that appeared before my book was published, I speculated on some of the factors contributing to the make-up of what I then called "psychological sensitives"—by which I meant people who seemed particularly susceptible to reporting extraordinary encounters involving apparent psychic or otherworldly phenomena.

Not long afterward, I received a letter from a researcher entirely unknown to me, a hypnotherapist named David Ritchey, and was astonished to learn that, quite independently, he had been sniffing along the same trail. And more than that, his preliminary findings and conjectures seemingly dovetailed almost perfectly with mine, and indeed, he had already gone further down this trail than I had and had begun to see connections that I hadn't myself previously been aware of. Needless to say, I was delighted to find such unexpected and timely support for some of my own hunches and not long after we arranged to meet in order to compare notes in person.

When we met, it was rapport at first sight, and David and I became fast friends. Indeed, we came to discover that we had quite a number of other interests and proclivities in common, quite apart from our preoccupation with the question of the nature of psychological sensitives, and soon determined that we even shared the same birthday—December 13th! Astrology aside, whatever the provenance of our affinities, they were obvious and led us to many enjoyable conversations in those early years of our friendship.

But one difference between us was also apparent. By the early 1990s, I was beginning to move on to other professional concerns whereas David was still hot on the trail of whatever factors conduced to what I was still calling "psychological sensitivity," so I naturally encouraged him to continue exploring this domain and offered to help him in any way I could. Well, he didn't need much help from me, as it turned out, because he had already formulated a research strategy of his own. And for the next ten years (!), he devoted himself to it with such a degree of unswerving dedication and painstaking attention to detail that one can only conclude that his work reflects a genuine spirit of *vocation*—a virtual calling that David was led to follow to its end with an almost fervent and totally admirable sense of professional commitment.

The book you now hold in your hand—*The H.I.S.S. of the A.S.P.*—is, then, David's definitive and groundbreaking study of just why some people (his term for them is "anomalously sensitive persons" [or ASPs]) are able to detect these alternate realities and of the various factors—neurological, environmental and psychological—that together tend to facilitate this type of sensitivity. The amount of work that went into fashioning this portrait of the ASP—all of it based on David's own original research and his copious and sedulous review of the findings of other investigators—has been prodigious, as you will soon become aware. The result is that David's ten-year odyssey has allowed him to produce such a richly textured and multi-faceted delineation of the origins and nature of the person who is sensitive to alternate realities that he has not merely given us a few clues to this former enigma, he has answered virtually every question about it. In short, a more masterly blend of original research and synthesis of the findings of others on this important topic is difficult to conceive.

But David has accomplished far more than this, for in drawing this portrait of the ASP, he has also humanized her (for most ASPs, he finds, are women, so I will use that pronoun here). Like the writings of the neurologist, Oliver Sacks, who has made us so keenly aware of both the humanity and rare talents of those whom others might have once seen only as victims of severe neurological impairment, David's depiction of the ASP shows her also to be a person of unusual giftedness and extraordinary sensitivities. Though she may indeed suffer from various illnesses and other unenviable conditions, the realities she perceives cannot be dismissed as fictive or hallucinatory, nor, as David's research shows, is it reasonable to discount, much less pathologize, her perceptions and abilities. There are realms beyond those of consensual reality, and what the majority regards as real is only normative, not definitive. The ASP, on the other hand, tends to perceive beyond normal boundaries, which have hitherto been unacknowledged by science, and her insights and sensitivities must ultimately be recognized and legitimated. David's work, though it carefully avoids advocacy, will clearly serve that laudable end.

So far I have only addressed the nature of David's seminal contribution, but not his style, which is worth a paragraph in itself. Though this book is a thoroughly serious, and even at times ponderous, consideration of the roots of the anomalously sensitive person, the title itself betrays David's characteristic antic inclinations. *The H.I.S.S. of the A.S.P.*! ...Really! I mean, David just can't resist the clever pun, and I'm sure he labeled his research questionnaire "The Holistic Inventory of Stimulus Sensitivities" (i.e., the HISS) for this express purpose. (I thought I was fairly ingenious in calling my version "The Psychological Sensitivity Inventory"—or PSI— but in this respect, my pathetic effort at whimsy would probably serve only to elicit David's disdain.) But in fact, David's book is, for the most part, written in the most accessible style, free of jargon, and full of humorous asides. Moreover, it features many amusing cartoons, specifically drawn for this book, and it is strewn with witty epigraphs and quotations, which leaven the text and provide many a chuckle for the reader. So be advised that David's own charm and delightful wit pervade the book and help to give it its own distinctive brand of irrepressible raillery at times, so that its seriousness of purpose will never prevent the occasional wry joke.

A potential problem for some readers will be David's use of a multitude of four-letter words (not of the vulgar sort, but of the abbreviation sort) and three-letter words like ASC, EMS, FMS, FPP, LSL, NRH, SOC, TPC, TPE and so on into the night. While it must be said in his defense that the choice to abbreviate served to shorten the text considerably (and he *has* provided a handy guide to those abbreviations), if you happen to be the sort of person who can't abide such things, you might be tempted to throw this book against the wall while figuratively hurling a host of expletives, of whatever length, at the author. Such behavior, however, while entirely understandable, would only be churlish. As an alternative, I recommend that you just deface your copy with a red marker and let it go at that. Besides, when you come to the statistical portion of the book (which mercifully has been set aside as a separate section at the end), you will find it nearly unreadable—unless, of course, you are a statistically-minded academician (for whom its inclusion was necessary), or you are, like David, an incorrigible obsessive-compulsive. So, in light of that, putting up with a plague of abbreviations is a bagatelle.

Just kidding, folks. This is really a richly rewarding book and it represents a monumental achievement in the study and understanding of those individuals who are anomalously sensitive. As such, it will be of profound and indispensable interest to all therapists, scholars and researchers who deal with such individuals, and to ASPs themselves in their search for both self-understanding and public recognition of their undeniable contribution to our appreciation of realities that transcend normal waking consciousness.

—Kentfield, California
June 2002

Preface

It is impossible to dissociate language from science
or science from language,
because every natural science always involves three things:
The sequence of phenomena on which the science is based;
the abstract concepts which call these phenomena to mind;
and the words in which the concepts are expressed.
To call forth a concept a word is needed;
to portray a phenomenon, a concept is needed.
All three mirror one and the same reality.
—*Antoine Laurent Lavoisier*

This book is about experiences…and it is also about the words used to categorize those experiences. When a specific class of experience is labeled with words that have skeptical, denigrative, or dismissive connotations— words such as "occult," "paranormal," "supernatural," "psychical,"

Many errors, of a truth, consist merely in the application of the wrong names of things.
—Baruch Spinoza

"metaphysical," and "New Age"—the reality of those experiences is called into question (even in the minds of those who have those experiences) and it is implied that they are unworthy of scientific investigation.

In my years as a clinical hypnotherapist, having worked with many clients who reported experiences of such things as Extra-Sensory Perception (ESP), past-life recall, spirit possession and alien contact, I became convinced that the *subjective experiences* were very real for the experiencers—this regardless of the reality status of the *objective phenomena* ("temporal or spatiotemporal objects of ordinary sensual experience and susceptible to scientific description and explanation"). I decided, therefore, that it was appropriate to direct some serious scientific scrutiny toward the nature of such experiences and toward the experiencers themselves.

One of my first research goals was "to find the right names for things." The value-neutral collective name that I eventually settled on was Stanislav Grof's term "Transpersonal Experiences (TPEs)," and I assigned to it the following meaning: "Experiences that occur beyond the ordinary differentiated boundaries of ego, space and time; experiences that suggest the essential interconnectedness (and/or absolute unity) of all that ever was, is, or will be; experiences that imply the existence of mind (as distinct from brain), of spirit, of soul."

The beginning of wisdom is to find the right names for things.
—Chinese Proverb

Moving further into the investigation, I soon discovered that many more terms that were pertinent to a study of Transpersonal Experiences—"Altered States of Consciousness (ASCs)," "dissociation," "hallucination," and "mind," among them—also had inappropriate value-laden connotations. Creating neologisms to replace those familiar terms, however, seemed to be an approach that would only give rise to additional confusion. Ultimately, the best solution appeared to be to assign to those terms, in the glossary of this book, meanings (sometimes non-standard) specific to their usage herein. As a reminder of this approach, such terms (and their abbreviations) appear in {{this non-standard typeface}} rather than in {{this standard typeface}}. Other terms, the *precise* (even if standard) meanings of which are especially important, are handled in the same way.

Every effort has been made to make the material in the text as accessible as possible to the layperson, but quite a few long words, obscure words, or technical words remain. Their inclusion was unavoidable because the subject matter encompasses many weighty academic fields

"When I use a word,"
Humpty Dumpty said,
in a rather scornful tone,
"it means just what I choose it to mean
—nothing more nor less."
—Lewis Carroll
(Through the Looking Glass)

such as neurology, psychology, biochemistry, philosophy and physics. As a result, the glossary is rather extensive.

Some other conventions used throughout *The H.I.S.S. of the A.S.P.* that merit mention here are:

- When medical or psychiatric terms are used in a clinical sense, they appear in "Title Case" format; when they are used in a purely descriptive sense, they appear in "lower case" format.
- Terms for which capitalized abbreviations are regularly employed throughout the book are capitalized (sometimes idiosyncratically) when the term is spelled out in full (e.g., "PsychoKinesis" which is abbreviated as "PK"). For easy reference, important abbreviations and their meanings are listed on the bookmark located in the back of this book.
- Names of the scales for the "Holistic Inventory of Stimulus Sensitivities (HISS)" questionnaire often appear as three-letter, capitalized abbreviations (e.g., "PHS"). When they are spelled out in full, their first letter is capitalized (e.g., "Physiological indicators"). Scale names and their abbreviations are also listed on the bookmark.
- Endnote numbers for references to sources have been omitted from the text to improve readability and flow. Links to the text are established by chapter number, page number and subject matter in "Sources" (which appears in the back matter).
- Pronoun genders, in formal quotations from other written material, appear in their original form. In my own writing, the conventions of "s/he" and "her/him" have been used. Because Anomalously Sensitive Persons (ASPs), the subject of this book, are predominantly female, the female pronoun has been placed in a position of precedence.

I am a Bear of Very Little Brain,
and long words bother me.
—Winnie-the-Pooh

Introduction

Begin at the beginning
...and go on till you come to the end:
then stop.

—*Lewis Carroll*
(Alice's Adventures in Wonderland)

*T*he *H.I.S.S. of the A.S.P.* is about the full spectrum of human
sensitivities—Physiological sensitivities, Cognitive sensitivities,
Emotional sensitivities, Altered States of Consciousness (ASC)
sensitivities and Transpersonal Experiences (TPE) sensitivities.
That's the broad perspective. From a narrower perspective, this book
is about Transpersonal Experiences (TPEs) and the people who have
them.[†]

The two perspectives are equally important—if they are treated
otherwise, one is likely to fall into the conventional trap of thinking
that Transpersonal Experiences are fictive, that they are not real.
This dismissal of the veridicality of Transpersonal
Experiences occurs because most people are unable to perceive the
putatively sensory stimuli *(phenomena)* that give rise to them—and
by consensus such experiences are therefore considered to be not a
part of objective reality. Individuals who respond to stimuli that are
not a part of consensus reality are said to be hallucinating and
hallucinations are generally held to be evidentiary of mental illness.

The concept of the Anomalously Sensitive Person (ASP) is
experientially rather than phenomenologically based. It thus avoids
the issue of cultural consensus about reality entirely—and sidesteps
the issue of psychopathology. The essence of the ASP hypothesis is
this:

[†] See either the Preface or the Glossary for the definition of Transpersonal Experiences.

Certain individuals—who will be spoken of as Anomalously Sensitive Persons (ASPs)—in addition to being anomalously sensitive to stimuli in the Transpersonal Experiences realm, are also anomalously sensitive to stimuli in the Physiological, Cognitive, Emotional and Altered States of Consciousness realms. These individuals are predisposed toward being anomalously sensitive by various Biological ("nature"), Trauma and Abuse ("nurture") and Temperament Type Preferences ("personality") factors.

Transpersonal Experiences are subjective experiences and, as such, are every bit as real as, say, love experiences, aesthetic experiences, or anger experiences. All experiences, whether the stimuli that engender them are transpersonal or otherwise, are simply the experiencers' interpretations of electro-chemical activity in the neurons and synapses of the brain. Neurologically, one *experience* has the same reality status as another. Many of the ASP's sensitivities (e.g., immunological, sensory, mnemonic) are objectively measurable and the data from the HISS ("Holistic Inventory of Stimulus Sensitivities") questionnaire show that anomalous sensitivity to stimuli in one realm is very likely to be accompanied by anomalous sensitivity to stimuli in all the other realms.

The experientially based discussion of Transpersonal Experiences (TPEs) that comprises the body of the text will, for many, probably raise more questions than it answers—so much the better. My primary objective in undertaking this project was, in addition to opening a few minds, more that of stimulating curiosity that might lead to further research by others, than it was that of providing definitive explanations.

Minds are like parachutes.
They only function when they are open.
—Sir James Dewar
(attributed)

The story of my explorations that follows begins in Part I (The Concepts) with the introduction of a hypnotherapy client who frequently had a variety of Transpersonal Experiences and my developing *Realizations* that sensitivity to TPEs appears to be accompanied by a host of other sensitivities. Next is a look at *Debunkers*, followed by an account of the early developmental stages of this research *Project*. The three subsequent chapters are devoted to a discussion of Predispositions toward sensitivities—*Biological* predispositions, *Trauma and Abuse* predispositions and *Temperament Type Preferences* predispositions. There are then five chapters about Indicators of sensitivities—*Physiological* indicators, *Cognitive* indicators, *Emotional* indicators, *Altered States of Consciousness* indicators and *Transpersonal Experiences* indicators. Part I concludes with thoughts about the *Future* of both the HISS and the ASP. Part II (The Evidence) is about the statistical analysis of the HISS data. It includes *A Statistical Primer* (for those who need one) and a summary of *The Findings* from the HISS data. Part II contributes substantially to the depth, meaning and credibility of the subject matter, but those who want no part of things mathematical can still get the gist of the book if they choose to skip it.

> *The important thing is to not stop questioning.*
> *—Albert Einstein*

PART 1

The Concepts

CHAPTER 1

Realizations

It's one thing not to see the forest for the trees,
but then to go on to deny the reality of the forest
is a more serious matter.
—*Paul Weiss*

Curiosity has its own reason for existence.
—*Albert Einstein*

"The patient I'm referring to you," said my psychiatrist colleague, "has received several different psychiatric diagnoses, been treated with a variety of psychotropic drugs and been institutionalized a few times, but she continues to be refractory. Her persistence in claiming that she has all sorts of paranormal experiences, suggests that a diagnosis of Schizotypal Personality Disorder, among others, is definitely in order. I'm making this referral outside the medical system because you appear to be knowledgeable about weird beliefs."

Knowledgeable I was, because, in my role as a clinical hypnotherapist, many clients had shared with me their experiences of such things as Extra-Sensory Perception (ESP), PsychoKinesis (PK), past-life recall, apparitions, spirit possession and alien contact.

"Weird" and "paranormal," however, were not terms that I used, in that they seemed unnecessarily pejorative. Moreover, I did not apply traditional psychiatric diagnoses to people who had such experiences because I felt that those experiences were not well enough understood to be definitively characterized as evidentiary of psychopathology.

Schizotypals Everywhere

Those whose stock-in-trade is psychiatric diagnoses, however, have plenty of support for their use of the label "Schizotypal Personality Disorder" in such cases. The *Diagnostic and Statistical Manual of Mental Disorders— Fourth Edition*

That's something for psychoanalysts
...if there are such people.
—Albert Einstein

(DSM-IV), in its list of key diagnostic criteria for Schizotypal Personality Disorder, includes: ideas of reference, unusual perceptual experiences and odd beliefs that are inconsistent with subcultural norms.[†]

Several other criteria need to be met for the diagnosis to be legitimately applied, but a contemporaneous article in the periodical *Perceptual and Motor Skills* seemed to exemplify the standard way of dealing with such experiences. In much abbreviated form, that article read:

> Belief in extra-sensory perception (ESP) is associated with a...bias for right-hemisphere processing. [This is especially] significant when viewed in the light of current theories of hemispheric asymmetries in schizophrenia. Belief in ESP has...been recognized as a variable relevant to schizophrenia, ...especially with respect to positive symptomatology [hallucinations, delusions and thought disorders]...[and] may therefore be construed as a behavioral feature [characteristic of] schizotypy....

[†] Endnote numbers for references to sources have been omitted from the text to improve readability and flow. Links to the text are established by chapter number, page number and subject matter in "Sources."

[S]ubjects scoring high on scales assessing schizotypy...show an increase in leftward lateral eye movements, a loss of the regular right-ear advantage in dichotic shadowing and a "sinistral shift" in handedness. A pathological overactivation of the right cerebral hemisphere [is]...the neurological basis of positive symptoms in schizophrenic patients. ...[and an] overactivation of the right hemisphere [also appears]...in normal subjects scoring high on scales...assessing positive symptoms of schizophrenia-like thoughts and behaviors.

[The primary] questionnaire [item] used to assess schizotypy reads "do you believe in telepathy?" ...[S]chizotypal personality disorder is characterized by... belief in clairvoyance, telepathy, or "sixth sense"... [B]oth pathological (schizophrenic) and institutionalized (parapsychological) belief systems share a common neurological basis [which]...comprise[s] a release of right-hemisphere function from left-hemisphere control. *[Brackets mine]*

Reproduced with permission of authors and publisher from: Brugger, P., Gamma, A,. Muri, R.., Shäfer, M., & Taylor, K. I. Functional hemispheric asymmetry and belief in ESP; towards a "neuropsychology of belief." *Perceptual and Motor Skills*, 1993, 77, 1299-1308. ©Perceptual and Motor Skills 1993

The statement made in the last paragraph seemed to be tantamount to defining schizotypy as "belief in ESP"—in other words, having such unconventional beliefs, in and of itself, supposedly constituted a mental disorder. That argument was allegedly bolstered by the neurologically based theory that belief in ESP results from an over-activation of the right cerebral hemisphere. Perhaps that theory was valid and perhaps it wasn't, but the pathologizing nature of the underlying definition of schizotypy seemed inappropriate.

Defining and pathologizing a belief in Extra-Sensory Perception as the primary symptom of a mental disorder appeared to me to be a way of brushing ESP under the rug and precluding, by dismissal, any study of ESP that might lead to a better understanding of it. Perhaps the adherents of this approach were not so much trying to understand ESP as they were trying to debunk it—so as to bolster an entrenched worldview that did not allow for the possible genuineness of such experiences. Maybe those who were doing the diagnosing, pathologizing and debunking believed that by defining ESP experiences as nothing more than symptoms of mental illness —something they believed they understood—they could keep their worldview intact and not have to deal with something they did not understand (and perhaps even feared).

LIZA

These thoughts were very much on my mind when I first met the referred client. Liza,[†] as I shall call her, was a young, attractive, intelligent woman with red hair, blue eyes and a very fair complexion. When it came to anomalous (a value-neutral term, meaning "unusual," used instead of the value-laden term "paranormal") experiences, Liza had much to relate. She reported one Near-Death Experience; several experiences of apparitions, spirit guides, past-life recall and Out-Of-Body journeying; and innumerable instances of PsychoKinesis (PK) and Extra-Sensory Perception (ESP) including psychic dreams, clairvoyance, telepathy and precognition. She stated, however, that she had no beliefs, one way or the other, about the objective reality of those experiences. Given that beliefs are central to the Schizotypal Personality Disorder diagnosis, it is small wonder that she presented a conundrum to those who were diagnostically oriented—she had the experiences, but hadn't invested herself in any beliefs about them.

Working with Liza gave me an opportunity to engage in a challenging theoretical exercise—one of determining how many different credible psychiatric diagnoses could be employed to pathologize her experiences and dismiss them as illusory. Her detailed case history included the following highlights:

- Liza often experienced what are generally labeled as "illusions," "delusions," and "hallucinations." The list of anomalous experiences already mentioned, is illustrative.
- She had "odd beliefs" and engaged in "magical thinking." One could argue that, despite her claim to the contrary, had she not believed that such things as ESP and PK were, in some sense, real, she would not have reported experiencing them.

[†] Pseudonym

- At times, she felt detached from herself, as if she were an outside observer. She also experienced episodes in which she perceived the external world as strange, distorted, or unreal.
- Occasionally, she spontaneously entered **Altered States of Consciousness (ASCs)** in which she experienced her mind as being absorbed into mystical realms of unity, light and energy.
- Interpersonally, she was extremely sensitive. Her relationships tended to be intense and unstable. She frequently experienced feelings of isolation and abandonment.
- She exhibited uncertainty about her self-image, her choice of friends and her goals.
- She exhibited a high level of emotionality, experiencing marked mood swings characterized by recurrent depression with occasional episodes of high energy and enthusiasm.
- She often experienced periods of considerable anxiety and worry, over which she had no control.
- She was subject to a variety of sleep disturbances including insomnia, nightmares, lucid dreams and myoclonic jerks (sudden, involuntary muscle contractions).
- At times, her thinking could become disorganized. She had periods of forgetfulness and inattentiveness. Despite her obvious intelligence, she also had difficulty with reading and with mathematics.
- Her speech tended to be digressive and abstract. She was inclined to express concepts in unusual ways and to use words in a novel manner.
- She had a variety of physiological symptoms that occurred episodically. These included fevers, headaches, flu-like symptoms, pains and gastrointestinal problems. She also experienced periods of restlessness, tremulousness and spatial disorientation.
- Unusual bodily sensations were commonplace for her—such things as tingling, numbness, rushes of energy, extremes of heat and cold, "pins and needles," and "electric currents."
- She was unusually sensitive to environmental stimuli, especially lights and sounds; she often experienced sensory synesthesias (the spontaneous **association** of a sensaton being activitated by external stimuli with another sensation of a different kind); and she appeared to have an exaggerated startle response.

Based on the above (and other) information, detailed research in the *DSM-IV* revealed that eleven psychiatric diagnoses in six different categories were excellent fits. They were:

- Personality Disorders: (1) Schizotypal Personality Disorder and (2) Borderline Personality Disorder;
- Dissociative Disorders: (3) Dissociative Disorder Not Otherwise Specified;
- Mood Disorders: (4) Bipolar II Disorder (With Rapid Cycling);
- Anxiety Disorders: (5) Posttraumatic Stress Disorder and (6) Generalized Anxiety Disorder;
- Disorders Usually First Diagnosed in Childhood: (7) Reading Disorder, (8) Mathematics Disorder and (9) Attention Deficit/ Hyperactivity Disorder (Predominantly Inattentive Type);
- Somatoform Disorders: (10) Somatization Disorder and (11) Conversion Disorder.

The conventional biomedical model considers each of these diagnoses to be a separate and distinct psychiatric disorder. Given their rates of occurrence in the general population, Liza's degree of comorbidity was extremely unusual. The probability of these eleven disorders occurring simultaneously in one individual is less than 2.3 x 10^{-17}. To put it another way, the odds are ten thousand to one against there being a single person on the entire planet having all eleven disorders—and yet I knew a couple of other people whose "symptomatology" was quite similar to Liza's.

Liza had also been diagnosed as having a host of chronic general medical conditions including: Systemic Lupus Erythematosus, Hypothyroidism, Chronic Fatigue Syndrome, Fibromyalgia, Chronic Epstein-Barr Virus, Lyme disease, recurrent Bronchitis/ Pneumonia and recurrent Streptococcus infections. Collectively, these eight different medical diagnoses were highly suggestive of a severely compromised immune system.

Eleven psychiatric diagnoses and eight chronic general medical diagnoses—Liza clearly had more than her share of problems, but statistically it was highly improbable that all of the diagnoses could be correct. Conversely, it also seemed absurd to select one—or two, or even three—of these diagnoses as *the* explanation for what was going on with her. The evidence definitely suggested the appropriateness of directing further inquiries toward finding a more encompassing condition or syndrome that could truly explain—not just explain away—most, if not all, of her symptoms.

BEYOND THE PERSONAL

Traditional psychiatric diagonsis was not my forte. It was not my primary interest, nor was it the reason Liza had been referred to me. My curiosity had been piqued, however. I wanted to understand what type of people had anomalous experiences and why, the contexts in which those experiences occurred and the reasons that mental health practitioners routinely pathologized and debunked them. Moreover, as a clinical hypnotherapist, my focus was on the clients' *experiences* rather than on the *phenomena* purported to underlie those experiences. Therapeutically, it had historically proven efficacious to work with the clients' experiences as if they were "really real"— to appropriately contextualize them, rather than to dismiss them as symptoms of a mental disorder. Furthermore, the clients' belief (or lack thereof) in the objective reality of the alleged underlying phenomena appeared to have little bearing on the successful outcome of the therapy.

Setting the stage for an in-depth investigation into these matters required addressing a few tangential issues first. Not the least of these was one of semantics—finding the proper words by which to refer to anomalous experiences, collectively. As previously mentioned, the term "paranormal" (and others such as "supernatural," "occult," and "metaphysical") had connotations that were too heavily value-laden. The term "anomalous," while appropriately value-neutral, was

First things first...
but not necessarily in that order.
—Anonymous

not sufficiently descriptive. Stanislav Grof's term, "Transpersonal Experiences," seemed to be the best choice. As it will be used throughout this book, the term "Transpersonal Experiences (TPEs)" means: "Experiences that occur beyond the ordinary differentiated boundaries of ego, space and time; experiences that suggest the essential interconnectedness (and/or absolute unity) of all that ever was, is, or will be; experiences that imply the existence of mind (as distinct from brain), of spirit, of soul."

Almost everyone will agree that the mind is somehow associated with the brain. However, when it comes to the question of whether or not the mind can in any way be considered to be separate and distinct from the brain, positions become polarized. Similarly, any attempt to distinguish between mind, spirit and soul leads to a philosophical quagmire. In order to avoid needless complications, I shall simply postulate that the mind, under the appropriate set of circumstances, can *appear* to be separate and distinct from the brain and, when it *appears* to be separate and distinct from the brain, it *appears* to take on qualities that some people attribute to the spirit or the soul. To put it another way, in any given instance, the more closely the mind appears to be associated with the brain, the more brain-like it appears to be and the less closely the mind appears to be associated with the brain, the more spirit-like or soul-like it appears to be. In this book then, the term "mind" will generally be used to refer to the "mind/spirit/soul" complex.

Developing a taxonomy of Transpersonal Experiences also proved to be helpful. Some lists of TPEs consist of hundreds of items. Upon analysis, however, it appeared that only eighteen—those that were most representative and relevant—truly needed to be considered. Logically, they could be organized into three general categories: (1) experiences of transpersonal perception, (2) experiences of transpersonal influence and (3) experiences of transpersonal manifestation of mind. Table 1.1, below, shows this categorical breakout and is followed by the definitions of the eighteen experiences.

Experiences of Transpersonal Perception	Experiences of Transpersonal Influence	Experiences of Transpersonal Manifestation of Mind
Déjà Vu Synchronicity Telepathy Precognition Psychic Dream Clairvoyance	Psychic Healing Electrical PsychoKinesis PsychoKinesis	Contact With Spirit Guides Out-Of-Body Experience Past-Life Recall Apparition Mediumistic Episode UFO Sighting Near-Death Experience Spirit Possession Alien Contact

Table 1.1 Three Categories of Transpersonal Experiences

Experiences of Transpersonal Perception:
- Déjà Vu—the strong feeling that some person, place, or situation has been experienced before, even though the experience is apparently occurring for the first time.

  It was déjà vu all over again.
  —Yogi (Lawrence Peter) Berra
  (Attributed)

- Synchronicity—the occurrence of a pattern of significant events, apparently causally unrelated, the connections among which seem to be too meaningful to be mere coincidence.
- Telepathy—transmission and/or reception of thoughts with another person without normal communication or clues.
- Precognition—accurate knowledge of an event that will take place in the future and that could not be predicted by logical means.
- Psychic Dream—a dream that matches in detail an event the dreamer did not know about, or have reason to expect, at the time of the dream.
- Clairvoyance (including clairaudience, clairsentience, claircognizance)—accurate awareness of events that are not available to usual sensory impressions.

Experiences of Transpersonal Influence:
- Psychic Healing—healing of an injury or illness through non-physical means such as prayer, meditation, laying on of hands, therapeutic touch, etc.
- Electrical PsychoKinesis—the influencing of electrical and/or electronic equipment (causing lights to go on and off, causing malfunctions in watches, calculators, computers, etc.) through no "natural" physical means.
- PsychoKinesis—the causing of changes in the location or state of a physical object (metal bending, fire-starting, things falling to the floor, etc.) through no "natural" physical means.

Experiences of Transpersonal Manifestation of Mind:
- Contact With Spirit Guides—mental contact with "spirits" or "higher beings" in which the individual receives information or guidance while remaining aware of what is happening.
- Out-Of-Body Experience—the sense that one's awareness or

mind has moved outside the physical body to a different location and the body can actually be seen from that location—other than during a Near-Death Experience (covered below).

- Past-Life Recall—the recollection of details and/or emotions of what apparently was another lifetime occurring before the experiencer was born into her/his current physical body.

- Apparition—a vision, while awake, of another person, living or dead, who is not physically, or objectively, present.

30

- Mediumistic Episode—communication of information or guidance by a "spirit" using the voice (trance channeling), or hand (automatic writing), of the experiencer, who is in an Altered State of Consciousness and

The medium is the message.
—Marshall MacLuhan

has little awareness afterwards of what was communicated.

- UFO Sighting—the observation of an Unidentified Flying Object ("UFO," "flying saucer," etc.) and/or its occupants without actual contact taking place.

- Near-Death Experience—coming very close to death (actually dying according to clinical criteria) and experiencing such classical NDE events as leaving the body, journeying through a tunnel, entering a world of light, perceiving a presence, etc., but ultimately surviving.

- Spirit Possession—the feeling that another mind (demon, spirit, soul of someone living or dead) is attempting to take (or has taken) over control of the experiencer's body and will.

- Alien Contact—actual contact with (what are often called) "extraterrestrial" beings (sometimes involving being taken aboard a UFO, frequently against the experiencer's will).

Within each of the categories, the individual experiences are organized by their frequency of occurrence as reported by subjects responding to the HISS questionnaire (to be discussed later). It is noteworthy that every type of experience of transpersonal perception was reported more frequently than every type of experience of either transpersonal influence or transpersonal manifestation of mind. This suggests the possibility of a psychosocial reporting bias being involved. Experiences of transpersonal perception are generally considered to be qualitatively less weird than experiences in either of the other categories—and may, therefore, be more freely reported. Experiences of transpersonal perception are actually quite commonly acknowledged. In a series of three studies with non-clinical populations, Douglas Richards found that 51%, 55% and 67%, respectively, of his samples reported having had such experiences.

It is inevitable that the unusual will sometimes occur.

—Aristotle

31

By convention, experiences of transpersonal perception are often referred to collectively as experiences of "Extra-Sensory Perception (ESP)" and experiences of transpersonal influence are often referred to collectively as experiences of "PsychoKinesis (PK)." Also by convention, experiences of both ESP and PK are often referred to collectively as "psi" (ψ, the 23rd letter in the Greek alphabet) experiences. Psi experiences can theoretically be independently verified under scientific laboratory conditions. Experiences of transpersonal manifestation of mind, on the other hand, cannot—and they are often referred to collectively as "psi-related" experiences. These terms will regularly appear throughout this book.

It also seemed important to deal, early on, with the reasons why reports of Transpersonal Experiences so often elicited a knee-jerk pathologizing and/or debunking response from so many mental-health professionals. Some of my findings about this behavior were quite intriguing and they will be presented in the next chapter.

CHAPTER SUMMARY

⇒   An article in a psychological journal arguing that a belief in Extra-Sensory Perception (ESP) was the primary diagnostic criterion for Schizotypal Personality Disorder, led me to suspect that those who pathologize paranormal experiences might be debunking (rather than diagnosing) as a way of keeping their worldviews intact.

⇒   Liza was a client who reported having multiple anomalous experiences. Eleven different psychiatric diagnoses could be credibly applied to her, each of which might be used to dismiss those experiences as illusory.

⇒   Liza had also received eight different diagnoses of chronic general medical conditions.

⇒   The statistical improbability of a single individual having eleven valid psychiatric diagnoses and eight valid chronic general medical diagnoses pointed to the likelihood of a more encompassing condition or syndrome being operative.

⇒   To avoid the connotative value-loading of terms such as "paranormal," "supernatural," "occult," and "metaphysical," the term "Transpersonal Experiences (TPE)" was selected to apply to: "Experiences that occur beyond the ordinary differentiated boundaries of ego, space and time; experiences that suggest the essential interconnectedness (and/or absolute unity) of all that ever was, is, or will be; experiences that imply the existence of mind (as distinct from brain), of spirit, of soul."

⇒   TPEs can logically be grouped into three general categories: (1) experiences of transpersonal perception, (2) experiences of transpersonal influence and (3) experiences of transpersonal manifestation of mind.

⇒   Experiences of transpersonal perception are often referred to as "Extra-Sensory Perception (ESP)" experiences and experiences of transpersonal influence are often referred to as "PsychoKinesis (PK)" experiences. Collectively, ESP and PK experiences are often referred to as "psi" experiences.

⇒   Psi experiences can theoretically be independently verified. Experiences of transpersonal manifestation of mind (often referred to as "psi-related" experiences) cannot.

CHAPTER 2

Debunkers

The discovery of the truth
is prevented more effectively,
not by the false appearance of things present
which mislead into error,
not directly by weakness of the reasoning powers,
but by preconceived opinion, by prejudice.
—*Arthur Schopenhauer*

An openly transgressed custom
brings sure punishment.
—*Mark Twain*

The difference between a skeptic and a debunker is significant. A genuine skeptic takes the position, as a good scientist should, that true knowledge, or knowledge in a particular area, is uncertain. A debunker, on the other hand, has an a priori commitment to invalidating the subject at hand. When it comes to Transpersonal Experiences (TPEs), it appears that the debunkers

*Men are most active
when evading real issues,
most powerful
when rejecting real values.*
—*Jean Toomer*

are committed to excluding the study of all of them from the mainstream of modern science. Theirs is definitely not a position of objective scientific neutrality, but rather seems to be driven by deep-seated, perhaps unconscious, emotion—and all indications are that the operative emotion is fear.

MOTIVATIONS FOR DEBUNKING

Transpersonal Experiences are unusual and in the realm of human emotion, "unusual," "different," "abnormal," and "weird" all have similar connotations. Differences establish "otherness," and...

> *Where there is other, there is fear.*
> *—Ancient Indian Upanishads*

Otherness can be and generally is, established on much more prosaic grounds than those of TPEs. There seems to be an evolutionary basis for this—at the old brain (limbic system) level of awareness, otherness implies danger (predators and such). In the distant past, those who didn't respond to otherness with fear and loathing didn't survive—their genes weren't passed on to succeeding generations. Otherness engenders fear and fear triggers the "fight-or-flight" response. When that other appears to be at a disadvantage, the fight response dominates and that other is aggressed against. In a "civilized" society, such aggression is most likely to take the form of ostracism.

Do you remember Miss Spellman?[†] Not Miss Spellman specifically, but somebody just like her. She was my second-grade teacher. She was a martinet. In our classroom, there were three left-handers. Each time one of them used the "wrong" hand, they received a vicious whack on the knuckles with a yardstick. Poor Vicki Knox[††] got so frightened, she would pee in her pants each time the teacher approached with weapon upraised. Miss Spellman presumably rationalized this abuse as ultimately being in Vicki's best interest, but there may have been more to it than that.

Even today, there are those who regard left-handedness, if not as a mark of the devil, at least as a sign of neurosis, rebellion, psychopathology, mental retardation, homosexuality, criminality… or, at best, as a bad habit or a social inconvenience. Illustratively,

[†] Pseudonym
[††] Pseudonym

note the left/right emphasis in the article on schizotypy (quoted in Chapter 1): "an increase in *leftward* lateral eye movements, a loss of the regular *right-* ear advantage in dichotic shadowing and a *'sinistral* shift' in handedness."

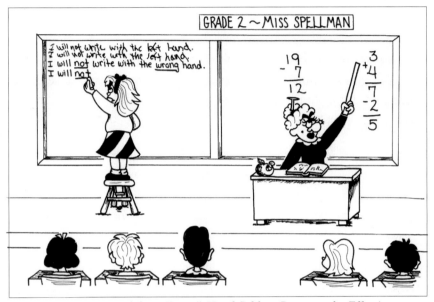

Punishment For Use of the "Wrong" Hand Seldom Proves to be Effective.

Even if all issues of religion and psychopathology are set aside, there is still a natural tendency for people in a large group to separate into tribes—to divide themselves into "us" and "them." Children quickly discover the security that is inherent in being part of a majority "us," as opposed to being part of a minority "us" (otherwise known as "them"). That's a powerful motivation to look for distinguishing characteristics that make an "other" a minority, to use those characteristics to concretize that otherness and then to vilify that otherness.

Left-handedness serves this purpose well because it is so obvious. Other obvious characteristics (all of which are associated with Non-Right-Handedness [NRH]) include epilepsy, Tourette's Disorder, cleft palate, harelip and clumsiness. Not so obvious differences that are also associated with Non-Right-Handedness include such things as learning disorders, speech impediments and intellectual or creative giftedness. Once otherness has been established, children prove to be very effective at locking it in with potent labels such as "geek," "dweeb," "nerd," "gay," "spaz," and "space-shot."

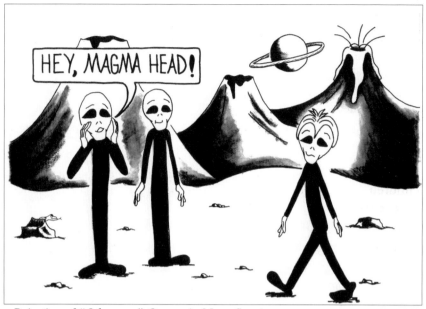

Rejection of "Otherness" Occurs in Many Species

Parents and teachers, unfortunately, are likely to be part of the problem rather than part of the solution. Consider, for example, the situation with children who exhibit creative genius, extraordinary imagination, or unusual facility with Altered States of Consciousness (ASCs). In Western society, adults are uncomfortable with and at a loss as to how to deal with, non-rational, non-objective, non-materialistic thought. A study of high creativity students and high I.Q. students by Getzels and Jackson revealed that whereas very successful high I.Q. students are labeled as "intellectually gifted," very successful high creativity students (without high I.Q.s) tend to be labeled as "overachievers." Those kids can get sent to the

> **SCHOOL'S OPEN.**
> **QUESTION AUTHORITY.**
> —*Composite Bumper Sticker*

counseling office to "resolve their psychological problems," and to reduce their achievement to a level more in line with their I.Q. The implication is that the I.Q. tests are right and the students are wrong. Even though the scholastic performance of the two groups of students is the same, teachers indicate a preference for having high I.Q. students, as opposed to high creativity students, in their classrooms.

In the same study, parents, when asked to define the gifted

child, ranked highest the characteristics of creativity, I.Q. and goal directedness. When asked to define the child they wanted in their family, they ranked highest the characteristics of emotional stability (adjustment), moral character and the ability to get along with others (conformity). The creative/intuitive child clearly cannot win a popularity contest in the classroom, on the playground, or at home. Creative/intuitive children may, indeed, be more difficult to get along with than conventional children, but this surely has nothing

Daring as it is to investigate the unknown,
even more so is it to question the known.
—Kaspar

to do with malice or evil. It is likely to stem, rather, from their independence, iconoclasm, different values and different ways of perceiving things. It has less to do with the children themselves than it does with the uncomfortable feelings they stimulate in others. Most people have something deep within them that yearns for reassurance that they are right. Those who are fundamentally different are perceived as a threat—their difference calling into question the certainty of that rightness—and they are reacted to with hostility. Creative/intuitive children are considered to be boat-rockers—their ideas and behaviors destabilize the status quo.

Adults generally operate with a bit more subtlety and finesse than do children. The labels used in childhood are replaced by something more sophisticated and politically correct. The term "eccentric," meaning "deviating from an established pattern or norm"—does the job nicely. A little emphasis on the word "deviating," with its connotation of deviancy and marginalization is effectively accomplished.

In Western society, eccentrics are relatively powerless—because of their small numbers, not because of any inherent insufficiency in their traits or characteristics. Illustratively, testing by Weeks and James revealed that eccentrics generally score very high on scales of: intelligence, imaginative-

It takes courage to be creative.
Just as soon as you have a new idea,
you are a minority of one.
—E. Paul Torrance

ness, assertiveness, forthrightness, venturesomeness, self-assuredness and self-sufficiency. They are also inclined to be creative, curious,

37

insightful, incorruptible, iconoclastic, non-conforming and anti-authoritarian. Strength being in numbers, such people could, indeed, collectively be a threat to the established order. The institutional imperative, therefore, demands that they be marginalized, isolated and suppressed.

Now, if something as mundane as left-handedness (or near-sightedness—do you remember the epithet "four-eyes?") can establish otherness, being known as a person who has (weird) Transpersonal Experiences is sure to do so (and at a higher order of magnitude).

38

> *One [person] with courage*
> *makes a majority.*
> *—Andrew Jackson*

Otherness is one thing, other-worldliness is quite another. Transpersonal Experiences directly challenge the prevailing worldview that is based on:

- Anthropocentrism—humans are the most significant entity in the Universe;
- Humanism—the human capacity for self-realization through reason is the basis for ascribing value, meaning, or purpose;
- Rationalism—reason is, in itself, a source of knowledge superior to and independent of, sense perception;
- Mechanism—natural processes (as in life) are mechanically determined and capable of complete explanation by the laws of physics and chemistry; and
- Materialism—physical matter is the fundamental reality and the highest values lie in material well-being and in the furtherance of material progress.

Experiences like PsychoKinesis, Out-Of-Body journeying, or contact with spirit guides lie far outside the boundaries of the paradigm defined by these criteria and those who are wedded to the prevailing worldview are consequently likely to experience fear when confronted with TPEs. One's worldview is not just a casually held philosophical principle. It is a core element in an individual's self-image and, in some cases, it is the underpinning that holds the mind together. Worldviews are not easily relinquished and strong institutional support exists for maintaining the status quo. People who report experiences, or present ideas, that challenge the prevailing worldview are punished.

In the past, when the Church was society's dominant belief-shaping institution, the punishment it meted out was loss of life by burning at the stake. Today, with Science as society's dominant belief-shaping institution, the punishment meted out is loss of respect by ridicule and rejection.

CHURCH AS INSTITUTIONAL DEBUNKER

The history of the Church, like the history of almost any institution, is a history of power politics. From its inception, the primary objective of the Church, in keeping with the institutional imperative, was to insure its own survival and continuation. Any group, individual, or idea that was perceived as a threat was either ignored, suppressed or eliminated, as the situation warranted.

Consider: At the Second Synod of Constantinople in 553 A.D., all references to reincarnation were expunged from the Bible and belief in reincarnation was proclaimed to be anathema. Consider also: The explosion of a super-nova in 1054 A.D., visible for 23 days and recorded throughout the world, was totally ignored (because it represented a flaw in the hypothesized perfection of the universe) by monks who were busily recording everything else in sight. Consider finally: The house arrest of Gallileo Galilei in 1633 for the heresy of supporting Nicholas Copernicus' heliocentric views of the universe (in 1992, he was finally forgiven for his transgressions).

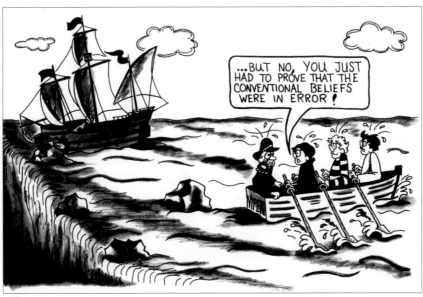

Challenging Conventional Concepts Can Occasion Consequences

People with a Gnostic (from the Greek *gnosis* meaning knowledge) orientation have been a major problem for the Church since its beginning. Gnostics hold that one's relationship with God appropriately involves direct and personal knowledge, or spiritual/religious/mystical experiences at first hand. Historically the Gnostic position undermined the Church's arrogation of the role of intermediary between man and God and therefore could not be tolerated—so it wasn't. For many years, the Gnostics were aggressively persecuted. In 1244 A.D., during the Albigensian Crusade, at Montsegeur in southern France, the last major organized group of Gnostics was eliminated.

40

The crusades very effectively dealt with organized resistance to domination by the Church. The Inquisition, in like manner, eliminated individual heretics—those who had the audacity to exhibit personal spiritual abilities. Most victims of the Inquisition were women. They were branded as witches and burned at the stake. Most perpetrators of the Inquisition were men. Their technique for demonstrating that a woman was a witch involved poking her with a long pin and, if she didn't howl in pain, her silence constituted proof. Witch status could also be determined by stripping a woman naked and examining her for signs of a mole or a blemish on the *left* side of the body.

The left side of the body was considered evil, so it followed that evil things were done with the left hand and that a left-handed person must be evil and in league with the devil. The English language is replete with pejorative terms related to left-handedness. Stanley Coren, in *The Left-Hander Syndrome,* states that the origin of the English word "left" comes from the Anglo-Saxon *lyft,* which means weak or broken. Included among the meanings of "left-handed" are crippled, defective, awkward, clumsy, inept, characterized by underhanded dealings, ambiguous, doubtful, questionable, ill-omened, inauspicious and illegitimate. In French, the word for left is *gauche,* which conveys the meanings crooked, ugly, clumsy, uncouth and bashful. The French word for right is *droit,* meaning straight and not twisted or perverse and from which comes the English word "adroit," meaning skillful, clever and adept. In Latin, the word for left is *sinister,* which implies evil, while the word for right is *dexter,* from which is derived the English word "dexterity," meaning grace, skill and ease. A left-handed compliment is an insult; a child from the left side of the bed is illegitimate; a left-handed marriage is an adulterous relationship; and a left-handed diagnosis is wrong. On the other hand, to be right means to be correct; to be somebody's right-hand man means to be especially important; at the last judgment, the sheep shall be set at God's right hand; and the right-hand path is the way of righteousness.

Presumably, not all of this prejudice was brought on by the simple physiological difference of left-handedness alone. While a Gnostic orientation was certainly the foremost marker of evil, behaviors and attitudes that were perceived as being characteristic of left-handers would have constituted additional evidence. For instance, such things as seizure disorders and speech impediments (an increased incidence of both is now known to be associated with Non-Right-Handedness) were said to be evidentiary of spirit possession.

Science as Institutional Debunker

It is comforting to think of all that as being in the past, a time when the Church was the dominant belief-shaping institution and people were emotional, ignorant and superstitious. It is reassuring to believe that today things are different, that Science is the dominant belief-shaping institution and that people are civilized, logical, rational, reasonable and in control. In truth, however, when confronted with things that are non-logical, non-rational, non-reasonable and non-controllable—things like Transpersonal Experiences (TPEs)— "civilized" people quickly revert to emotionality, ignorance and superstition. Human beings are, by nature, emotional creatures. Many who are scientifically oriented would prefer to deny their own inherent emotionality and are likely to insist that they do not fear the unknown—but denial is a commonly used, very powerful, often unconscious, psychological defense mechanism.

Science has clung tenaciously to the worldview it was responsible for creating and has used its authority to suppress major paradigm shifts. Scientists fill the roles of the experts who know the

Authority is the greatest enemy of truth.
—Albert Einstein

truth about the way things really are—and, for many, the possibility that they could be wrong is unthinkable. Not only do they share (often without admitting so) all the fears of the common folk, they also have too much else at stake—"the 4Ps": power, prestige, position and pelf (money)—to countenance change.[†]

More than a few scientists are inclined to be driven by theory rather than by data. Data make them uncomfortable unless those data conform to an existing theory. Such an approach, however, can lock them into a most disquieting pattern of circular reasoning: "The phenomenon in question doesn't exist because our theories show that it can't exist...but the data demonstrates that it does exist...but the data must be wrong because we know that the theories are right...but we can't find the problem...but ...."

Some historical "facts" that have fit this pattern are: The Earth is flat; the Earth is the center of the universe; rocks (meteorites) cannot fall from the sky (because there are no rocks in the sky); gorillas and panda bears don't exist;

> *Most men can seldom accept even the simplest and most obvious truth, if it be such as would oblige them to admit the falsity of conclusions which they have delighted in explaining to colleagues.*
> —Leo Tolstoy

germs don't exist (so hand-washing by surgeons is unnecessary); heavier-than-air flight is impossible; and humans are physiologically incapable of running a four-minute mile.

Absent an encompassing accepted theory, the data are likely to be rejected, discounted, or ignored. Moreover, human nature being what it is, those who find themselves in the uncomfortable position of being con-

> *Don't believe the results of experiments until they are confirmed by theory.*
> —Sir Arthur Eddington
> (said with irony)

fronted by data that undermine their theories, will often use disconfirming evidence to actually strengthen their beliefs—and create rationalizations for the inconsistencies.

[†] Interestingly, a 1960 Brookings Institute study suggested that decision makers consider withholding from the public information concerning discoveries of scientific anomalies (such as the existence of extraterrestrial intelligences) so as to avoid political change and a possible devastating effect on the scientists themselves.

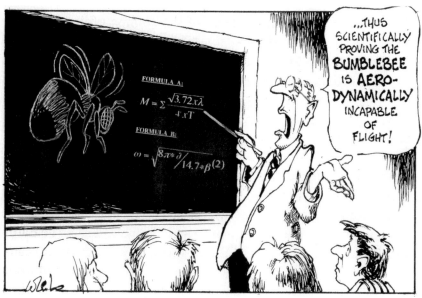

Scientists Can "Prove" Many Things

Discomfort of this sort is called "cognitive dissonance." There are three basic strategies for dealing with cognitive dissonance: (1) change one's beliefs, (2) apply pressure to those who present information that challenges one's beliefs and (3) devalue those who present such information. History has shown that scientists rarely adopt the first strategy—paradigm shifts generally occur

> *Ignorance*
> *more frequently begets confidence*
> *than does knowledge.*
> *—Charles Darwin*

only after the adherents of the old belief die off and those who are promoting the new belief move into positions of power. That leaves only options (2) and (3)—and the tactics used in applying those options can, at times, be most unsavory…ridicule, ostracism, ad hominem attacks and deception among them.

As irrational and unreasonable as such tactics might sometimes appear, they are usually quite effective—they instill fear in those who would challenge the status quo and fear is a most effective weapon.

> *Science advances one obituary at a time.*
> *—Max Planck*
> *(Paraphrased)*

This is not to say that debunkers are completely lacking in substantive arguments. They have a couple that, at least on the surface, actually appear to be quite good.

Principal Arguments of Debunkers

There is a significant body of scientific evidence supporting the veridicality of psi experiences (experiences of transpersonal perception and transpersonal influence). That evidence is difficult to dispute. Debunkers, therefore, tend to focus their attacks on psi-related experiences (experiences of transpersonal manifestation of mind), assuming, perhaps, that the debunking of one type of TPE will, by association, debunk the others. Psi-related experiences are an easy

44

target because they are subjective experiences that cannot be independently verified. The debunkers claim that such experiences are nothing more than fantasies, illusions, delusions, or hallucinations (see Chapter 10 for further discussion of hallucinations). Theirs is not an unreasonable hypothesis, but it is only a hypothesis, not the absolute fact that many purport it to be. Unfortunately, in arguing their case, they often resort to the distasteful tactics referred to above. Two versions of their position will be examined in what follows.

The Theory of the Fantasy-Prone Personality

Sheryl Wilson and Theodore Barber, in a 1983 study, showed that *highly hypnotizable persons,* who make up about 4% of the population and who are heavily represented among famous mediums, psychics and religious visionaries:

- have a history of a profound fantasy life;
- have the ability to hallucinate in all sensory modalities;
- have vivid personal memories with little childhood amnesia;
- exhibit physical concomitants to fantasies and other perceptual stimuli;
- report numerous Transpersonal Experiences including ESP, Out-Of-Body Experiences, mediumistic trance, automatic writing, apparitions and psychic healings;
- frequently experience classical hypnogogic imagery;
- tend to be female;
- are socially aware and function much like any other group of educated American women; and
- should not be pathologized, in that they are as well adjusted as the average person.

At first glance, this study seems to present a balanced, even-handed profile of the highly hypnotizable person. Unfortunately, Wilson and Barber chose to use the label "Fantasy-Prone Personality (FPP)" (see the first and second points in the list above) to categorize such people. That label has considerable pejorative loading and potential for abuse. In keeping with their assertion that these people should not be pathologized, they might more appropriately have chosen a value-neutral label, or even one with a somewhat positive loading such as "hypermnesic" (see the third point in the list above).† Of course, they also could have just left it at "highly hypnotizable person."

In any event, Steven Lynn and Judith Rhue, in later work, after pointing out that Wilson and Barber's construct of "fantasy-proneness" is indistinguishable from Hilgard's earlier "imaginative involvement" and Telegren and Atkinson's earlier "psychological absorption" constructs (both relatively neutral terms), climbed aboard the FPP bandwagon. Among their contributions to the field were the suggestions that the FPP could be pathologized as:

- lonely and isolated *[schizoid?]*;
- exhibiting the primary symptoms of *pseudoneurotic schizophrenia;*
- exhibiting qualities characteristic of *hysterics*;
- perceiving themselves as unique, creative individuals *[narcissistic?]*;
- having their adaptive imaginative tendencies overlap with more pathological *autistic* ideational functioning;
- being likely to have *severe adjustment problems* in adult life; and
- exhibiting *schizotypal* or *borderline* tendencies.

A later update by Joe Nickell gratuitously and purely anecdotally added five more items to the list of FPP characteristics:
- having seen UFOs;
- having New Age or mystical involvements;
- having been involved in a religio-philosophical limbo or quest for meaning;

---

† The term "hypermnesic" means "having an unusually vivid or complete memory of historical events or stimuli." As will be shown, debunkers use the label "Fantasy-Prone Personality" to dismiss experiences of transpersonal manifestation of mind as fantasies. Imagine what would happen to their argument if these highly hypnotizable persons had been given the label "Hypermnesics," instead.

- having been brought up Roman Catholic; and
- being involved in the arts as a vocation or avocation.

Lynn and Rhue's 52 item "Inventory of Childhood Memories and Imaginings (ICMI)" was allegedly designed to identify individuals with a Fantasy-Prone Personality. It has some shortcomings. Of the 52 items, only 20 address fantasy-proneness. Eight address Transpersonal Experiences; seven address normal, unremarkable childhood behaviors (e.g., "When I was a child, I enjoyed running and jumping."); four address hypermnesia; three address simple curiosity and/or exploratory impulses; three address sleep behaviors; two address philosophical interests; two address psychosomatism; and one addresses psychological abuse—and the questions aren't limited to childhood as the questionnaire's title suggests. As Ken Ring puts it, the ICMI is not just about fantasy-proneness, it's about the kitchen sink, as well.

The ICMI and the concept of fantasy-proneness, as debunkers and pathologizers currently use them, seem to be cynical instruments of tautological disinformation accompanied by a conveniently pejorative label—and, as such, are deployed to categorically deny the ontological validity of Transpersonal Experiences. The apparent sequential steps in the circular argument based on the FPP concept are these:

(1) Highly hypnotizable persons, relative to the norm, report an increased incidence of Transpersonal Experiences.

(2) Highly hypnotizable persons, relative to the norm, have a profound fantasy life and therefore, by definition, have Fantasy-Prone Personalities.

(3) Transpersonal Experiences don't conform to the tenets of consensus reality, so (since they are experienced by persons with Fantasy-Prone Personalities) they are, by definition, fantasies.

(4) Fantasies are, by definition, not real.

(5) Transpersonal Experiences, since they are (in accordance with the above reasoning) fantasies, are not real.

It's a rather clever maneuver that has succeeded in convincing a lot of people who have neither the time nor the inclination to deconstruct the logic of the theory. The argument is a relatively obscure one—few people other than researchers and clinicians know about fantasy-proneness. The debunkers' other principle argument—that of the "False Memory Syndrome (FMS)"—however, has found its way into the mainstream and is creating a great deal of controversy.

The Theory of False Memory Syndrome

Proponents of the False Memory Syndrome (FMS) theory assert that memories of forgotten (repressed or dissociated) events that are recovered during psychotherapy (especially when hypnosis is used) are not memories at all, but are, rather, fantasies that have been created as a result of the therapeutic set and setting. As of this writing, most of what has become a high-profile debate has centered on claims of childhood sexual abuse. Everybody involved—the alleged victims, the alleged perpetrators and the alleged therapists—is suing everybody else. It's a great moneymaker for the alleged lawyers and nothing but heartbreak for all the other parties. Hundreds, perhaps thousands, of families have been utterly devastated. FMS is a very serious problem, especially as it relates to false memories of childhood sexual abuse.

False memories can and do arise in any type of situation where Altered States of Consciousness (ASCs) occur (and, most likely, also in situations where they don't). The dynamics involve state-dependent memory, the Perky Effect and suggestibility (see Chapter 10

> *It isn't so astonishing the number of things I can remember, as the number of things I can remember that aren't so.*
>
> *—Mark Twain*

for a further discussion of all), but not all memories recovered in an ASC are necessarily false memories. Some are false, some are quite ordinary and some are not only accurate, but also unusually vivid and complete (hypermnesic).

It appears that it won't be long before lawsuits are filed claiming the implantation of false memories during hypnotherapy used to explore experiences of transpersonal manifestation of mind—the most likely scenarios being those related to past-life experiences, spirit possession experiences and alien contact experiences. While childhood sexual abuse experiences can, at least in theory, be independently verified, psi-related experiences such as these cannot. The overarching issue, then, will center on the fundamental

It's a poor sort of memory that works only backward.
—Lewis Carroll
(Through the Looking Glass)

nature of reality. Is there a single consensus reality, or are there multiple subjective realities? Are these experiences "really real," or are they hallucinations? The majority, of course, gets to decide—and the majority will be represented by its dominant belief-shaping institution, the scientific establishment. The decision will most likely be made, however, not on the basis of science, but on the basis of emotions and/or politics.[†]

The key to false memories is the centrality of ASCs in their occurrence. In certain ASCs, all bets are off as far as conventional rules of perception and memory are concerned. A number of replicable experiences relating directly to the issue of False Memory Syndrome, are readily elicited through classical hypnosis:

- Positive Hallucinations—the perception of something that does not have a corresponding stimulus in consensus reality;
- Negative Hallucinations—the failure to perceive something that does have a stimulus in consensus reality;
- Amnesia—the loss of memory for one or more events or stimuli;
- Hypermnesia—unusually vivid or complete memory of historical events or stimuli; and
- Post-Hypnotic Suggestion—after reorientation to normal waking consciousness, having amnesia for, but responding to, cues or stimuli that were suggested while the experiencer was in an Altered State of Consciousness.

[†] In 1896, the young psychiatrist, Sigmund Freud, presented his first major paper entitled "The Aetiology of Hysteria." It proposed what he believed to be an irrefutable cause of the neuroses suffered by many of his patients—sexual abuse in childhood. The backlash among his colleagues was swift and decisive. In order to avoid ostracism by the psychoanalytic establishment, Freud recanted and offered, instead, a rather convoluted theory about infants' fantasies of sexually seducing their parents.

Amnesia, hypermnesia and post-hypnotic suggestion are examples of state-dependent learning and state-dependent remembering (i.e., dependent on recreation of the State of Consciousness (SOC) in which the learning originally occurred). If the appropriate SOC is recreated, the memories arising therein, if uncontaminated, can be both extraordinarily vivid and extraordinarily accurate. Conversely, given that hallucinatory experiences (both positive and negative) and suggestibility (both auto- and hetero-) are associated with Altered States of Consciousness, ASCs can also result in the creation of false or

49

Always doubt what you believe.
—Epictetus

distorted perceptions and/or memories. Thus, a conundrum—those who are particularly facile at accessing ASCs are both: (1) more able accurately to recall genuine historical events than the norm and (2) more subject to false or distorted memories than the norm.

It can be seen, then, that a memory of a Transpersonal Experience that is recovered in an ASC, even if there is no supporting evidence in consensus reality for the veracity of that experience, is not necessarily a false memory. The claim that these memories (or the experiences themselves) are, of necessity, false, arises out of the traditional pathologizing psychiatric model having no place for the individual who is especially adept at accessing ASCs and who is able to perceive (what might be called) "alternate realities" (see Chapters 10 and 11 for further discussion).

While the theoretical mechanisms (as originally explicated) underlying the constructs of both the Fantasy-Prone Personality and the False Memory Syndrome are basically sound, the problems lie in their pejorative labeling and in the use of the concepts to categorically dismiss the validity of any

Great spirits
have always encountered
violent opposition from
mediocre minds.
—Albert Einstein

and all memories or experiences involving ASCs. That involves distortion and deception—and illustrates the primary difference between skepticism and debunking.

CHAPTER SUMMARY

⇒ "Otherness" (which can be as mundane as left-handedness) can stimulate fear and trigger the "fight or flight" response. When that other appears to be at a disadvantage, the fight response dominates and that other is aggressed against. In a civilized society, such aggression usually takes the form of ostracism.

⇒ Admitting to having Transpersonal Experiences (TPEs) is a dramatic form of otherness. Such experiences challenge the prevailing worldview, which is based on anthropocentrism, humanism, rationalism, mechanism and materialism. A challenge to one's closely held worldview can be extremely threatening.

⇒ There is strong institutional support for maintaining the prevailing worldview. In the past, the Church was society's dominant belief-shaping institution. Today, Science has taken on that role. Both institutions have a stake in debunking TPEs.

⇒ Debunkers have an a priori commitment to invalidating all TPEs. The tactics of debunking often include ridicule, ostracism, ad hominem attacks and deception.

⇒ Using the "Fantasy-Prone Personality (FPP)" theory to support their position, debunkers define highly hypnotizable persons as having Fantasy-Prone Personalities and then argue that because such people have more Transpersonal Experiences than the norm, those experiences are, by definition, fantasies.

⇒ Debunkers use the "False Memory Syndrome (FMS)" theory to suggest that memories, which are recovered in an Altered State of Consciousness (ASC), are not memories at all, but are, rather, fantasies that are an inevitable concomitant of ASCs.

⇒ Those who are particularly facile at accessing ASCs are both: (1) more able accurately to recall genuine historical events than the norm and (2) more subject to false or distorted memories than the norm.

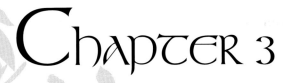

Chapter 3

The Project

If you wish to see the truth,
Then hold no opinions for or against anything.
—Sengtsan

Opinion in good men is but knowledge in the making.
—John Milton

Some people are more likely than others to have Transpersonal Experiences (TPEs) and those who are likely to have them are greatly outnumbered by those who are not. TPEs are sufficiently unusual and the non-experiencing majority is sufficiently large, that Science, society's current belief-shaping institution has declared TPEs to be "not real." This declaration, however, raises some questions about the nature of reality. Might it be that different people have different perceptions of the nature of reality and might it be that some of those perceptions are no less valid than is the consensus perception? A mundane experience helped to shape my thinking on this issue.

The Monk and the Hot Dog Vendor

A few years ago, on the corner of the main intersection in the town where I lived, there was regularly stationed a hot dog vendor. One day I observed an adolescent boy sidle up to him and loudly order, "Make me one with everything!" A Buddhist monk (saffron robes, shaved head and all) happened to be standing nearby. "Might the boy's words," I mused, "have a very different meaning for the monk than they do for the hot dog vendor?"

52

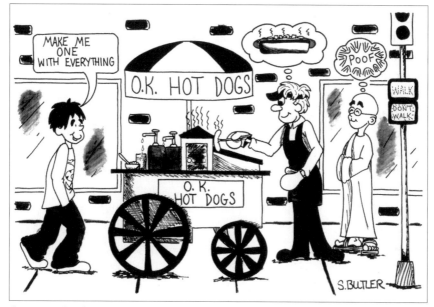

Semantic Confusion at the O.K. Hot Dog Cart

Presumably the hot dog vendor would have heard those words within the context of a personal reality that was simple, tangible and concrete. The monk, on the other hand, might have heard them within the context of a personal reality that was complex, metaphysical and cosmological in nature. I found myself wondering if the pathologizers might diagnose the monk as suffering from a mental disorder and decided that the answer was probably "yes." Within the monk's own culture, however, he would presumably have been considered quite normal. How strange that the definition of mental illness should be a function of local consensus—that a person who is "sane" in Azerbaijan could instantly become "crazy" upon relocating to Zimbabwe. The *DSM-IV* addresses this difference in viewpoints by stating that beliefs need to be "inconsistent with *subcultural* norms," to qualify as being "odd beliefs" for diagnostic purposes, but not many people in Zimbabwe are going to read the fine print in the *DSM-IV.*

The opinion of the majority within a specific group seems to be rather an arbitrary basis on which to determine mental health status. Cultural conditioning, of course, does play a role in the shaping of people's beliefs and perceptions, but it seemed that there had to be something more fundamental going on—something having to do with individual human differences.

I had learned from my clients that their Transpersonal Experiences (TPEs) were subjectively very real for them—and that their belief (or lack thereof) in the objective reality of transpersonal *phenomena* had little to do with whether or not they had such experiences. I had also learned that the supposedly differentiated types of TPEs were not really all that unlike one another. An alien-contact experience had many characteristics in common with a spirit-possession experience; a spirit-possession experience had many characteristics in common with a Near-Death Experience; a Near-Death Experience had many characteristics in common with an Out-Of-Body Experience; an Out-Of-Body Experience had many characteristics in common with a clairvoyant experience; etc.—and Extra-Sensory Perception experiences appeared to be associated, in one way or another, with all of them. Rather than these being a host of separate and discrete experiences, it seemed that they might all be different facets of a single meta-experience, part of a larger, encompassing whole—and that people who experienced one type of TPE were likely to experience other types as well. If that were the case, a valid explanation for any one type of TPE would likely be valid for all other types of TPEs as well.

The objective reality status of the specific transpersonal phenomenon purported to underlie each individual Transpersonal Experience, then, became of considerably less import in my investigation than was the nature of the processes through which individuals developed subjective perceptions of their own (perhaps idiosyncratic) realities. Perceptions arise within the mind and are, therefore, presumably a concomitant of consciousness (see Chapter 10 for further discussion). From that, it appeared to follow that perceptions of realities in which Transpersonal Experiences occur are most likely associated with "non-ordinary" States of Consciousness (SOCs). "Ordinary" States of Consciousness result in ordinary perceptions, "non-ordinary" States of Consciousness (generally spoken of as "Altered States of Consciousness [ASCs]") result in "non-ordinary" perceptions. I was a hypnotherapist and hypnosis is said to involve Altered States of Consciousness. Clients came to me to experience ASCs and it was in ASCs that they were most likely to recall having had TPEs. ASCs being a key factor in the recall of the experiences, ASCs were presumably also a key factor in the clients' having had the experiences in the first place, given the likelihood of that recall being state-dependent.

54   The relationship between TPEs and ASCs was a point that had been clearly made in Wilson and Barber's study of highly hypnotizable persons (see Chapter 2). That study also addressed issues having to do with fantasies, hallucinations, sensory perceptions, memories, hypnogogia and gender—all of which suggested that neurological differences might be a central issue. Perhaps, as suggested by the article on schizotypy (quoted in Chapter 1), such neurological differences really did involve a "bias for right-hemisphere processing," and perhaps such neurological differences really were reflected in "a 'sinistral shift' in handedness"—but it struck me as unlikely that those neurological differences were necessarily indicative of psychopathology.

On further reflection, it appeared that such variants in neurophysiological structuring, in addition to accounting for differences in Transpersonal Experiences and differences in Altered States of Consciousness, might also account for cognitive differences, emotional differences and certain physiological differences (especially sensory and immunological differences through the mind/body connection). What is more, it seemed likely that there would also be factors in the nature (Biological), nurture (Trauma and Abuse having been shown to affect neurology) and personality (Temperament Type Preferences) realms that could predispose an individual toward manifesting those differences. The use of the word "differences," however, presented a terminological problem because of its potentially pejorative connotation of "otherness." The word "sensitivities," ostensibly a value-neutral term, therefore appeared to be a better choice.[†]

The study, then, would be designed to cover the broad spectrum of human *sensitivities,* with emphasis on Transpersonal

---

[†] Because it can mean either "highly responsive to" or "easily hurt or broken," the word "sensitive" is also potentially subject to value-loading (either positive or negative) by those who have an agenda, but it seemed to be the best option.

Experiences sensitivities—and would also cover the full range of sensitivities (from the very low to the very high) with particular attention directed toward those individuals whose levels of sensitivities were unusually high. Again, the use of the word "unusual," presented a terminological problem because it, too, had potential for pejorative value loading—so the term "anomalous" was selected as a value-neutral substitute. "Anomalous sensitivity," then, became the term that would be used in speaking of levels of sensitivity that were exceptionally high (relative to a specified norm)—and those individuals who exhibited anomalous sensitivities would be referred to as "Anomalously Sensitive Persons (ASPs)."

THE HISS

Querying a large number of subjects with a questionnaire and using statistical methodologies to analyze their responses seemed to be the best way to explore levels of sensitivities. That appeared to be the best approach to help me maintain objectivity and prevent my personal opinions from influencing the results.

> *Opinion is ultimately determined by the feelings and not by the intellect.*
> *—Herbert Spencer*

The questionnaire methodology having been decided upon, the first step was to gather together those previously extant questionnaires that addressed some of the relevant issues and to select from among them those that were most germane.[†] It was then necessary to find people who could be cajoled into filling out those questionnaires.

In the early stages of exploration, only a few subjects were employed—the preliminary objective being simply to understand why individuals answered each question as they did and to determine what relevance their responses had in their everyday lives. Eight people, each of whom I knew well and to whom I had ready access for further questioning, agreed to participate. My guess (which later proved to be correct) was that two would be high scorers, two would be low scorers and four would be "middle-of-the-roaders."

[†] See Appendix G, "Other Questionnaires," for a listing of those questionnaires.

After the results of the first round of testing had been analyzed, the next step was to edit, condense and reformat all the material into a single questionnaire with consistent wording and style throughout. This questionnaire came to be called the "Holistic Inventory of Stimulus Sensitivities (HISS)." The preliminary version of the HISS, consisting of approximately 750 questions, was then administered to the original eight subjects—all of whom eventually ended up answering almost 2000 questions. If a willingness to answer questions turns out to be one of the criteria for gaining admission through the Pearly Gates, these people will have a distinct advantage over the rest of us.

56

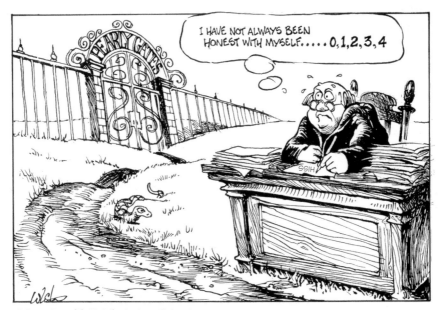

"Questionable" Admission Criteria

Analysis of the results of the second round of testing led to additional editing, condensing and reformatting of the material. This resulted in the version of the HISS that was finally used for the research project being 221 questions long.[†] For responding to most items, the subject is instructed to circle a number from "0" to "4." Depending on the nature of the item, the number circled indicates either the degree to which the statement applies to the respondent or the frequency with which the respondent has had an experience. Average time required for completion of the HISS is approximately forty minutes.

[†] See Appendix A, "The HISS Questionnaire," for the version of the HISS used in the study.

For scoring purposes, the questionnaire items were grouped into scales, the three first-level (most comprehensive) scales being Predispositions (PRE) toward sensitivities, Indicators (IND) of sensitivities and Other (OTH). These first-level groupings of scales all encompass second-level scales. Subsidiary to Predispositions (PRE) are Biological (BIO), Trauma and Abuse (TAB) and Temperament Type Preferences (TTP). Subsidiary to Indicators (IND) are Physiological (PHS), Cognitive (COG), Emotional (EMO), Altered States of Consciousness (ASC) and Transpersonal Experiences (TPE). Subsidiary to Other (OTH) are Explanatory (EXP) and Internal Checks (CHK). All second-level scales encompass third-level scales and in some cases, third-level scales encompass fourth-level scales.† Figure 3.3., below, illustrates the organization of the first-, second- and third- level HISS scales.

57

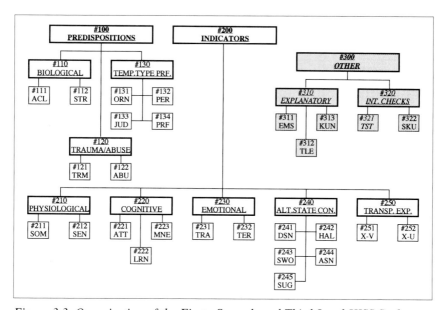

Figure 3.3. Organization of the First-, Second- and Third-Level HISS Scales

---

† See Appendix B, "Index of HISS Scales," for scale numbers, names and name abbreviations. See Appendix C, "Composition of HISS Scales" for a listing of the responses that comprise each scale. See Chapter 14, "The Findings," for a discussion of the more important findings relative to each scale. Note that scale names are nothing more than convenient labels under which to group questions with a common theme. They are not intended to suggest definitive theoretical constructs, nor are they intended to be used for diagnostic purposes.

All told, there ended up being 50 scored HISS scales. Scores for the third- and fourth-level scale are the mean (arithmetic average) of the scores for the individual questionnaire items included within each. In most cases, scores for each first- and second-level scales are the mean of the scores for the lower-level scales encompassed by each. All final scale scores, then, have a possible numerical range of zero to four.

BROAD-BRUSH FINDINGS

Ultimately, valid completed HISS questionnaires were received from 295 subjects. Throughout this book, those subjects will be referred to collectively as the HISS "Reference Group." The Reference Group, composed of 183 females (62%) and 112 males (38%), had a mean age of 41 years and a mean education level of 15.7 years.

In the Reference Group, scores for women were substantively higher than were scores for men. Illustratively, women's mean score on the first-level Predispositions (PRE) scale was 1.14 as compared to men's mean score of 0.98; women's mean score on the first-level Indicators (IND) scale was 1.44 as compared to men's mean score of 1.24; and women's mean score on the second-level Transpersonal Experiences (TPE) scale was 0.95 as compared to men's mean score of 0.81.

Scores on the HISS scales showed no significant correlation with either age or education level. They did, however, show clear-cut differences by occupation—artists having the highest scores and career military personnel having the lowest. Other factors of a demographic nature that were associated with high HISS scores were: Non-Right-Handedness, hypopigmentation (red/blond hair, blue/gray eyes, very fair/fair complexion), being one of a multiple birth (twins, triplets, etc.) and an other-than-conventional sexual orientation.

The correlations among the scores on the various HISS scales were very strong. Between the scores on the first-level PRE scale and the scores on the first-level IND scale, for example, the correlation was such that the probability of it occurring by chance alone was less than one in a trillion. The implication of this is that if an individual reported a high (or, conversely, a low) level of Predispositions toward sensitivities, s/he was very likely to report a high (or, conversely, a low) level of Indicators of sensitivities. Likewise, the correlations between the scores on any two second-level scales in the IND grouping—Physiological (PHS), Cognitive (COG), Emotional (EMO), Altered States of Consciousness (ASC) and Transpersonal Experiences (TPE)—was such that the probability of chance occurrence was also less than one in a trillion. This suggests that if an individual reported a high (or, conversely, a low) level of sensitivity in any one realm, s/he was very likely to report a high (or, conversely, a low) level of sensitivity in all of the other realms.

59

The ASP

On all scales, low scorers far outnumbered high scorers. For example, with the maximum possible score on any scale being 4.0, on the first-level PRE scale, 93% of the subjects scored less than 2.0; on the first-level IND scale, 85% of the subjects scored less than 2.0; and on the second-level TPE scale, 89% of the subjects scored less than 2.0. The average score for all of the subjects on all of the eight second-level PRE and IND scales was 1.25. The distribution of scores, then, did not form a "normal" (or "bell-shaped") curve. An "anomalously high" score on any given scale was defined as one that was two or more standard deviations above the mean score on that scale.[†] On a normal curve, two or more standard deviations above the mean would suggest a score in the top two percent. With this non-standard distribution, the percentage was somewhat higher.

It followed from the above criterion that a *quintessential* Anomalously Sensitive Person (ASP) would be an individual who scored two or more standard deviations above the mean on every one of the HISS scales. The quintessential ASP, however, would be an extreme rarity—so rare, in fact, that none were found within the Reference Group. From a practical perspective, therefore, it seemed advisable to think in terms of a *basic* ASP and to define the Anomalously Sensitive Person (ASP) as an individual who scored two or more standard deviations above the mean on both the first-level PRE and the first-level IND scales.

Seventeen subjects (5.8% of the Reference Group) had anomalously high scores on the first-level PRE scale and seventeen subjects (5.8% of the Reference Group) had anomalously high scores on the first-level IND scale. Ten subjects (3.4% of the Reference

---

[†] See Chapter 13, "A Statistical Primer," and Chapter 14, "The Findings," for more information about score distribution as well as about means and standard deviations.

Group) had anomalously high scores on both of these scales and therefore qualified as basic ASPs. Of the ten basic ASPs in the Reference Group, eight were female, eight were Non-Right-Handed, six were hypopigmented, seven had been one of a multiple birth, three had an other-than-conventional sexual orientation and eight had artistic, investigative, or social occupations. When the term "ASP" is used throughout this book, it is intended to refer to these ten basic ASPs. Perhaps one can generalize from these ten to ASPs in the population at large, perhaps not—but such a generalization would only be speculative and would not be statistically supportable.

60

One of these basic ASPs, a woman I shall call "Claire,"[†] was interviewed and studied in some depth. Claire is a divorced woman in her sixties with four adult children and is in a Social (human services) occupation. She is extremely intelligent and has received extensive graduate-level education. Born in central Europe, she was delivered to a 22-year-old mother and not one of a multiple birth. She was the second of six children and was born three years after her next older sibling. Both her parents were of European ethnicity and she came from long lines of accomplished artists on both sides of the family. She is moderately hypopigmented (light brown hair, hazel eyes and fair complexion), fully right-handed and conventionally heterosexual.

Claire's PRE score was 2.57 standard deviations above the mean and her IND score was 2.70 standard deviations above the mean. Of all the subjects in the Reference Group, she had the sixth highest score on the PRE scale, the fifth highest score on the IND scale and the sixth highest score for the two scales combined. The second-level scales on which Claire did not meet the quintessential ASP criterion of two standard deviations above the mean were: Biological (BIO) predispositions, Cognitive (COG) indicators and Transpersonal Experiences (TPE) indicators.

The pattern of Claire's scores can most easily be comprehended by viewing them graphically. The "Tally of Applicable Individual Life Sensitivities (TAILS)" graph presented in Figure 3.4., next page, shows her scores in standard deviations ("Z" Scores) from the Reference Group mean for the first-level PRE and IND scales and their respective second-level sub-scales. Solidly shaded columns represent scores that exhibit a *very* noteworthy (two or more standard

---

[†] Pseudonym

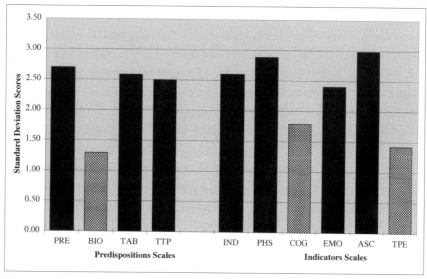

Figure 3.4. *"Tally of Applicable Individual Life Sensitivities (TAILS)"—Claire*

deviations) difference from the mean, crosshatched columns represent scores that exhibit a noteworthy (one or more, but less than two standard deviations) difference from the mean and unshaded columns (if there were any) would represent scores that exhibit no noteworthy (less than one standard deviation) difference from the mean.

The next several chapters of this book will examine ASPness from the perspective of the three second-level scales in the Predispositions (PRE) grouping, the five second-level scales in the Indicators (IND) grouping and the three third-level scales (Electro-Magnetic Sensitivity [EMS], Temporo-Limbic Epilepsy [TLE] and Kundalini Arousal [KUN]) in the Explanatory (EXP) grouping. Each chapter will open with a look at what an anomalously high score on the scale under consideration means and will be followed by an explication of Claire's responses, with comments from her as to how the elements involved play out in her life. The main body of each of these chapters will consist of a discussion of the factors that might underlie high scoring responses to the questions included in that particular scale.

CHAPTER SUMMARY

⇒ The consensus that Transpersonal Experiences (TPEs) are "not real" raises some questions about the nature of reality. Is there only one objective reality, or might there be other subjective realities and, if so, might the nature of those subjective realities be shaped by the States of Consciousness (SOCs) in which they are experienced?

⇒ The supposedly differentiated TPEs have many characteristics in common and might all be different facets of a single meta-experience.

⇒ Differences in SOCs are, perhaps, neurologically based and, in addition to accounting for differences in TPEs, may also account for cognitive differences, emotional differences and certain physiological differences. Moreover, factors of the nature, nurture and personality sorts may predispose an individual toward manifesting those differences.

⇒ The ostensibly value-neutral term "sensitivities" will be substituted for the more value-laden term "differences." The ostensibly value-neutral term "anomalous" will be substituted for the more value-laden term "unusual." Those who have anomalously high levels of sensitivities (their scores being two or more standard deviations above the the Reference Group mean on both the first-level PRE and the first level IND scale) will be referred to as "Anomalously Sensitive Persons (ASPs)."

⇒ The questionnaire that was developed to explore sensitivities came to be called the "Holistic Inventory of Stimulus Sensitivities (HISS)." In the version used for this study, it consists of 221 questions.

⇒ The scales used to score the HISS are divided into three first-level groupings: Predispositions (PRE) toward sensitivities, Indicators (IND) of sensitivities and Other (OTH). Second-level scales within the Predispositions (PRE) grouping are: Biological (BIO), Trauma and Abuse (TAB) and Temperament Type Preferences (TTP). Second-level scales within the Indicators (IND) grouping are: Physiological (PHS), Cognitive (COG), Emotional (EMO), Altered States of Consciousness (ASC) and Transpersonal Experiences (TPE). Second-level scales within the Other (OTH) grouping are: Explanatory (EXP) and Internal Checks (CHK).

⇒ Valid completed questionnaires were received from 295 subjects who are collectively referred to as the HISS "Reference Group."

⇒ Women scored higher on the HISS than did men. Other demographic variables associated with high HISS scores included Non-Right-Handedness, hypopigmentation, being one of a multiple birth and an other-than-conventional sexual orientation.

⇒ Correlations among the scores on the various HISS scales were very strong. In most cases, the probability of their chance occurrence was less than one in a trillion.

⇒ Low scorers on the HISS far outnumbered high scorers. Ten (3.4% of the Reference Group) subjects scored two or more standard deviations above the Reference Group mean on both the first-level PRE scale and the first-level IND scale—thereby meeting the criteria for basic ASPness.

⇒ Claire is an ASP who was interviewed and studied in some depth. Her PRE score was 2.57 standard deviations and her IND score was 2.70 standard deviations above the Reference Group mean.

64

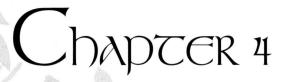

CHAPTER 4

Biological Predispositions Toward Sensitivities

If the brain was so simple we could understand it,
we would be so simple we couldn't.
— *Lyall Watson*

[In England]
The rule of the road is a paradox quite,
Both in riding and driving along;
If you keep to the left, you are sure to be right,
If you keep to the right you are wrong.
—*Henry Erskine*

An anomalously high scorer on the HISS Biological (BIO) predispositions scale is likely to be a Non-Right-Handed, hypopigmented female who has an other-than-conventional sexual orientation and was born as one of a multiple birth. S/he would also be likely to report developmental learning disorders, developmental speech disorders, low body temperature, low blood pressure, chronic sinusitis and chronic body pain.

Claire's score on the BIO scale was not anomalously high.

As previously noted, she is a fully right-handed, moderately hypopigmented female who is conventionally heterosexual and had a solo birth. She reported early learning and speech disorders, low body temperature, high (not low) blood pressure, chronic sinusitis and chronic body pain.

Questions included in the BIO scale were suggested primarily by the Anomalous Cerebral Laterality (ACL) work of Norman Geschwind and Albert Galaburda, neurologists at Harvard Medical School and also by the work of Brad Steiger with his "Star People Questionnaire." Discussion of the latter is quite brief, so it will be covered first.

Star People Questionnaire

The "Star People Questionnaire" was developed by Brad Steiger to explore evidence for the possible occurrence of interbreeding between extraterrestrials and humans. Given the "far-out" nature of this hypothesis and given that many of the characteristics (e.g., compelling eyes, highly charismatic) said to identify "Star People" were not objectively quantifiable, I was originally disinclined to give any serious consideration to this work. Credit must be given where credit is due, however. It turned out that some of the characteristics (e.g., low body temperature, low blood pressure, chronic sinusitis, chronic body pain) were quite down-to-Earth and appeared to merit inclusion in the HISS—especially since they dovetailed nicely with other more conventional hypotheses (especially "Wilson's Syndrome," discussed in Chapter 7), as well as with the work of Geschwind and Galaburda.

Anomalous Cerebral Laterality

Geschwind and Galaburda's research explored the relationships found to exist between left-handedness, developmental learning disorders, immunological disorders and a host of other phenomena. They hypothesized that a common factor—an anomaly in neurophysiological structuring they called "anomalous cerebral dominance"—underlay the connections.

The concept of cerebral dominance has to do with which hemisphere of the cerebrum (the upper part of the brain) has primary responsibility for certain functions performed by the central nervous system. Neurological research into cerebral dominance issues has historically centered on dominance for handedness and dominance for language. Most people exhibit standard cerebral dominance in which the left hemisphere is strongly dominant for both handedness and language—the right hemisphere being dominant for other functions such as certain spatial and musical abilities, attention and many aspects of emotion. Because motor control is contralateral (i.e., the left hemisphere controls the right side of the body and the right hemisphere controls the left side of the body), right-handedness is much more prevalent than is left-handedness.

Anomalous cerebral dominance is any pattern of cerebral dominance that differs from the norm. There is no specific cutoff point that defines a shift from standard to anomalous dominance. It is a matter of degree on a continuum.

In standard cerebral dominance, the two cerebral hemispheres exhibit an asymmetry in size. Portions of the left hemisphere, especially in the area of the planum temporale (the upper surface of the back portion of the temporal lobe) are larger than are their equivalents in the right hemisphere and the left Sylvian fissure (which lies above the temporal lobe) is longer than the right (see Figure 4.1., below). Approximately 30% of the population has (some degree of) anomalous cerebral dominance. For them, the standard asymmetry is reduced, non-existent, or even occasionally reversed—and the corpus callosum (the bundle of fibers that connects the two cerebral hemispheres) is enlarged.

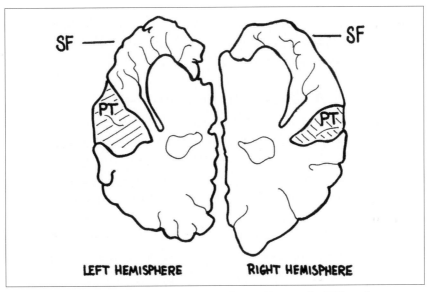

Figure 4.1. Standard Enlargement of the Planum Temporale (PT) and Elongation of the Sylvian Fissure (SF) in the Left Hemisphere

The intent of Geschwind and Galaburda's hypothesis was to account for a number of related phenomena, including:

- Left-handedness occurs more frequently in men than it does in women;
- Developmental disorders of language, speech, cognition and emotion are much more common among men than they are among women;
- Generally, women have better verbal skills than do men and men have better spatial skills than do women;
- Left-handedness and ambidexterity are both associated with developmental learning disorders;
- Both males and females who are left-handed and/or who have developmental learning disorders, frequently exhibit superior right hemisphere functioning; and
- Certain diseases, such as various immune disorders, are more common among left-handed people than they are among the general population.

68

Right hemisphere dominance can come about as the result of: (1) genetic programming that creates a mirror image of the dominance norm (this occurs in approximately 10% of people and is more common in women than it is in men), (2) early and extensive damage to the left cerebral hemisphere, for which the right hemisphere attempts to compensate, or (3) a delay in the development of the left hemisphere (where the individual's genetic programming has specified normal left hemisphere dominance) that permits enhanced development of the right hemisphere. In keeping with Geschwind and Galaburda's definition, only the last of these—a delay in the development of the left hemisphere, permitting enhanced development of the right hemisphere—qualifies as the "anomalous cerebral dominance" addressed in their hypothesis.

DAM

—Acronym for

"Mothers Against Dyslexia"

The brains of females, they suggested, develop earlier than do the brains of males and, in both sexes, the right hemisphere develops earlier than does the left. As a result, the female brain, overall and the right hemisphere of the brain in both sexes, will be less affected by factors that delay brain development. Given that female brains are naturally Less Strongly Lateralized (LSL) (one-sided or asymmetrical) than are male brains, *anomalies* in cerebral dominance will appear less frequently in females than in males. When such anomalies do occur (whether in men or in women), they will manifest as a relative weakening of the left h e m i s p h e r e accompanied by a

> *There is no female mind.*
> *The brain is not an organ of sex.*
> *As well speak of a female liver.*
> *—Charlotte Perkins Gilman*

69

relative strengthening of the right hemisphere—and the brain with anomalous cerebral dominance will be more symmetrical than the asymmetrical norm. In other words, the structure (and most likely the functioning as well) of the brain with anomalous cerebral dominance becomes more female-like and less male-like.

Since the neural substrates (bases) for handedness are separate from those for language and since the effects of developmental delays occur earlier (and for a shorter period of time) on the substrate for handedness than on the substrate for language, delayed left hemisphere development does not lead to a consistent and predictable shift in dominance. Dominance for either handedness, language or both will be random. In other words, the more nearly symmetry is achieved in a particular region of the brain, the more likely it is that random dominance will occur for the function primarily associated with that region.

The upshot of all this is that approximately one third of the population has random dominance (occasionally involving definite shifts to the right hemisphere) for either handedness, language or sometimes both—and random dominance for language is more common than random dominance for handedness. About 10% of the population is frankly left-handed. Of the 30% of the population meeting the criteria for anomalous cerebral dominance, then, only one third is left-handed. Figure 4.2., next page, illustrates this distribution graphically.

Delays in left hemisphere development appear to lead not so much to shifts in absolute dominance, as they do to relative degrees of reduced lateralization. Ambidexterity is more common than is full left-handedness. Strong right hemisphere dominance for language is almost nonexistent. The term "Anomalous Cerebral Laterality (ACL)," then, would seem to be more accurate than the term "anomalous

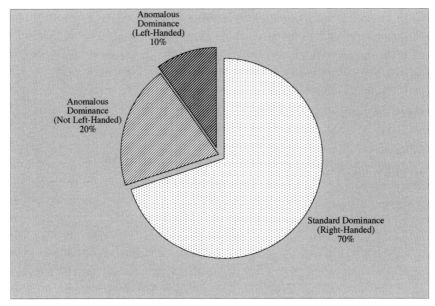

Figure 4.2. Distribution of Cerebral Dominance and Handedness in the General Population

cerebral dominance"—and this is the term that will be used throughout the rest of this book. Also, because ambidexterity (in varying degrees) is more common in **Anomalous Cerebral Laterality** than is full left-handedness, the term "Non-Right-Handed (NRH)" is more accurate than is the term "left-handed"—and this term will also be used wherever practicable. (However, since much of the work in the field has focused specifically and perhaps too narrowly on left-handedness, the term "left-handed" will continue to appear frequently, as well.)

As it will be used herein, the term "**Anomalous Cerebral Laterality (ACL)**"[†] implies:

- from a structural perspective—an enlargement of portions of the right cerebral hemisphere and/or diminution of portions of the left cerebral hemisphere, such that standard hemispheric asymmetry ceases to exist; and

---

[†] Anomalous Cerebral Laterality can be considered to be a special instance of a Less Strongly Lateralized brain—one that results from delays in the development of the left cerebral hemisphere. The meaning of the term "Less Strongly Lateralized (LSL)," then, can include, but is not limited to, instances of "Anomalous Cerebral Laterality (ACL)."

- from a functional perspective—a greater than normal participation of the right cerebral hemisphere in functions normally under the purview of the left cerebral hemisphere (notably language and motor control for handedness).

Since handedness and language are the functions most obviously affected by degrees of laterality and since ACL apparently runs in families, the following four characteristics can be considered to be likely markers for an individual's having Anomalous Cerebral Laterality:

- Non-Right-Handedness;
- right-handedness with Non-Right-Handed first-degree biological relatives (i.e., parents, siblings, offspring);
- right-handedness with developmental learning disorders; and
- right-handedness with first-degree relatives having developmental learning disorders.

Studies of Left-Handers

A number of different researchers have demonstrated that many phenomena are strongly correlated with left-handedness. The same phenomena, however, are even more strongly correlated with developmental learning disorders. Left-handedness, per se, is only one aspect of the broader domain of cerebral laterality issues—a convenient marker for a brain that is Less-Strongly-Lateralized (LSL) than the norm. Neurological structuring anomalies involving the language function (and cognition) are more difficult to identify than those involving the handedness function, but their influence on psychological, behavioral and experiential factors appears to be more significant. While it is true that in studies of phenomena associated with left-handedness, 20% to 30% of the subjects turn out to be left-handed (as compared to a 10% incidence of left-handedness in the general population) the other 70% to 80% are nevertheless right-handed.

> *Only left-handers are in their right minds.*
> *—Anonymous*

This finding that right-handers outnumber left-handers by a factor of three to one in studies of phenomena associated with left-handedness clearly suggests that factors other than handedness are also involved.

The list of correlates of left-handedness (as a marker for ACL) is enormous, chaotic and confusing. In what follows, an attempt has been made to organize the especially pertinent items into relatively coherent categories.

- <u>Cognitive Anomalies:</u> Dyslexia, stuttering, delayed speech, Attention-Deficit/Hyperactivity Disorder, Tourette's Disorder, Asperger's Syndrome;
- <u>Biochemical Anomalies:</u> Sex hormones (especially testosterone), stress hormones (cortisol, norepinephrine, etc.), monoamine oxidase, dopamine, serotonin, melatonin;
- <u>Chromosomal Abnormalities:</u> Down's Syndrome (an extra chromosome, No. 21), Turner's Syndrome (a missing X chromosome), Klinefelter's Syndrome (an extra X chromosome);
- <u>Physiological Anomalies:</u> Neural tube defects, scoliosis, cleft palate, harelip, hypopigmentation;
- <u>Autoimmune Disorders:</u> Gastrointestinal disorders (especially Celiac Disease, Regional Ileitis and Ulcerative Colitis), Diabetes Mellitus (especially the Type I, insulin-dependent, variety), Thyroiditis (especially Hashimoto's Disease— hypothyroidism), Rheumatoid Arthritis, Myasthenia Gravis, Lupus Erythematosus;
- <u>Other Immune Disorders:</u> Hormone dependent cancers (including breast cancer and prostate cancer), hypopigmentation-related cancers (including basal cell carcinoma, squamous cell carcinoma and malignant melanoma), migraine headaches, atopic disorders (including asthma, eczema and hay fever), food allergies;
- <u>Neurological and Psychological Anomalies:</u> Alzheimer's Disease, Autistic Disorder, mental retardation, seizure disorders (especially early febrile convulsions and later Temporal Lobe Epilepsy), vestibular and occulomotor disorders (including strabismus, nystagmus and esotropia), psychoses (including Schizophrenia), dissociative disorders (including Dissociative Identity Disorder[†]), mood disorders (including Bipolar Disorder,[††] Seasonal Affective Disorder,

---

[†] Formerly called "Multiple Personality Disorder."
[††] Formerly called "Manic-Depressive Disorder."

depression and suicide), sleep disorders, memory disorders, heightened sensitivity to psychotropic drugs, chemical dependence (including drugs, alcohol and nicotine), high level of hypnotizability;

- <u>Enhanced Talents and Abilities:</u> Creative giftedness (especially in art, music and writing), exceptional athletic abilities (especially in baseball, tennis and fencing), other special talents (especially in mathematics, spatial relations and chess);

- <u>Miscellaneous Phenomena:</u> Homosexuality, elevated incidence of childhood abuse, premature aging, accident-proneness, decreased life expectancy, twinning, birth complications (including prematurity, low birth weight, minor anoxias, instrument deliveries, breech births and Rh incompatibilities) and anomalous birth patterns.

According to the theory of Anomalous Cerebral Laterality (ACL), the origins of most, if not all, of these elements lie, at least in part, in the biochemical realm.

BIOCHEMICAL FACTORS

In the general population, although there are more Non-Right-Handed (NRH) males than females, genetics appears to play a stronger role in the NRH of females than in the NRH of males. In other words, NRH females are more likely to have NRH first-degree relatives than are NRH males. That being so, Geschwind and Galaburda directed their research toward locating the other factor(s), presumably environmental, they hypothesized as being operative in ACL—especially as pertains to the NRH of males.

Their most likely candidate proved to be high levels of intra-uterine sex hormones, primarily testosterone. The evidence indicated that high levels of intra-uterine testosterone (and/or a high level of sensitivity to normal levels of testosterone) inhibited the development of the left cerebral hemisphere and thus created the opportunity for enhanced development of the right cerebral hemisphere—thereby setting the stage for NRH.

Anomalous hormonal influences, they stated, could also affect physiological and immunological development. The operative mechanism involves, in the earliest stages of embryonic development, a structure called the "neural tube," and its associated "neural crest"— and an anomalous hormonal environment can lead to anomalous migration of cells from these structures.[†] High levels of intra-uterine testosterone are associated with a number of factors including: maternal predispositions, advanced maternal age, season of conception, latitude of birth, birth order and parity (the number of children previously born). Additional roles of the neural crest, in the development of non-neural tissues, show up in ACL by way of immune disorders[††] and hypopigmentation.[†††]

The distinction between hormones and neurotransmitters is a fine one. Technically, hormones (produced primarily in the glands of the endocrine system) are chemicals that help to regulate the functioning of cells throughout the body; neurotransmitters (produced primarily in the brain) are chemicals that help to carry signals across neuronal synapses. For the sake of simplicity and convenience in this discussion, the distinction between the two will be deliberately blurred and the term "neurohormones" will be used. Neurohormones can be thought of as hormones that are produced by, or act upon, nervous tissue. Melatonin is one of them. The neurohormone melatonin is often confused with the pigment

74

[†] The neural tube is the embryonic site from which ultimately emerges the central nervous system. Soon after the neural tube forms, it develops three specialized enlargements that eventually become the forebrain, the midbrain and the hindbrain. The remainder of the tube becomes the spinal cord. During the normal folding up of the neural tube, some cells remain outside the tube and form the neural crest, from which the peripheral nervous system eventually forms. In very early developmental stages, embryonic cells are not yet specialized — they are free to take on any form and function. Somewhat later, their commitment to a specialized function is determined by their interaction with various biochemicals. Neurons generally don't remain at the site of their origin in the neural tube/neural crest, but rather tend to migrate outward, often to considerable distances. After their migration, the neurons then begin their growth and maturation.

[††] Anomalous migration of cells from the neural crest affects the development of connective tissues in the thymus gland — a major component of the immune system.

[†††] There is an elevated incidence of hypopigmentation among those who are NRH. There is also a high incidence of early gray or white hair (indicating a lack of pigmentation) among those with cognitive anomalies, autoimmune disorders and other immune disorders. Nearly every pigmented cell in the body originates in the neural crest. Indications are that melanin-bearing (pigmented) cells act as guides in the development of neural (and possibly other) structures. Many anomalies of obvious neural crest origin — neural tube defects, scoliosis, cleft palate and harelip among them — are frequently accompanied by hypopigmentation.

melanin, but they are different compounds.† In any event, melatonin, as well as melanin, plays a very important role in the phenomenology of ACL.

Melatonin is the primary, but not the only, chemical messenger of the pineal gland. It is synthesized from two other compounds— the amino acid tryptophan and the neurotransmitter serotonin. The mammalian pineal gland is extremely sensitive to environmental light, temperature, stress and a host of other factors that affect psychological and somatic equilibrium. As part of the brain, the pineal gland has reciprocal links with the thalamus, the hypothalamus, the hippocampus and the amygdala (see Figure 4.3., below). As part of the endocrine system, the pineal gland has reciprocal links with the pituitary gland (located deep within the brain), the thymus gland (located in the chest), the thyroid and parathyroid glands (located at the base of the neck) and the adrenal glands (located on top of the kidneys), as well as the reproductive organs and the pancreas.

75

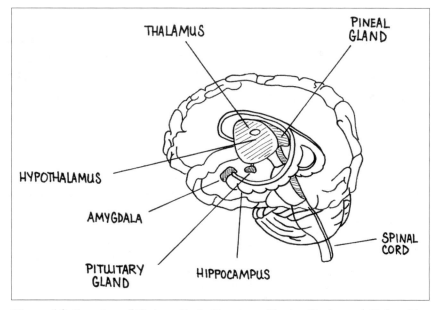

Figure 4.3. Location of Various Brain Structures Having Reciprocal Links with the Pineal Gland

---

† Not entirely different, however. Melatonin was so named because its chemical structure is similar to that of both the pigment melanin and the neurotransmitter serotonin. It also has some functional similarity to melanin—laboratory experiments have shown that melatonin can influence coat color in mammals and skin color in amphibians.

Light inhibits the synthesis of melatonin and darkness enhances it. There is an inverse relationship between the production of melatonin and the production of serotonin—when melatonin levels go up, serotonin levels go down and vice versa. Nobody knows for certain exactly what the interplay between melatonin and serotonin is all about. One researcher might argue that a high level of melatonin is responsible for a given phenomenon, while another might claim that a low level of serotonin is responsible. It makes sense, therefore, to speak more loosely of "the melatonin/serotonin relationship." This relationship (further discussed in Chapters 9 and 10) appears to be a key factor in Emotional sensitivities and in Altered States of Consciousness sensitivities (and thus in Transpersonal Experiences sensitivities as well).

The melatonin/serotonin relationship, by way of the pineal gland's reciprocal links with other organs, has an important place in: (1) bodily communications (i.e., the homeostasis of both the endocrine and the neurotransmitter systems), (2) bodily rhythms (i.e., the sleep-wake cycle and other cycles) and (3) immune system responsiveness. These three factors all have significant implications for the aging process. Some researchers have suggested that a decreasing level of melatonin informs cell DNA that the body is aging—and actually contributes to the manifestation of various indicators of the aging process. As a result, in the mid-1990s, melatonin became *the* hot nutritional supplement.

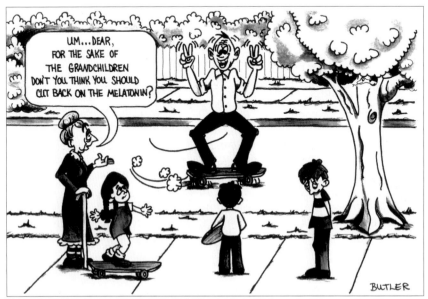

Because of Its Reported Anti-Aging Properties, Melatonin Became the Hot Nutritional Supplement of the mid-1990s.

Elevated levels of stress hormones (cortisol, norepinephrine, etc.) are another neurohormonal factor associated with Anomalous Cerebral Laterality. Stress hormones can inhibit the production of melanin pigment and studies have shown that elevated levels of stress hormones are, indeed, correlated with hypopigmentation. Moreover, stress hormones have been shown to be immuno-suppressive and there are a number of illnesses (e.g., peptic ulcers, ulcerative colitis, hypertension, hypothyroidism, rheumatoid arthritis, neurodermatitis and asthma) that have been known, for more than half a century, to be stress related. The list is continually growing.

77

There are many different types of stress; all of them can stimulate the production of stress hormones. Norman Shealey, in his book *Sacred Healing,* suggested the following categories of stress:

- Physical stress—including cuts, fractures, fatigue and excess heat or cold;
- Chemical stress—including drugs, alcohol, nicotine, caffeine and food additives;
- Electro-magnetic stress—including radios, televisions, telephones, computers, microwaves and power transmission lines;
- Mental stress—including worry, frustration and confusion;
- Emotional stress—including fear, guilt, anger, anxiety and depression;
- Spiritual stress—including moral, existential and transpersonal challenges.

Desynchronization of bodily rhythms can contribute to stress and result in significant negative consequences for both physiological and psychological health. Light is the most important environmental factor influencing all bodily rhythms—including those mediated by the melatonin/serotonin relationship. Temperature, electrical and magnetic fields and other factors, are secondary. Bodily rhythms, the most powerful of which are the circadian (about-a-day-long) rhythms, are established and modulated by what is colloquially called the "biological clock."[†] The biological clock controls, among other

---

[†] The human biological clock is thought to be located in a specific component of the hypothalamus called the "suprachiasmatic nucleus," which has two important characteristics that support this view: (1) it has clear rhythms of its own, independent of the rhythms of any surrounding tissues and (2) it functions as the receiving station for information flowing from the eyes to the hypothalamus — specifically information about light and dark.

things, sleep/wake cycles, hormonal cycles and cycles having to do with temperature, blood pressure, pulse, white blood cell count and drug and allergen sensitivity. In the absence of light, or other normal cues, for regular resetting to a 24-hour schedule, the biological clock begins to free-run (generally on a 25-hour schedule) and bodily rhythms become desynchronized. Abnormal cues arising from life in an industrialized, civilized society—artificial lighting, Electro-Magnetic Radiation, high-speed aircraft travel, shift work and stressful lifestyles, among them—can be extremely disruptive to biological rhythms.

MISCELLANEOUS PHENOMENA

Some other correlates of left-handedness (as a marker for ACL) merit additional discussion before moving on:

- Chromosomal abnormalities—It is highly unlikely that these are directly affected by the relatively subtle environmental factors implicated in ACL. They are, after all, genetic in nature by definition. The most likely environmental cause for them would be the presence of major toxins in utero. Chromosomal abnormalities are, nevertheless, correlated with left-handedness.
- Twinning—There is no simple genetic explanation for the elevated incidence of left-handedness in either identical or fraternal twins. The explanation may lie in an ACL-related environmental factor—perhaps hormones—but there is currently no strong evidence to support this speculation.
- Homosexuality—Recent research (apparently yet to be replicated) has shown that one tiny region of the brain—the interstitial nuclei of the anterior hypothalamus—in homosexual men is more like that of women than it is like that of heterosexual men. Since this is a difference in neurological structuring, it may reflect delayed cell migration from the neural crest and thus be a result of anomalously high testosterone levels in utero—the factor that is so central to the ACL hypothesis.

A review of the list of correlates of left-handedness (presented earlier in this chapter) reveals that Geschwind and Galaburda's work suggests the existence of an association between Biological factors and both Trauma and Abuse factors and Temperament Type Preferences factors (both of which are Predispositions toward sensitivities). It also suggests the existence of an association between Biological factors on the one hand and Physiological factors, Cognitive factors, Emotional factors and Altered States of Consciousness factors (all of which are Indicators of sensitivities) on the other. Steiger's work suggests the existence of an association between Biological factors and Transpersonal Experiences factors (also an Indicator of sensitivity). These associations will all be discussed in depth in subsequent chapters.

CHAPTER SUMMARY

⟹   Research by Geschwind and Galaburda explored relationships that exist between left-handedness, developmental learning disorders, immunological disorders and a host of other phenomena. They hypothesized that those relationships arise out of an anomaly in neurological structuring—"Anomalous Cerebral Laterality (ACL)"—that is caused by delays in left hemisphere development and in which standard hemispheric asymmetry is reduced.

⟹   In instances of ACL, there is a greater than normal participation of the right cerebral hemisphere in functions normally under the purview of the left cerebral hemisphere (notably language and motor control for handedness). This results in (among other things) an elevated incidence of developmental learning disorders and of Non-Right-Handedness (NRH).

⟹   ACL is a special instance of a brain that is Less Strongly Lateralized (LSL) than the norm. The brains of females are naturally LSL than are those of males, but *anomalies* in cerebral laterality appear more frequently in males than they do in females.

⟹   Many phenomena that are strongly correlated with left-handedness are even more strongly correlated with developmental learning disorders. Studies of the correlates of left-handedness (as a marker for ACL) show an elevated incidence of: cognitive anomalies, biochemical anomalies, chromosomal abnormalities, physiological anomalies, autoimmune disorders, other immune disorders, neurological and psychological anomalies, enhanced talents and abilities and miscellaneous phenomena.

⟹   Anomalously high levels of intra-uterine sex hormones, especially testosterone, are hypothesized to be causative environmental factors in NRH and ACL.

⟹   Sensitivities to the melatonin/serotonin relationship and to stress hormones, appear to play important roles in the phenomenology of ACL.

CHAPTER 5

Trauma And Abuse
Predispositions Toward Sensitivities

Fortune is not satisfied with inflicting one calamity.
—*Publilius Syrus*

The question is this: are we to be controlled
by accidents, by tyrants, or by ourselves ...?
—*Burrhus Frederic Skinner*

An anomalously high scorer on the HISS Trauma and Abuse (TAB) predispositions scale is likely to report various experiences of trauma throughout his/her life, as well as experiences of abuse in childhood. Trauma includes accidents, injuries, illnesses and psychological shocks (e.g., being raped, seeing a loved one killed, being in a fire); Abuse includes sexual abuse, mental abuse and abusive punishments.

Claire reported a very high level of psychological shocks and a high level of accidents, injuries, illnesses, hospitalizations and surgeries. She also reported a very high level of sexual abuse, a high level of mental abuse and a moderate level of abusive punishment in childhood.

TRAUMA

Literature in the field of neurology posits that a history of trauma—as exemplified by automobile accidents, concussive head injuries, hospitalizations and surgeries, febrile illness, hypoxia and childhood abuse—is frequently associated with Temporal Lobe Epilepsy. Literature in the field of psychiatry posits that a history of childhood abuse (especially sexual abuse) is frequently associated with psychological dissociation. Literature in the field of transpersonal psychology posits that a history of childhood abuse (especially sexual abuse) is frequently associated with Transpersonal Experiences.

Those who are sociologically oriented tend to consider childhood abuse—whether sexual, mental, or punishment—to be different from other types of trauma. Perhaps that is because it, more than the others, has obvious psychosocial underpinnings and is presumably therefore more amenable to theraputic intervention. From a neurological perspective, specifically that of Temporal Lobe Epilepsy, however, trauma is trauma—and childhood abuse is simply one subset of trauma. The neurological implications of trauma vis-à-vis Temporal Lobe Epilepsy will be discussed in Chapter 11. For the time being, this discussion will focus solely on the implications of trauma for psychological dissociation.

Psychological dissociation presumably involves Altered States of Consciousness (ASCs). As already mentioned, there are strong indications that ASCs are a key factor in Transpersonal Experiences (TPEs). The findings of correlations between trauma (including abuse) and dissociation, on the one hand and trauma (including abuse) and TPEs on the other, can easily lead one to conclude that trauma causes dissociation and that dissociation gives rise to TPEs. That may well be the case, but it does not necessarily follow from the data. Correlations, no matter how strong they might be, prove nothing about cause and effect. Establishing cause and effect requires that the researcher manipulate the independent variable—in this case the level of trauma—and, given the ethical issues involved, it is unlikely that this was done in any of the published studies. Based on the available data, one *could* argue that Transpersonal Experiences cause dissociation and then make a case for dissociative behaviors setting the stage for trauma and abuse (perhaps by signaling a vulnerability). That explanation, seemingly blaming the victim as it does, is politically incorrect (and probably wrong as well), but there is nothing in the available data to suggest otherwise.

When it comes to the study of TPEs, the special role granted by some to childhood sexual abuse, as a differentiated form of trauma, is probably ill advised. Consider:

- While it is true that in the population at large, women are more likely, than are men, to have experienced sexual abuse and to be diagnosed as having Dissociative Identity Disorder and;

- while it is also true that the data from the HISS Reference Group show that women exhibit a higher level, than do men, of Trauma and Abuse, Altered States of Consciousness and Transpersonal Experiences;

The little world of childhood, with its familiar surroundings, is a model of the greater world. The more intensively the family has stamped its character on the child, the more it will tend to feel and see its earlier miniature world in the bigger world of adult life.
— Carl Gustav Jung

83

- nevertheless, the data from the HISS Reference Group show that women exhibit a higher level, than do men, of *all* Predispositions toward sensitivities and *all* Indicators of sensitivities; and

- thus, women are more likely, than are men, to be Anomalously Sensitive Persons and, as ASPs, they may be *constitutionally* more disposed to have Transpersonal Experiences.

Perhaps it is sufficient to say that, while childhood sexual abuse may appropriately have a separate and distinct place in the world of social psychology, in the domain of Transpersonal Experiences it is simply one of many different types of trauma—and that the relationship between trauma in general, Altered States of Consciousness (frequently labeled "dissociation") and Transpersonal Experiences is what is relevant for the purposes of this book.

DISSOCIATION

The *Diagnostic and Statistical Manual of Mental Disorders—Fourth Edition (DSM-IV)* definition of "dissociation" is: "a disruption in the usually integrated functions of consciousness, memory, identity, or perception of the environment." Similarly, Bennett Braun in his BASK model, defines dissociation as: "a process whereby an individual separates Behaviors, Affects, Sensations and/or Knowledge from the mainstream of waking consciousness." Despite a warning in the *DSM-IV* that "...dissociative states are a common and accepted expression of cultural activities or religious experiences in many societies [and] dissociation should not be considered inherently pathological...," dissociation is generally assumed to be evidentiary of significant psychological problems. One author, for example, states, "Except when related to brain injury, dissociation always seems to be a response to traumatic life events." Given that the term "dissociation" is often used inappropriately to refer to any type of Altered State of Consciousness (of which there are many), that statement only serves to confound the issue. The potential stimuli for ASCs are multitudinous and varied—trauma is just one of them. This matter will be taken up again in Chapter 10.

Despite the pathologizing spin frequently given to dissociation, Frank Putnam argues that it is both an intelligent and a creative survival strategy in that it serves to facilitate seven major functions:

- automatization of certain behaviors;
- efficiency and economy of effort;
- resolution of irreconcilable conflicts;
- escape from the constraints of reality;
- isolation of catastrophic experiences;
- cathartic discharge of certain feelings; and
- enhancement of herd sense (e.g., the submersion of the individual ego for the group identity, greater suggestibility).

Dissociation as a defense mechanism becomes maladaptive and pathological only when the ability to discriminate between merely stressful stimuli and truly traumatic stimuli is lost—that is, when dissociation is mobilized unnecessarily as a disproportionately extreme response to stressors. One hazard of using dissociation as a coping mechanism is that it is so effective that those who dissociate often do not develop other useful defenses—such as denial, resistance, rationalization, or projection.

Both Braun and Kluft in their models of Dissociative Identity Disorder state that the dissociative defense mechanism is not available to everyone—only about 25% of people in the general population have the inborn capacity to dissociate. Since this is roughly the same percentage as those who are born with Less Strongly Lateralized (LSL) brains, consideration should be given to the possibility that there might be a significant overlap between the two groups. Stacking the deck in favor of this speculation is a 1991 study by Kunzendorf and Marsden that found an elevated level of dissociative experiences among ambidextrous students.

Psychological dissociation can result in amnesia. Dissociative amnesia is different from the psychoanalytical concept of repression. Ernest Hilgard clarifies this distinction when he speaks of repression (in the Freudian sense) as being a horizontal barrier (in keeping with the metaphor of the unconscious being "deeper") against unacceptable impulses, in contrast to the dissociative amnesic barrier which is a vertical one preventing the exchange of memories between different States of Consciousness (SOCs) with potentially equal cognitive status. This amnesic process can be spoken of as "state-dependent memory"—meaning that an experience associated with one specific State of Consciousness maintains that association over time and that its availability to recall may be dependent on recreation of the same SOC in which the experience originally occurred. This association is exemplified by the drunk who, when sober, is unable to recall his intoxicated behavior, but, when again intoxicated, is then able to do so.

This separation of behavior, affect, sensation, or knowledge from the mainstream of waking consciousness presumably means that what has been separated (dissociated) has been relegated to the subconscious mind. That being the case, "the subconscious mind" appears to be just another name for amnesia. The subconscious mind, then, is appropriately thought of not as a static thing, but as a dynamic process—one that potentially involves any State Of Consciousness other than ordinary waking consciousness. Since experience is state-dependent and since there is (at least some degree of) amnesia between ordinary waking consciousness and all other States Of Consciousness, it follows that an individual does not have just one subconscious mind, but has as many subconscious minds as there are possible SOCs—presumably an infinitude. It follows, as well, that different people will have different degrees of barrier permeability between their various States Of Consciousness—that is, in the general population, proneness to dissociation will be spread out over a continuum. Finally, heightened proneness to dissociation having been characterized as a heightened sensitivity to stressors, it follows that dissociation-proneness (more generally, sensitivity to Altered States of Consciousness) and sensitivity to Transpersonal Experiences are likely to go hand-in-hand.

Links to FPP and FMS

The use of the concept of the Fantasy-Prone Personality (FPP) (see Chapter 2) for debunking purposes is grounded in the common tendency to pathologize Altered States of Consciousness (ASCs). Wilson and Barber's original study dealt with highly hypnotizable persons and, since dissociation can be thought of as a form of self-hypnosis, their research was therefore presumably dealing with people who had an inborn capacity to dissociate (i.e., who were highly sensitive to ASCs).

It follows, then, that a person with a Fantasy-Prone Personality, in addition to being highly hypnotizable and having a history of a profound fantasy life, is likely to be female and is likely to report having an elevated incidence of Transpersonal Experiences. Despite Wilson and Barber's original statement that FPPs should not be pathologized and despite acknowledgement that the FPP construct was indistinguishable from Hilgard's earlier "imaginative involvement" and Telegren and Atkinson's earlier "psychological absorption" constructs (both value-neutral), the FPP concept was co-opted for pathologizing and debunking purposes. That having been said, it must be conceded that the theory of the Fantasy-Prone Personality does allude to the same connections between femaleness, Altered States of Consciousness and Transpersonal Experiences that are demonstrated by the HISS data and that are central to the ASP hypothesis—it's just that the FPP concept has given these connections a pejorative spin.

Similarly, the theory of False Memory Syndrome (FMS) alludes to connections between experiences of trauma and abuse (especially childhood sexual abuse, which is female-predominant), dissociation (various ASCs) and cognitive/mnemonic anomalies.

These connections are also demonstrated by the HISS data and are, again, central to the ASP hypothesis—but likewise without the pejorative spin.

The experience of Trauma and Abuse, as suggested in the above material, is closely intertwined with one's levels of sensitivities. It also is related to one's Temperament Type Preferences (personality). Common sense suggests that one might speculate about Trauma leading to an Introverted rather than an Extraverted Orientation, an iNtuitive rather than a Sensate strategy for Perceiving and a Feeling rather than a Thinking strategy for Judging. Cause and effect again being indeterminable from the data, however, it could be that these Temperament Type Preferences are such as to set the stage (by signaling a vulnerability) for experiences of Trauma and Abuse. Temperament Type Preferences, the third and last of the HISS Predispositions toward sensitivities, will be discussed in the next chapter.

CHAPTER SUMMARY

⇒ The relevant literature in various fields asserts that a history of Trauma and Abuse is associated with: (1) Temporal Lobe Epilepsy, (2) psychological dissociation and (3) Transpersonal Experiences.

⇒ The data from the HISS Reference Group show that women have a higher level, than do men, of *all* Predispositions toward sensitivities (including Trauma and Abuse) and *all* Indicators (including Altered States of Consciousness [ASCs] and Transpersonal Experiences [TPEs]) of sensitivities.

⇒ The term "dissociation" is often used inappropriately to refer to any type of ASC. There are many different types of stimuli for ASCs—trauma is just one of them.

⇒ ASCs can result in state-dependent memory. An experience associated with one State of Consciousness (SOC) maintains that association over time and its availability to recall may be dependent on recreation of the SOC in which the experience originally occurred.

⇒ The theory of the Fantasy-Prone Personality (FPP) alludes to the same connections between femaleness, ASCs and TPEs that are demonstrated by the HISS data. The theory of the False Memory Syndrome (FMS) alludes to the same connections between trauma, ASCs and cognitive/mnemonic anomalies that are demonstrated by the HISS data. Both theories put an unnecessarily pejorative spin on the information.

CHAPTER 6

Temperament Type Preferences Predispositions Toward Sensitivities

I have often thought that the best way
to define a man's character would be
to seek out the particular mental or moral attitude which,
when it came upon him, he felt himself
most deeply and intensely active and alive.
At such moments there is a voice inside which speaks and says:
"This is the real me!"

—*William James*

There is very little difference between one man and another;
but what little there is, is very important.

—*William James*

An anomalously high scorer on the HISS Temperament Type Preferences (TTP) predispositions scale is likely to have an Introverted rather than an Extraverted Orientation, an iNtuitive rather than a Sensate strategy for Perceiving and a Feeling rather than a Thinking strategy for Judging—and to *exhibit* a Preference for her/his Judging rather than her/his Perceiving function. This is an uncommon personality type found in only one percent of the population. The relevance of these dichotomous variables underlying TTP predispositions toward sensitivities will be explained shortly.

Claire has a strong Orientation toward Introversion and a very strong iNtuitive strategy for Perceiving. Her strategy for Judging is moderately Feeling and she exhibits a moderate Preference for her Judging function over her Perceiving function. Despite her ability to interact well in group situations, she is a very private person and thinks of herself as having deep, empathic friendships with a few individuals rather than superficial friendships with many. She is a daydreamer with an active imagination and considerable innovative talents. By making lists and bringing loose ends rapidly to closure she strives to maintain order in her external world.

THE MYERS-BRIGGS TYPE INDICATOR

The "Myers-Briggs Type Indicator (MBTI)" (and a variation thereof, the "Kiersey Temperament Sorter [KTS]") is a widely used personality test. The HISS Temperament Type Preferences (TTP) scale and the four sub-scales it encompasses are modeled on the MBTI and measure similar, but not necessarily identical, personality traits. Much of the discussion that follows is based on research by others with the MBTI and KTS; some is based on my own research with the HISS. Distinctions among the various test instruments may be blurred—especially since MBTI/KTS terminology will consistently be used for clarity—but since a strong correlation exists between KTS scores and HISS TTP scores (see Chapter 14, "The Findings" and Appendix E, "Double-Checking" for additional information), this should not present a problem.

The MBTI categorizes people according to four different sets of dichotomous variables. Its primary scales are continua between the extremes of each set, namely: (1) an Orientation toward either Extraversion or Introversion, (2) a Perceiving strategy based on either Sensation or iNtuition, (3) a Judging strategy based on either Thinking or Feeling and (4) an exhibited Preference for either the Perceiving function or the Judging function. The underlined upper-case letters in these terms are the abbreviations commonly used to refer to each attribute. The various combinations of these eight characteristics result in a total of sixteen possible personality types.

The qualities said to be associated with each of the characteristics are as follows:

- Orientation—People who are oriented toward Extraversion (<u>E</u>) are sociable, they value breadth, are revitalized by contact with others and experience loneliness in solitude; those who are oriented toward Introversion (<u>I</u>) are territorial, they value depth, are drained by contact with others and experience loneliness in crowds. 91
- Perceiving—People whose Perceiving strategy is based on Sensation (<u>S</u>) are practical and fact oriented, they value perspiration, realism and the past; those whose Perceiving strategy is based on iNtuition (<u>N</u>) are innovative and possibility oriented, they value inspiration, speculation and the future.
- Judging—People whose Judging strategy is based on Thinking (<u>T</u>) are objective and principle oriented; those whose Judging strategy is based on Feeling (<u>F</u>) are subjective and value oriented. This is the only one of the variables with a gender bias—60% percent of men prefer a Judging strategy based on Thinking, whereas 60% of women prefer a Judging strategy based on Feeling.
- Preference for Function—People who prefer their Perceiving (<u>P</u>) function over their Judging (<u>J</u>) function try to keep options open, are process oriented and are motivated by the play ethic; those who prefer their Judging (<u>J</u>) function over their Perceiving (<u>P</u>) function seek closure, are outcome oriented and are motivated by the work ethic.

As a man is, so he sees.
—William Blake

Table 6.1., below consolidates a considerable amount of information about the sixteen different types. It provides the abbreviation for each type name, a descriptive term for the type and the percentage of each type in the general population.

MBTI TYPES									
iNtuitives					*Sensates*				
Type	**Descriptor**	**Percent**			**Type**	**Descriptor**	**Percent**		
		Tot.	Ext.	Int.			Tot.	Ext.	Int.
iNtuitive Feelers					*Sensate Thinkers*				
ENFJ	Teacher	5	5		ISTP	Crafter	5		5
INFJ	Counselor	1		1	ESTP	Promoter	14	14	
ENFP	Champion	5	5		ISTJ	Inspector	5		5
INFP	Healer	1		1	ESTJ	Supervisor	14	14	
Total: iNtuitive Feelers		12	10	2	*Total: Sensate Thinkers*		38	28	10
iNtuitive Thinkers					*Sensate Feelers*				
ENFJ	Field Marshall	5	5		ISFP	Composer	5		5
INTJ	Mastermind	1		1	ESFP	Performer	14	14	
ENTP	Inventor	5	5		ISFJ	Protector	5		5
INTP	Architect	1		1	ESFJ	Provider	14	14	
Total: iNtuitive Thinkers		12	10	2	*Total: Sensate Feelers*		38	28	10
Total: iNtuitives		**24**			**Total: Sensates**		**76**		
Total: Ext. iNtuitives			20		*Total: Ext. Sensates*			56	
Total: Int. iNtuitives				4	*Total: Int. Sensates*				20

Table 6.1 Frequency Distribution of the sixteen MBTI Types in the General Population.

THE INTROVERTED INTUITIVE (IN--)

The two most salient personality characteristics associated with being an Anomalously Sensitive Person (ASP) appear to be an iNtuitive strategy for Perceiving and an Orientation toward Introversion. Given that the IN--s (INFJ, INFP, INTJ and INTP collectively) are the types most likely to be ASPs, the ensuing discussion will focus primarily on them.[†]

All ten ASPs in the HISS Reference Group use an iNtuitive strategy for Perceiving and almost all are Oriented toward Introversion (eight are Introverts, two are ambiverts and none are Extraverts). IN--s are a very small minority in the general population, collectively comprising only 4%, whereas their antithetical types, the Extraverted Sensate (ES--) types (ESTJ, ESTP, ESFJ and ESFP collectively) make up 56% of the population. The others—the Introverted Sensate

---

[†] In accordance with convention, when reference is made to a personality type and not all of its variables are specified, the abbreviation for that type will substitute hyphens for the letters of the unspecified variables. Hence, "IN--" refers to all Introverted iNtuitive types (INFJ, INFP, INTJ and INTP collectively.)

(IS--) types (ISFJ, ISFP, ISTJ and ISTP collectively) and the Extraverted iNtuitive (EN--) types (ENFP, ENFJ, ENTP and ENTJ collectively)—each make up 20% of the population. This distribution is shown graphically in Figure 6.1., below.

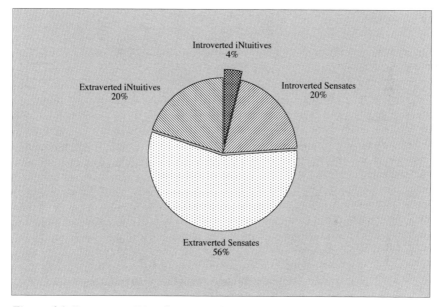

Figure 6.1. Percentage Distribution of the IN--, IS--, EN-- and ES-- Psychological Types in the General Population.

Intuition's vital role with respect to ASPness, is a result of its contribution to an individual's sensitivity, inspiration and insight. An iNtuitive strategy for Perceiving appears to go hand-in-hand with a high level of Altered States of Consciousness (ASCs) sensitivities and, as was pointed out in Chapter 3, ASC sensitivities can be considered to be the hallmark of the ASP.

The importance of Introversion's role in ASPness has to do with its creating a sense of independence that buffers one against societal pressures toward conformity. Moreover, relative to the norm, Introverts tend to have elevated levels of stress hormones. Stress hormones heighten sensitivity to stimuli—not only gross stimuli, by which ASPs can be overwhelmed, but also subtle stimuli to which others might be oblivious.

When sensitivity and independence are juxtaposed in the same individual, some confounding of usual cultural stereotypes can oc-

Public opinion, [is]
a vulgar, impertinent, anonymous tyrant
who deliberately makes life unpleasant
for anyone who is not content
to be the average man.
—William Ralph Inge

cur. Women are "supposed to be" sensitive; men are "supposed to be" independent. What then is to be made of a man who is sensitive or a woman who is independent? One possibility, of course, is to pathologize that person, but...

One who lets sacred cows lie will
never uncover the ideological bull.
—Ted Goertzel

Whether or not they are pathologized, IN--s are often perceived as being a threat to the status quo. This is so because they tend to be:

- intelligent and well-educated;
- aware, insightful, intuitive, spiritual and psychic;
- skilled in the metaphorical use of thought and language, excellent and persuasive writers and highly charismatic;
- oriented toward truth, honor and integrity and are unlikely to engage in activities involving the manipulation or deception of others;
- independent and seldom influenced by the opinion, approval, or disapproval of others; and
- non-conforming, unconventional, irreverent, iconoclastic and anti-authoritarian.

THE iNTUITIVE FEELER (-NF-) & iNTUITIVE THINKER (-NT-)

Emotional acuity (further discussed in Chapter 9) is likely to be highly developed in the ASP. Emotional acuity is something different from emotionality—it is the ability to have subtle and nuanced emotional responses to a variety of stimuli. It is an important element, not only in Emotional sensitivities, but also in creativity and Transpersonal Experiences sensitivities, as well. This does not mean that in order to be an ASP, one's score on the HISS must necessarily indicate the use of a Feeling rather than a Thinking strategy for Judging. What is being measured by the HISS Judging scale is not emotional acuity, per se; it is, rather, the credence that one gives to one's emotional acuity and the degree to which one exhibits that emotional acuity to the external world.

The iNtuitive Feeler (-NF-) is inclined to make judgments based on her/his emotions. The iNtuitive Thinker (-NT-), with the same emotional experience and the same degree of emotional acuity, is inclined to make judgments based on her/his intellect. People who are ASPs, it is true, more often employ a Feeling strategy than a Thinking strategy for Judging (all ten ASPs in the HISS Reference Group use a Feeling strategy), but then ASPs tend to be females (as are eight of the ten ASPs in the Reference Group) and, as previously mentioned, females are more likely than males to use Feeling as their strategy for Judging. This is probably, at least in part, a reflection of females being Less Strongly Lateralized than are males (see Chapter 4). Chances are, however, that an Introverted male who has a highly developed iNtuitive strategy for Perceiving and uses a Thinking strategy for Judging, could learn to further develop his Feeling strategy for use in those situations where it would better serve his needs.

Those who primarily use a Feeling strategy for Judging tend to be overtly more subjective, personal and emotional than those who primarily use a Thinking strategy. Conversely, those who primarily use a Thinking strategy for Judging tend to be overtly more objective, impersonal and analytical than those who primarily use a Feeling strategy. There are a number of differences between iNtuitive Feelers (- NF-s) and iNtuitive Thinkers (-NT-s) relative to their respective personality styles, motivations, special interests and typical professions. These differences are summarized in Table 6.2., next page.

Typical of iNtuitive Feelers are such people as Betty Friedan, Mahatma Gandhi, Martha Graham, Eleanor Roosevelt, Margaret Sanger and Mother Theresa. The ranks of iNtuitive Thinkers include the likes of Elizabeth Arden, Albert Einstein, Ernest Hemingway, Pablo Picasso, Frank Lloyd Wright and Leonardo da Vinci.

INTUITIVE FEELER		INTUITIVE THINKER
Warm Personable Supportive Idealistic Spiritual	**Personality Style**	Individualistic Iconoclastic Theoretical Innovative Creative
Intimacy Authenticity Values Self-actualization Making a Difference	**Motivated By**	Truth Excellence Uniqueness Possibility Challenge
People Service Charity Human Potential Meaning of Life	**Special Interests**	Learning Concepts Strategies Possibilities Exploration
Nursing Counseling Teaching Ministry Writing	**Typical Professions**	Science Mathematics Engineering Entrepreneurship Architecture

Table 6.2 Comparison of iNtuitive Feelers and iNtuitive Thinkers

JUDGING (---J) & PERCEIVING (---P)

People who prefer their Judging (---J) function (Feeling or Thinking) to their Perceiving (---P) function (iNtuition or Sensation) like to have clear-cut answers, to avoid ambiguity and to come to closure. Conversely, those who prefer their Perceiving function to their Judging function like to explore tangential possibilities, are intrigued by paradoxes and contradictions and want to keep their options open as long as possible.

Anomalous sensitivity is more about Perceiving than it is about Judging. ASPs will tend to rely more heavily on their Perceiving function than they will on their Judging function—and their Perceiving function will almost assuredly be based on an iNtuitive strategy. Among the ten ASPs in the HISS Reference Group, six exhibited a preference for their Judging function, two exhibited a preference for their Perceiving function and two exhibited no preference. These findings would seem to belie the previous statement about ASPs' reliance on their Perceiving function.

There is, however, with respect to Introverts, a subtle twist in score interpretation that needs some explanation. The MBTI was designed to measure those characteristics that an individual *exhibits* to the external world. If an Introvert were to openly exhibit her/his dominant, preferred function, that would involve her/him in an uncomfortable degree of Extraversion vis-à-vis that function (i.e., Perceiving or Judging). Doing so would cost that person dearly in terms of peace, quietude and tranquility. Therefore, the world is allowed to see only the auxiliary function. An Introvert whose dominant function is actually one of Perceiving will *exhibit* to the outside world her/his auxiliary Judging function as if it were dominant—and will score, on the MBTI (or HISS), toward the Judging end of the Judging/Perceiving continuum. In other words, despite preferring the Perceiving function, s/he will test and will appear to others, as preferring the Judging function.

97

The implication of this for ASPness is that if an individual is both Introverted and iNtuitive (whether with Feeling or with Thinking as a strategy for Judging), that individual's exhibiting a preference for the Judging function over the Perceiving function is evidentiary of a motivation to achieve closure on stimuli arising in *external* (or objective) reality. Such closure serves to clear the mental decks so that stimuli arising from the individual's *internal* (or subjective) reality can more readily be attended to. For these people, then, an *exhibited* preference for the Judging function actually emphasizes the role of their Perceiving function—iNtuition—by reducing the constraints on perception that are a concomitant of external reality.

The INFJ & INTJ

The hypothesis being presented here is suggesting that an iNtuitive strategy for Perceiving (innovative and possibility oriented, valuing inspiration, speculation and the future) is the most important personality characteristic vis-à-vis ASPness. An Introverted Orientation (territorial, valuing depth, drained by contact with others, experiencing loneliness in crowds) is second most important. A Feeling strategy for Judging (subjective and value oriented) is third most important. An exhibited preference for the Judging function (seeking closure, outcome oriented, motivated by the work ethic) is fourth most important. In other words:

(1) All those who use an iNtuitive strategy for Perceiving will be more ASP-like than all those who use a Sensate strategy for Perceiving.

(2) Among those who use an iNtuitive strategy for Perceiving, all those with an Orientation toward Introversion will be more ASP-like than all those with an Orientation toward Extraversion.

(3) Among those Introverts who use an iNtuitive strategy for Perceiving, all those who use a Feeling strategy for Judging will be more ASP-like than all those who use a Thinking strategy for Judging.

(4) Among those Introverts who use an iNtuitive strategy for Perceiving and a Feeling strategy for Judging, all those with an *exhibited* preference for their Judging function (an actual preference for their Perceiving function) will be more ASP-like than all those with an *exhibited* preference for their Perceiving function (an actual preference for their Judging function).

This reasoning leads to the conclusion that INF-s (J first and P second) are the types most likely to be ASPs and that INT-s (J first and P second) are the types next most likely to be ASPs. The type least likely to be an ASP is the direct antithesis of the INFJ—that is the ESTJ (the Extraverted Thinker with Sensing as her/his auxiliary function).[†] That's the theory—and the data from the HISS Reference Group back it up very nicely (see Chapter 14).[††] Because the differences between the INFJ and the INFP and similarly the differences between the INTJ and the INTP are quite subtle (and not particularly relevant to this discussion), further explication of the personality types most likely to be ASPs will focus on the INFJ and the INTJ.

[†] The theoretical ranking of all sixteen types with respect to ASPness is: INFJ > INFP > INTJ > INTP > ENFP > ENFJ > ENTP > ENTJ > ISFJ > ISFP > ISTJ > ISTP > ESTP > ESFJ > ESTP > ESTJ.

[††] Others who have studied relationships between Myers-Briggs personality types and various Transpersonal Experiences have found that Extraverts perform better than do Introverts on demonstrations of psi under scientifically controlled laboratory conditions. Their findings appear to contradict those of the HISS, at least in the transpersonal realm, but that may not actually be the case. The HISS is not measuring publicly demonstrated psi, it is measuring privately reported psi. Given that those who are Introverts are loath to publicly exhibit their actual preferred function (whether it be one of Perceiving or of Judging) and given that a preference for an iNtuitive Perceiving strategy is of overriding importance in Transpersonal Experiences sensitivities, the INFJ and the three other top-scoring IN-- types are unlikely to do well at public demonstrations of psi.

The Introverted iNtuitive with Feeling (INFJ) type (see earlier in this chapter for the defining characteristics) is the most spiritual, metaphysical, or psychic of all the types. To her/him, Transpersonal Experiences may not seem anomalous at all—they are just a part of what is. S/he forms powerful empathic, intuitive, telepathic connections with other people, deals well with complex social interactions, has a strong humanitarian bent and is focused on the positive possibilities inherent in human relationships. Her/his life is about values, integrity, service and self-actualization. S/he has a vivid imagination and is able to produce complex aesthetic works of art, especially in music or writing. Her/his greatest potential weaknesses lie in her/his tendencies toward vulnerability, transience and impracticality. Her/his most likely vocational choices include nursing, social work, ministry, counseling, teaching, music and creative writing.

99

The Introverted iNtuitive with Thinking (INTJ) type (see earlier in this chapter for defining characteristics) is the most independent and self-confident of all the types. For her/him, tradition, convention and authority are utterly irrelevant. S/he lives in a future-oriented, introspective reality and focuses her/his attention on potentials and possibilities. S/he is the supreme pragmatist who sees consensus reality as something quite arbitrary and made-up—it is simply a tool that can be used for the refining of ideas…or it can be ignored. While s/he considers her/himself to be a logical thinker, her/his form of logic has little in common with more conventional concepts of rationality. S/he needs only to have a vague intuitive sense of a hypothesis' internal consistency to accept it as logical. If an idea (rule, belief, concept, approach) makes sense to her/him, it is adopted; if not, it is simply discarded.

> *Every great advance in science has issued from a new audacity of imagination.*
> —*John Dewey*

S/he is creatively focused on the future with a decisive, single-minded, goal-oriented approach and expects all things, all people and all events to serve a positive purpose. Her/his greatest potential weaknesses lie in her/his inattentiveness to societal norms and her/his difficulty in dealing with the complexities of interpersonal relationships. Her/his most likely vocational choices include science, mathematics, engineering, entrepreneurship, architecture and art.

Given that Introverted iNtuitives (IN--s) are the types most likely to be ASPs, it follows that they are also the types most likely to have Anomalous Cerebral Laterality (ACL). ACL implies developmental learning disorders, so it comes as something of a surprise to discover that the ranks of the highly educated are heavily weighted with INFJs and INTJs. While it is true that many of these people have difficulties in the early years of their education—both with the subject matter and with the way in which it is presented—IN--s are characteristically tenacious and determined. After riding out the turbulent years of primary and secondary education, upon reaching college and graduate school, they often find themselves in environments where their particular styles of learning, their particular modes of intelligence, their particular brands of individuality, can flourish.

...And flourish they do! Studies have shown that the percentage of students who are both Introverted and iNtuitive increases markedly with increasing levels of education. Interestingly, though, there is no change in the Thinking/Feeling distribution with educational level—a reflection, perhaps, of the overriding importance of an iNtuitive strategy for Perceiving at the higher levels. Testing has confirmed the association of intellectual strengths—both aptitude and achievement—as well as educational level, with the personality characteristics of Introversion and iNtuition. INTJs, INTPs and INFPs (in that order) exhibit the highest aptitude scores and INTJs and INFJs (in that order) exhibit the highest achievement scores, of all the types.

The ethereal realms of genius are heavily populated with INFJs and INTJs, as well. Scratch a humanitarian genius and you will probably find an INFJ. Scratch a scientific genius and you will probably find an INTJ. Scratch an artistic genius and you will probably find one or the other of these types.

"Genius" is defined as "extraordinary intellectual power, especially as manifested in creative activity." On the surface, genius would appear to be a gift that would elicit respect, but many people, in addition to being somewhat envious of genius, can be spooked by it. Genius, because it is uncommon, is a marker for "otherness" (discussed in Chapter 2) and as such, is often feared and rejected (or at least

> *First and last, what is demanded of genius is the love of truth.*
> *—Goethe*

marginalized). Artistic genius, scientific genius and even humanitarian genius, while they might engender awe and a certain amount of grudging regard, seldom garner acceptance. Acceptance is the reward for conformity and genius, by definition, is non-conforming.

This discomfort with genius goes back a long way in history and is reflected in the word's linguistic origins and meanings. In the dictionary, the very first definition of "genius" is: "An attendant spirit of a person or place." That spirit is not just any sprit; it is a "genie." "Genie" is an Anglicization of the Arabic word "jinn," meaning: "One of a class of spirits that according to Muslim demonology inhabit the earth, assume various forms and exercise supernatural powers." That definition is suggestive of genius being perceived as a transpersonal manifestation of mind. Since IN--s, in addition to being the types most likely to be geniuses are, as ASPs, also the types most likely to have Transpersonal Experiences, perhaps that's not too far off the mark—but being known as one who has TPEs (especially of the spirit possession variety) is likely to result in ostracism.

Genius, in truth, means little more than the faculty of perceiving in an unhabitual way.
—William James

101

As previously mentioned, the genies of the INFJ are most likely to manifest in the humanitarian realm and the genies of the INTJ are most likely to manifest in the scientific realm. The genies of both personality types can also manifest in the creative realm and in the transpersonal realm, but these manifestations will assume different forms for the different types. The creative experiences and the Transpersonal Experiences of the INFJ are likely to be relatively subjective, personal, emotional and attached; those of the INTJ are likely to be relatively objective, impersonal, analytical and detached. In the creative realm, the experiences of the INFJ will tend toward the purely personal, such as poetry, whereas the experiences of the INTJ

Individuality of expression is the beginning and end of all art.
—Johann Wolfgang von Goethe

will tend toward the functional and utilitarian, such as architecture. Similarly, in the transpersonal realm, it is likely that the experiences of the INFJ will incline toward such things as telepathy, psychic healing and contact with spirit guides, whereas the experiences of the INTJ will tend toward such things as synchronicities, PsychoKinesis and UFO sightings.

As of this point in the book, the three Predispositions toward sensitivities—Biological, Trauma and Abuse and Temperament Type Preferences—have been examined and it has been shown that they are all interrelated. In the next five chapters, the (Indicators of) sensitivities themselves—Physiological, Cognitive, Emotional, Altered States of Consciousness and Transpersonal Experiences sensitivities—will be examined and it will be shown that they too are closely intertwined.

CHAPTER SUMMARY

⟹ The Myers-Briggs Type Indicator is a widely-used personality test with primary scoring scales based on four sets of dichotomous variables: (1) an Orientation toward either Extraversion or Introversion, (2) a Perceiving strategy based on either Sensation or iNtuition, (3) a Judging strategy based on either Thinking or Feeling and (4) a Preference for either the Perceiving function or the Judging function. The various combinations of these eight characteristics result in a total of 16 possible personality types.

⟹ The two most salient personality characteristics associated with being an Anomalously Sensitive Person (ASP) appear to be an iNtuitive strategy for Perceiving and an Orientation toward Introversion. iNtuition is vital for its contribution to an individual's sensitivity, inspiration and insight; Introversion is important in creating a sense of independence from society's conventional norms. Introverted iNtuitives (IN--s), who comprise just 4% of the population, are often perceived as a being a threat to the status quo.

⟹ Emotional acuity is highly developed in the ASP and will be more obvious in those who use a Feeling strategy for Judging than it will be in those who use a Thinking strategy for Judging.

⟹ ASPs generally prefer their Perceiving function over their Judging function—and their primary strategy for Perceiving will almost assuredly be iNtuition. ASPs, however, tend to be Introverts and Introverts avoid showing their preferred function to the external world, so ASPs are likely to test and appear to others, as preferring their Judging function.

⟹ INF-s (J first and P second)—that is, the Introverted iNtuitive Feelers—are the types most likely to be ASPs. INT-s (J first and P second)—that is, the Introverted iNtuitive Thinkers—are the types next most likely to be ASPs. The type least likely to be an ASP is the direct antithesis of the INFJ—the ESTJ (that is, the Extraverted Thinker with Sensation).

⟹ A humanitarian genius will probably be an INFJ, a scientific genius will probably be an INTJ and an artistic genius will probably be either an INFJ or an INTJ.

⟹ INTJs, INTPs and INFPs (in that order) show the highest scholastic aptitude scores and INTJs and INFJs (in that order) show the highest scholastic achievement scores, of all the types.

⇒　The creative experiences and the Transpersonal Experiences (TPEs) of the INFJ are likely to be relatively subjective, personal, emotional and attached; those of the INTJ are likely to be relatively objective, impersonal, analytical and detached.

CHAPTER 7

Physiological Indicators of Sensitivities

Health that mocks the doctor's rules,
Knowledge never learned in schools.
—*John Greenleaf Whittier*

Genius is the capacity to see ten things
where the ordinary man sees one,
and where the man of talent sees two or three,
plus the ability to register that multiple perception
in the material of art.
—*Ezra Pound*

An anomalously high scorer on the HISS Physiological (PHS) indicators scale is likely to report high levels of sensitivities in both the Somatic and the Sensory realms. Somatic sensitivities include Immune system sensitivities, Psychogenic sensitivities, Substance sensitivities and Electro-Magnetic Radiation sensitivities. Sensory sensitivities include Aesthetic sensitivities and Overload sensitivities.† Somatic sensitivities, on the downside, can involve susceptibility to immune and autoimmune disorders; on the upside, they can enhance the efficacy of psychogenic health and healing. Sensory sensitivities, on the downside can involve the possibility of being overloaded by environmental stimuli; on the upside, they can result in an awareness of subtleties that enhances creative potentials.

Claire has suffered from a number of health problems—migraine headaches, sinusitis, hypothyroidism and a variety of unusual medical conditions including Lyme Disease, Chronic Epstein-Barr Virus, Chronic Fatigue Syndrome and Fibromyalgia. She has also been diagnosed as having an autoimmune disorder—a variant of Rheumatoid Arthritis—perhaps triggered by Lyme Disease.

Many of her physiological problems have had strong neurological concomitants. Headaches, for example, have been accompanied by auras, synesthesias and temporary blindness. Other illnesses have been accompanied by twitching and shaking, dizziness and loss of balance, tickling and itching, numbness and insensitivity and unusual sensations of heat and cold.

In addition to migraine headaches, she exhibits other physiological symptoms in response to psychological stress—asthma, hives, muscle spasms and TemporoMandibular Joint (TMJ) pain. She has had various allergic reactions (most notably to insect stings) and unusual reactions to both caffeine and alcohol. She is very sensitive to loud noises, bright lights, temperature, humidity, textures, tastes and smells.

Despite Claire's tendencies toward ill health, she also reports significant self-healing abilities. She seems to be inclined to think of those abilities as little more than the converse of becoming ill. Healing for her, she says, is principally a matter of attention and intention. For instance:

> I've dealt with skin conditions and such, but that's probably just a matter of self-hypnosis. Warts are easy. I've gotten rid of warts, but anyone can do that. I also did it with a growth on my leg that a

† As stated previously, scale names are nothing more than convenient labels under which to group questions with a common theme. They are not intended to suggest definitive theoretical constructs, nor are they intended to be used for diagnostic purposes. See Appendix C, "Composition of HISS Scales," for further information.

dermatologist wanted to remove surgically—I just made it go away. It was nothing more than focusing my attention and intention. It was that simple.[†]

Her very acute sensory abilities provide her with the ability to discriminate among the subtleties of various tastes, smells, textures, colors and sounds. Focusing on her sense of smell, she said:

> I often use my sensory abilities in doing counseling work. For example, I believe I can sometimes smell emotional states on people. If somebody is schizophrenic, for instance, to me they have a certain smell. It's more than just their emotions, it's their whole state. The smell is not so much specific to the individual as it is to the state—the schizophrenic odor is applicable to schizophrenics in general. It is consistent from one schizophrenic to the next.

107

HEALTH AND LONGEVITY IMPLICATIONS

The pineal/hypothalamus/pituitary link and the pituitary/thyroid/thymus/adrenal link are key elements in understanding the immunological implications of Anomalous Cerebral Laterality (and hence of ASPness). Many significant correlations between immune system dysfunctions and factors associated with ACL are well known. Consider, for example, that there is an increased frequency of allergies among stutterers, of celiac disease among autistic children (and autoimmune thyroid disorders in their parents), of migraine headaches among dyslexics and food allergies and atopic disorders among hyperactive children. Consider, as well, that all three forms of skin cancer—basal cell carcinoma, squamous cell carcinoma and malignant melanoma—have an elevated frequency of occurrence among people who are hypopigmented.

What is more, hormone dependent cancers—including two thirds of all breast cancers and most prostate cancers—show indications of being related to a dysfunction of the pineal gland. Women with breast cancer and men with prostate cancer cycle melatonin abnormally. Sighted women (who receive melatonin-suppressing light through the eyes) are twice as likely to get breast cancer as are blind women. There

---

[†] This and other quotations from Claire are transcribed from interviews that occurred during November of 1999 and September and October of 2001.

is also a compelling body of research showing that fields of Electro-Magnetic Radiation (further discussed in Chapters 11 and 14) interfere with melatonin production—and low melatonin levels can result in immune system weaknesses, thus potentially increasing susceptibility to cancer.

108

In ACL, the immune system appears to be both overactive and insufficiently differentiative (i.e., it has difficulty distinguishing between that which is "self" and that which is "not-self"—between normal, healthy tissue and "other"). The hallmarks of ACL immune system dysfunction are allergies and autoimmune disorders. An overactive immune system, in responding to antigens from outside the body ("not-self")—ragweed, for example—can result in an allergy; an overactive immune system, in responding to antigens that are a normal part of the body ("self")—healthy tissues such as joint cartilage, for example—can result in an auto-immune disorder (such as Rheumatoid Arthritis). Conversely, an underactive immune system, one that fails to recognize an outside antigen as not-self—a bacterium, for example—can result in infection; an underactive immune system that fails to recognize an abnormal antigen that is an unhealthy part of the body, can result in cancer.[†] Table 7.1, below, may prove helpful in understanding these concepts.

	Over-active Immune System	Under-active Immune System
Self (Endogenous Antigens)	AUTOIMMUNE	CANCER
Not-Self (Exogenous Antigens)	ALLERGY	INFECTION

Table 7.1 Typical Immune System Dysfunction

Many people with ACL appear to be suffering from an occult (difficult to diagnose) syndrome characterized by a motley assortment of symptoms, including: low body temperature, low blood pressure,

[†] Geschwind and Galaburda speculated that the increased frequency of allergies and autoimmune disorders (that result from immune system overactivity) might be accompanied by a decreased frequency of infections (that result from immune system underactivity). They also speculated that the immune system overactivity associated with ACL might result in a decreased frequency of certain types of cancers—those that are neither hormone- nor pigment-related. There is currently no data available to support those speculations.

sore throat, fatigue, muscle weakness, muscle pain, arthritis, headache, depression, anxiety, forgetfulness and sleep disturbances. A number of different labels have been attached to this collection of symptoms, including: Wilson's Syndrome, Chronic Epstein-Barr Virus, Chronic Fatigue Syndrome, Fibromyalgia, Candidiasis, Myalgic Encephalomyelitis and environmental sensitivity. In the 1800s, the term "Neurasthenia" was in vogue. Whatever the name, the precipitating factor appears to be exposure to significant stressors in one or more of the categories (i.e., physical, chemical, electromagnetic, mental, emotional and spiritual) discussed in Chapter 4.

109

Those who have studied these symptoms in the context of the label "Wilson's Syndrome," claim that stress, in those who are especially susceptible, interferes with the function of the thyroid gland, lowers the metabolic rate, disrupts enzyme functions and results in hypersensitivities. Eighty percent of Wilson's Syndrome sufferers, they state, are women. Both hypopigmentation and Scotch, Irish, Welsh, Russian, or American Indian ethnic origins are associated with increased vulnerability. Those who are part Irish, part American Indian are said to be the most susceptible.

Immune system problems obviously have an adverse effect on life expectancy and there are a number of other factors associated with ACL that appear to reduce longevity as well. Among these are birth complications, chromosomal abnormalities, physiological anomalies, neurological anomalies, accident proneness, risk-taking behaviors and

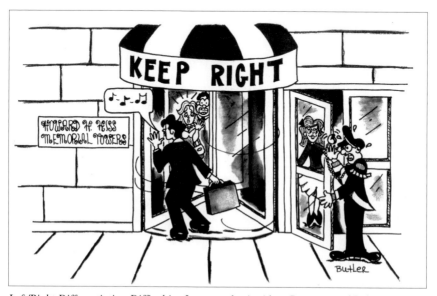

Left/Right Differentiation Difficulties Increase the Accident-Proneness of Left-Handers

an elevated level of drug, alcohol and nicotine use.[†]

The results of a 1991 life expectancy study by Halpern and Coren, involving 987 deaths, are quite striking. In this group, the mean age of death for women was 77 years; for men, it was 71 years—a difference of 6 years. The mean age of death for right-handers was 75 years; for left-handers, it was 66 years—a difference of 9 years. Right-handed women were found to live an average of 77 years, 8 months; left-handed women lived an average of 72 years, 10 months—a difference of 4 years, 10 months. Right-handed men were found to live an average of 72 years, 4 months; left-handed men lived an average of 62 years, 3 months—a difference of 10 years, 1 month. These data are summarized in Table 7.2., below. What all this means is that handedness is a more significant factor in longevity than is sex and it has a greater implication for the longevity of men than it does for women.

	Right-Handed	Left-Handed	All
Males	72 yr., 4 mo.	62 yr., 3 mo.	71 yr.
Females	77 yr., 8 mo.	72 yr., 10 mo.	77 yr.
All	75 yr.	66 yr.	74 yr.

Table 7.2 Life Expectancy by Handedness and Sex

In short, the **Anomalously Sensitive Person (ASP)** is more likely than the norm to suffer both injuries and illnesses. Indications are, however, that the **ASP** might also have the *potential* ability to effect recovery from injuries and illnesses more readily and effectively than the norm. The **ASP's** facility with **Altered States of Consciousness** sets the stage for self-healing abilities—for effective psychoneuroimmunological functioning, for the "placebo effect."

The term "psychoneuroimmunology" refers to the complex interactions that occur between one's psychology, one's neurology and one's immunology. At the most basic level, it can be said that if one's psychology is truly oriented toward healing, one's immune system will cooperate and effect that healing—provided one has the right neurology (and/or training). The right neurology appears to be

---

[†] Studies of accident-proneness have shown that: (1) tools, equipment, automobiles and the like are designed for the safety and convenience of the right-handed majority rather than the left-handed minority; (2) left-handers are more likely than right-handers to have coordination difficulties and (3) left-handers are more likely than right-handers to be distractible. The bottom line is that left-handers are approximately six times more likely to die in accidents than are right-handers.

that of the ASP—specifically, neurology involving a brain that is Less Strongly Lateralized (LSL) than the norm.

Studies of the placebo effect have demonstrated that a patient's belief in the effectiveness of a treatment makes that treatment more potent. The placebo effect is enhanced by anxiety reduction, suggestion of efficacy and expectancy. Good placebo responders:

- are highly hypnotizable;
- are able to move easily between different States of Consciousness;
- see conceptual relationships that others tend to miss;
- minimize doubt/skepticism by inhibiting analytical thinking; and
- tend to embroider or elaborate on the potential benefits of a treatment.

In short, good placebo responders are able to make real the suggested benefits of the treatment. "Make real" is something very different from the idea of "pretend to be real." In the appropriate Altered State of Consciousness (ASC), the benefits *become* real, the immune system accepts them as real and the rest of the body follows suit. Imagination and belief are both vitally important to the

If you can dream it, you can do it.
—Walt Disney

efficacy of this process. The introduction of doubt or skepticism by medical personnel, family and friends, or an experimental observer, can totally undermine the power of the placebo response. *That* effect has been called the "experimenter effect." The experimenter effect occurs frequently in any setting where the capabilities of the human mind are being explored.

Among the many medical conditions in which the utility of the placebo effect has been demonstrated are: coronary artery disease, hypertension, migraine headache, cancer, multiple sclerosis, Parkinsonism, diabetes, arthritis, gastrointestinal problems, asthma, hay fever and other allergies, dermatitis, warts and acne. Not surprisingly, the origins of many of these conditions have been shown to have significant emotional components.

Stigmata are perhaps the most dramatic demonstration of the influence of Altered States of Consciousness (ASCs) on the status of the body. Classical spontaneous stigmata are psychogenically created physical wounds, often mimicking (what the individual believes to have been) the wounds suffered by Christ during His crucifixion. Similar effects have been demonstrated in laboratory experiments: Deeply hypnotized subjects, when touched with a pencil eraser, having been told that it is a lighted cigarette, have reacted with pain and alarm. Their bodies often later respond to the "trauma" by developing inflammation and blistering.

112   The ability to access ASCs can be useful not only in the healing process, but also in protecting oneself from stressful stimuli involved in the onset of illness. Consider this: The rate of cancer in paranoid schizophrenics is significantly higher than the norm; in catatonic schizophrenics it is significantly lower than the norm. Findings for the incidence of asthma and allergies are similar. Paranoid schizophrenics are hypersensitive to stimuli and stressors; catatonic schizophrenics are often in an ASC that appears to function as a self-protective buffer. The evidence is not sufficiently strong to justify recommending catatonic schizophrenia as a way of life, but it does rather dramatically illustrate that ASCs have potential health benefits.

Current explorations into the use of ASCs for the promotion of health and healing include the methodologies of Transcendental Meditation and the Relaxation Response. These are techniques directed toward activating the parasympathetic nervous system as opposed to the sympathetic nervous system—toward encouraging relaxation rather than arousal. Significant beneficial physiological responses to both approaches have been demonstrated, including: decreased respiratory rate and oxygen consumption, decreased heart rate and blood pressure, decreased muscle tension, decreased blood lactate, increased galvanic skin response and increased low frequency coherent brainwaves.

Another piece of this puzzle appears to be purely biochemical in nature. The HISS data indicate that ASPs have a heightened sensitivity to substances that affect the central nervous system—caffeine, alcohol, marijuana and, presumably, the entire spectrum of psychotropic (acting on the mind) drugs. Studies have shown that the brains of left-handers exhibit greater changes in response to the administration of various drugs—including an antihistamine, a number of sedatives, an antidepressant, an antipsychotic, several experimental drugs and even aspirin—than do the brains of right-handers. The Anomalous Cerebral Laterality (ACL) explanation for this may be that, even if the action of a specific drug were identical in terms of molecular events in two different locations, the systemic effect could differ depending on which hemisphere of the brain is predominantly affected. In an ACL person, with a relatively enlarged right hemisphere, the net effect of the drug will reflect the presumably greater responsiveness of that hemisphere. Conversely, the action of another type of drug might be different in terms of the molecular events occurring in two different locations—and this would explain why ACL people sometimes exhibit paradoxical responses to certain drugs (e.g., Ritalin, a stimulant, reduces hyperactivity).

113

COMING TO THEIR SENSES

Heightened levels of Sensory sensitivities are associated with both an elevated level of stress hormones and with Introversion (as discussed in Chapters 4 and 6). ASPs are easily overloaded by gross sensory stimuli originating in the environment—loud noises, bright lights, noxious odors and large crowds, for example. On the other hand, ASPs are inclined to be aware of subtle stimuli to which others are oblivious. Such awareness, in addition to enhancing the breadth and depth of an individual's personal experience of the world, can have practical vocational utility. Heightened visual sensitivity, for example, would be of value to an artist and heightened auditory sensitivity would be of value to a musician. Heightened olfactory sensitivity would presumably be a prerequisite for employment as a fragrance tester for a perfume manufacturer and heightened gustatory sensitivity would presumably be a prerequisite for employment as a professional tea taster.

Particularly interesting in the sensory realm are synesthesias. A synesthesia is the spontaneous association of a sensation being activated by an external stimulus with another sensation of a different kind. Hearing a sound in association with the visual perception of a color, for example, would qualify, as would smelling an odor in association with the tactile perception of a texture. A synesthetic perception stimulates a powerful emotional response, causes the experiencer to fully enter into the perception and results in an experience that is both meaningful and memorable. Analogies, metaphors and images that originate in the mind become actualities and, as such, have sufficient tangible substance that they can be apprehended by the cerebral cortex and ultimately be accepted as belonging to the external world.

Both Aesthetic sensitivities and Synesthetic sensitivities appear to be important factors in fostering creativity. Creativity is an extremely complex and nebulous subject, but an attempt will be made to deal with it in the next chapter.

114

Chapter Summary

⇒ In Anomalous Cerebral Laterality (ACL) (and hence in ASPness), the immune system appears to be both overactive and insufficiently differentiative. The hallmarks of ACL immune system dysfunction are allergies and autoimmune disorders.

⇒ Many ACL people suffer from a syndrome variously labeled as: Wilson's Syndrome, Chronic Epstein-Barr Virus, Chronic Fatigue Syndrome, Fibromyalgia, Candidiasis, Myalgic Encephalomyelitis and environmental sensitivity. The precipitating factor appears to be exposure to significant stressors.

⇒ Factors involved in the decreased life expectancy of people with ACL include: immune and autoimmune disorders, birth complications, chromosomal abnormalities, physiological anomalies, neurological anomalies, accident-proneness, risk-taking behaviors and an elevated level of drug, alcohol and nicotine use. The life span of left-handers is nine years shorter than is that of right-handers.

⇒ Because of their facility with Altered States of Consciousness (ASCs)—and hence with psychoneuroimmunology and the Placebo Effect—Anomalously Sensitive Persons (ASPs) are likely to have enhanced self-healing abilities.

⇒ ASPs are easily overloaded by gross sensory stimuli and are also unusually aware of subtle stimuli.

⇒ ASPs are likely to experience sensory synesthesias—the spontaneous association of a sensation being stimulated by an external stimulus with another sensation of a different kind.

CHAPTER 8

Cognitive
Indicators Of Sensitivities

What does a fish know
about the water in which it swims all its life?
—Albert Einstein

We know the human brain is a device
to keep the ears from grating on one another.
—Peter De Vries

An anomalously high scorer on the HISS Cognitive (COG) indicators scale is likely to report a high level of sensitivities in the Attention, Learning and Mnemonic realms. The HISS inquires directly about such things as organization, distractibility, learning difficulties and memory—and as will be discussed, Cognitive sensitivities, by inference, also have a significant role in coordination/ athleticism and in creativity. Cognitive sensitivities, on the downside, are likely to result in difficulty with reading, spelling and mathematics, a high level of distractibility, poor orientation in both time and space and a poor memory for certain types of information; on the upside, they may lead to specific linguistic and/or mathematical skills, the ability to hyper-focus attention when appropriate and the remembering of some types of information with extraordinary clarity and detail.

Claire's lapses of attention are well known among her friends and many would prefer not to ride in a car when she is at the wheel. Under some circumstances, she is easily distracted and will often start tasks but not finish them. Under other circumstances, she can hyper-focus for many consecutive hours. She has a poor sense of both time and direction and frequently drops objects or bumps into things. Rote memorization, handling change or balancing a checkbook and following verbal instructions are all challenges for her. She can also be quite forgetful: when she is speaking, her mind frequently goes blank; she often will move from one room to another and then forget why she has done so; and at times, she will experience that which is familiar as being unfamiliar. On the other hand, perhaps paradoxically, she can relive events in memory as if they were happening again; she has vivid mental "flashbacks"; and she accurately remembers numerous events that occurred before she was three years old.

Claire is well aware of both her shortcomings and her strengths in the Cognitive realm and had this to say:

> In school, besides being a star at geometry, I was also a star at algebra. That's apparently unusual…to be really good at both. But then, when it comes to basic arithmetic, well…that's another story. And there's not much to be said for my calculus ability either. I did, however, score a perfect 800 on the math Scholastic Aptitude Test.
>
> I also scored 800 on the verbal Scholastic Aptitude Test. I guess my greatest learning strength has always been in the verbal area. I'm strong in vocabulary, in analogies, in metaphors—and I make good use of language in the therapeutic context. Also, I do well at Scrabble and crossword puzzles.
>
> I can be either highly focused or easily distracted—it all depends on what I'm doing. If I'm engrossed in something that really interests me, I can hyper-focus for hours at a time and nothing can distract me—I can deal with a possible distraction without ever acknowledging its existence. If I've been writing,

116

for example and a potential distraction occurs, I can continue writing mentally even if I have to leave my desk and go deal with that other thing. It never hooks my attention. It's as if I have a dual consciousness operating.

On the other hand, there are times when I hate what I'm doing and, despite the appearance of my being fully absorbed, I'm very alert for distractions—anything that can be used as an excuse to abandon the task. It's a "saved by the bell" kind of thing. It's as if I have a specific focusing mechanism. When the circumstances are such that the mechanism is engaged, I "can't be distracted even when I'm distracted." When that mechanism is not engaged, most likely because I'm not really interested in what I'm doing, the slightest thing can totally distract me.

My memory for detail has always been excellent. When I was young, I essentially had total recall and a photographic memory. As I got older, my head got filled up with too many things to be able to sustain that, but I still have a pretty phenomenal memory. Sometimes I'm not able to connect on a person's name, but I'll inevitably remember some detail about them, something like their dog's name, or what they were wearing the last time I saw them and I can cover nicely that way. I've had many instances of unusually vivid memory—not always accurate, I'm sure, but vivid nonetheless—and more often than not it is accurate. Numbers...I have a problem with numbers and with dates and with sequencing. When I'm trying to figure out which of two events occurred first, counting on my fingers is often necessary.

I used to be very absent-minded and forgetful. I'd be someplace and not remember whether I had gotten there by train or by car...or I'd know I had come by car, but wouldn't have any idea where I had parked. My son delights in telling a true story about the time I headed out the door to work without my skirt on. I've worked very hard at correcting that forgetfulness and have been pretty successful. Maybe

117

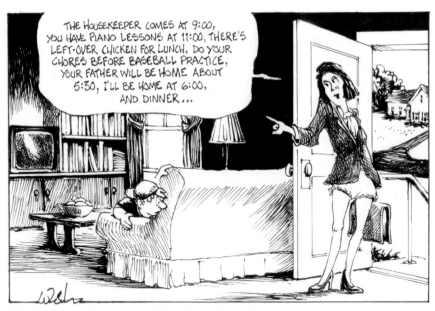

THE HOUSEKEEPER COMES AT 9:00, YOU HAVE PIANO LESSONS AT 11:00, THERE'S LEFT-OVER CHICKEN FOR LUNCH, DO YOUR CHORES BEFORE BASEBALL PRACTICE, YOUR FATHER WILL BE HOME ABOUT 5:30, I'LL BE HOME AT 6:00, AND DINNER...

The Contrasts Between an ASP's Strengths and Weakness Can Be Dramatic

I've managed to make some new neuronal connections, or something like that.

While she didn't say much about her creative abilities, those who know her well would say she is very creative—that she thinks creatively and lives creatively. Her reticence may have something to do with her perceiving "creative" as something she is, rather than as something she does—a result, perhaps, of her having grown up in a family of very creative individuals, a family in which creativity was taken for granted. She did acknowledge having been told in school that she was quite talented in music, drawing and painting—talents she did not pursue—and that she currently uses writing as a creative outlet.

When asked about her coordination/athleticism, Claire simply laughed—but finally admitted to a few talents:

When I was in the eighth grade, my school didn't have remedial gym—but they had to set up a special sub-group in my gym class. It consisted of a retarded kid, a kid who couldn't walk and me.

I rode horseback well (perhaps a reflection of the empathy I felt for horses), I got an "A" in badminton in college and I was good at yoga. Also, I do well at square dancing—perhaps because I have a good sense of rhythm. But all those things were a long time ago. Now, when I feel the need for exercise, I get it by removing the top from my car and driving very fast.

She responded to questions about her spatial abilities similarly. After initially denying having any at all, she ultimately acknowledged some.

119

> What spatial abilities? When I had some neurological testing done, I was utterly unable to put the blocks together to form the requisite pattern. And mentally rotating a three-dimensional image? … Hah! Then there have been things like wondering if my car will fit in a parking space and having no way of knowing other than trying. That got to be real expensive! Recently, though, I've been getting much better.
>
> Well…in school I was brilliant in geometry—but only in plane geometry, not in solid. I can do spatial things well only if they are two-dimensional. For example, I am very good at both Scrabble and crossword puzzles.

LANGUAGE AND LEARNING DISORDERS

Geschwind and Galaburda's theory of Anomalous Cerebral Laterality (ACL) had its genesis in their study of people with developmental learning disorders—dyslexia, stuttering, delayed speech, Attention-Deficit/Hyperactivity Disorder, Tourette's Disorder and Asperger's Syndrome (a mild form of autism) among them. Each of these disorders is separately coded in the *DSM-IV,* but for the purposes of this book it is their similarities, not their differences, that are important. The symptoms of developmental learning disorders include:

- Perceptual impairments: perceptual reversals in reading and writing; spatial orientation problems, including difficulty in differentiating left from right and up from down; poor tactile discrimination; problems with differentiating figure from background, both visually and auditorially; impaired orientation in time; poor eye-hand coordination; general awkwardness and clumsiness.

- <u>Disorders of speech and communication</u>: various aphasias (especially anomic aphasia—difficulty in naming things); delayed speech development; stuttering, speech hesitation and/ or lisp; auditory discrimination problems; difficulty in speaking/answering on demand.

  What's in a name? that which we call a rose, By any other name would smell as sweet.
  —William Shakespeare (Romeo and Juliet)

- <u>Disorders of thought processes</u>: disorganized thinking; problems with abstract reasoning and/or analogies; preoccupation with inner thoughts; thought perseveration.
- <u>Academic difficulties</u>: problems with reading, writing, spelling and mathematics; poor organization and time management abilities; difficulty with rote memorization; problems with both short-term and long-term memory; difficulty in following complex oral instructions.
- <u>Disorders of attention and concentration</u>: frequent daydreaming and/or a highly active imagination; a high level of distractibility; impaired concentration ability; short attention span; frequently losing things.

While learning disorders are correlated with neurological anomalies related to handedness, the problems associated with such disorders appear to be primarily attributable to neurological anomalies related to language. Language is an extremely important factor in the functioning of modern humans.

Two different areas of the left hemisphere are associated with two different aspects of the language function. Broca's area, in the frontal lobe, is primarily responsible for the production of speech. Wernicke's area, in the temporal lobe, is primarily responsible for

120

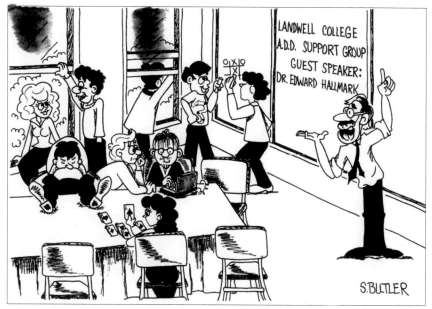

Attention Deficit Disorder Continues to Confound the Experts.

the comprehension of language. Figure 8.3., below, illustrates their locations. Wernicke's area appears to be much more affected by cerebral laterality anomalies than does Broca's area.

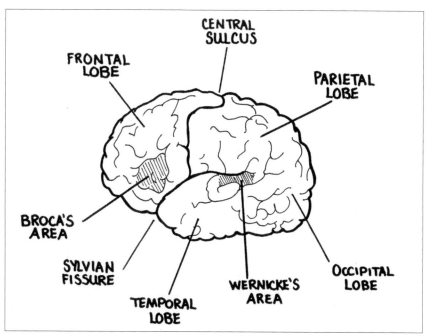

Figure 8.3. Surface View of the Left Cerebral Hemisphere Showing the Location of Broca's Area and Wernicke's Area

In a brain that is Less Strongly Lateralized (LSL) than the norm, one, or both of these language-related functions have spread, at least partially, into the neurological structures of the right hemisphere. The neuronal connections between the structures are thus more dispersed and effective mental functioning requires a greater than normal flow of information between the two hemispheres. The exchange of information occurs by way of the corpus callosum and other neural pathways. This need for increased inter-hemispheric communication results in left-handed men having a larger corpus callosum than do right-handed men. Similarly, the corpus callosum in women (who are LSL than men) is generally larger than it is in men.

Despite increased inter-hemispheric communication, greater dispersion of the neurological structures associated with language apparently reduces the overall efficiency and effectiveness of neuronal connectivity. Degradations in the accuracy of language-based functions such as learning, attention and memory can result. Moreover, the spreading of the language function into the right hemisphere tends to be accompanied by a weakening of visuo-spatial skills, which are normally associated with the right hemisphere.

Let go and let Dog.
—Dyslexics Anonymous
Slogan

Apparently the language function is of such overriding importance as to permit it to co-opt neuronal structures normally used for visuo-spatial functions.

All of this is further complicated by paradoxes. While learning disorders can accompany a LSL brain, so too can genius; while attention deficits can accompany a LSL brain, so too can the ability to hyper-focus; while forgetfulness can accompany a LSL brain, so too can extraordinary memory abilities; and while poor eye-hand coordination can accompany a LSL brain, so too can athletic and artistic giftedness.

INTELLIGENCES AND PARADOXES

In contemporary Western society, conformance to and mastery of learning style norms has historically been considered to be indicative of intelligence. This view has centered on logical-mathematical and linguistic abilities, those skills normally measured by conventional I.Q. tests. Such tests are designed to gauge a person's strengths in recognizing and recalling information and, to a certain extent, in solving problems. They don't address creativity, innovation, or invention at all. Thus, they measure the weaknesses, as opposed to the strengths, of those with LSL brains—those whose primary intellectual abilities involve the accessing of new concepts, not in the retrieving of old data.

The "three Rs"—reading, 'riting and 'rithmetic—are the central elements of learning in a traditional Western educational system. Not only are children required to learn the "three Rs," they are required to learn them in a specific way—one that involves structure, discipline, orthodoxy and convention. When children have difficulty meeting standard learning demands they are often labeled as being "learning disordered." The "three Rs" being the stuff of conventional I.Q. tests, these children also frequently test as having low I.Q. scores, thus lending support to the learning disorder diagnosis. Given cultural consensus, a low I.Q. score is taken to mean a low level of intelligence, but that conclusion can be erroneous. Albert Einstein, for example, exhibited significantly delayed speech (diagnosis: Expressive Language Disorder) as a child and was, by his own admission, a "second-rate mathematician." Few people today, however, would suggest that Einstein was a man of low intelligence. Clearly, there's more to all this than meets the eye.

123

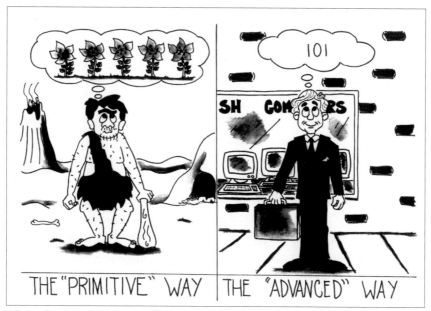

"Primitive" and "Advanced" Conceptualizations of the Number Five

124

Quite a few great theoretical mathematicians, many of whose brains were presumably **Less Strongly Lateralized** than the norm, struggled with basic arithmetic as children. Strange as that may seem, it makes sense when it is recognized that, whereas arithmetic involves linear sequential thinking (generally thought to be "advanced"), higher mathematics involves holistic simultaneous thinking (generally thought to be "primitive"). What is more, holistic (or analog) thinking lends itself much more readily to the creative process than does linear (or digital—especially binary) thinking.

In a like vein, there's the all-too-frequently occurring situation in which a child receives poor grades in arithmetic, not because s/he is incapable of determining the correct answer, but because s/he is unable to explain the proper sequential steps by which one is "supposed to" arrive at that answer. An educational strategy of that sort, even when the student is not accused of cheating, is likely to nip potential genius in the bud.

A similar situation exists with respect to linguistic intelligence. Indications are that many novelists, playwrights and poets (perhaps most poets) have **LSL** brains. This results in their having difficulty with the meaning (or objective qualities) of words—as opposed to the sense (or subjective quality) of words. Anomic aphasia, (difficulty in naming things), which is associated with the **LSL** brain, exemplifies this tendency. Naming things serves to categorize them, to pigeonhole them, to objectify them. It allows the speaker to distance her/himself from that which is being named and from the experience associated with that thing; it allows for externalization and

> *To name an object is to take away the pleasure given by a poem.*
> —*Stéphane Mallarmé*

analysis; it minimizes the concrete qualities of the thing by creating an abstraction. This is a strategy of separation and differentiation. The linguistic abilities of those with **LSL** brains, however, lie not in the objective, analytical realm of differentiating things by naming them, but in the subjective, emotional realm of linking things together through the use of jokes, puns, alliteration, onomatopoeias, rhymes, similes and metaphors.

As previously stated, differences in mathematical and linguistic learning styles of the sort being discussed here, especially if they are accompanied by low I.Q. scores, are often the bases for learning disorder diagnoses. Many people who have been diagnosed as having learning disorders, however, demonstrate a very high level of ability in one or more areas—usually in athletics, art, music, mathematics, chess, spatial relations, or visualization/manipulation of mental images. Studies of extremely precocious students show that more than 50% of them are Non-Right-Handed (NRH) (and presumably LSL), or, if right-handed, they have first-degree biological relatives who are NRH. NRH, then, in addition to being correlated with learning disorders, is also (seemingly paradoxically) correlated with intellectual precociousness. Moreover, studies of some of the world's greatest geniuses—Winston Churchill, Leonardo daVinci, Thomas Edison, Albert Einstein, George S. Patton, Nikola Tesla and William Butler Yeats among them—show that many evidenced symptoms of learning disorders.

125

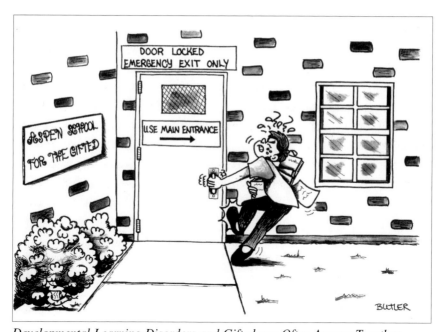

Developmental Learning Disorders and Giftedness Often Appear Together

A possible explanation for this apparent paradox may be that people with Anomalous Cerebral Laterality (ACL) are neurologically awkward longer than others. They continue to build neurological complexity and specialization well beyond the age when their peers have ceased further development. In other words, what is conventionally labeled a "developmental learning disorder," is actually a delay in the completion of neurological development.

Development may occur at a normal rate, but it continues for a longer time, thus resulting in something extra.

The diagnosis of "Attention Deficit/Hyperactivity Disorder (ADHD)" is closely related to diagnoses of other learning disorders. ADHD children are the ones who are unwilling to sit still for hours in an uncomfortable chair while listening to a boring lecture, who are intensely curious and ask many questions only tangential to the subject matter and who are attracted by more novel and challenging stimuli. In short, they have difficulty putting up with a dull, unstimulating, frustrating, curiosity-suppressing environment.

Reason can answer questions,
but imagination has to ask them.
—Ralph W. Gerard

126

ADHD also appears to arise out of a LSL brain, but a reduced attention span is not necessarily indicative of a disorder. Gifted, talented, creative children have a greater intensity—and increased levels of emotional, imaginal, intellectual, sensual and psychomotor excitability—than the norm. This is a part of their natural developmental pattern—natural, perhaps, but not normal and normalization is usually the goal in an institutional environment. What is generally overlooked is that many ADHD children can focus their attention quite well when engaged in something they personally consider to be challenging, stimulating and exciting—often to the extent of hyper-focusing. It is then that their boundless creative energies become very productively directed.

ADHD children are likely to be emotional, but in contemporary Western society, emotion, especially in males, tends to be negatively valued. Emotionality is sometimes treated as if it were the direct antithesis of intelligence. Perhaps that is, in part, why the ADHD label is more frequently applied to boys

If it ain't broke, don't fix it.
—Anonymous

than it is to girls. Those with LSL brains, whether male or female, have learning styles that are based more on emotions than the norm. Their interests tend to lie in the "hows and whys" of things rather than in the "whats and whens." They are drawn to the dynamics, not to the data—and when their curiosity is engaged by a dynamic, they want to explore its ramifications fully, rather than be overloaded with more data. It comes as no surprise, then, that when the natural flow of their energies is suppressed, they can develop resentments and begin to act out.

A LSL brain is also associated with a style of remembering that is more emotional than the norm and, again, what gets remembered are the dynamics, not the data. Memories, in the LSL brain, tend to be concrete (i.e., the recall of many traits of one instance) rather than abstract (i.e., the recall of a few traits shared by many instances). The breadth and inclusiveness of such memories make them hard to hold onto—because what is being remembered is not anything in particular but everything in general. One ASP from the Reference Group, for example, in recalling a visit to a restaurant, was able to describe the pattern of the tablecloths, the smell of the room, the demeanor of the waitress and somebody's spilling a glass of water. She had no idea, however, at what stage in her life the event took place, in what part of the country the restaurant was located, or what the name of the restaurant might have been. Interestingly, circumstances were such that her memories could be validated … and it turned out that she was 18 months old when that restaurant visit occurred!

The three stages of memory—acquisition, retention and retrieval—are all strongly influenced by an emotional style of thinking. When memory is emotionally based, the affective and aesthetic qualities of the original stimulus play an important role in determining the effectiveness with which each stage operates. Emotional gestalts related to memories can be so powerful, so vivid, so tangible and so real, that the person doing the remembering relives the original experience as if it were occurring again.

A few researchers, such as Howard Gardner in *Frames of Mind,* have directly addressed the issue of traditional I.Q. testing ignoring many abilities that are generally not recognized as intelligences. Gardner argued that logical-mathematical and linguistic abilities should not be considered the only indicators of intelligence— they are but two of a multitude of human talents and do not deserve special status. His suggestion was that either they both be spoken of as "talents," or that other talents also be granted the status of "intelligences." Opting to call them all "intelligences," he posited the existence of seven:

127

- logical-mathematical intelligence;
- linguistic intelligence;
- musical intelligence;
- visuo-spatial intelligence;
- bodily-kinesthetic intelligence;
- intra-personal intelligence; and
- inter-personal intelligence.

128   Logical-mathematical intelligence and linguistic intelligence are reflective of left-hemisphere strengths; the others are reflective of right hemisphere strengths. Left-hemisphere thinking is analytical reasoning of the type measured by I.Q. tests. It uses rationality to move toward a single goal; it is sequential; it is reductionistic; it excludes from its field of consideration as many extraneous stimuli as possible. Terms that have been used to describe left-hemisphere thinking include: conscious, intellectual, convergent, auditory, sequential, deductive, objective and masculine.

Right-hemisphere thinking involves a richness of ideas and originality. It is characterized by movement away from set patterns and goals; it is simultaneous; it is holistic; it includes in its field of consideration as many stimuli as possible. Terms that have been used to describe right-hemisphere thinking include: subconscious, intuitive, divergent, visual, holistic, inductive, subjective and feminine.

Silvano Arieti, in *Creativity,* speaks of left-hemisphere thinking as "secondary process thinking," and of right-hemisphere thinking as "primary process thinking." Secondary process thinking, he states, perceives differences and recognizes discrete entities—it uses a strategy of separation and differentiation. Primary process thinking, on the other hand, perceives similarities and recognizes patterns—it uses a strategy of incorporation and unification. Secondary process thinking, by itself, has no originality,

I like radio more than television—
the pictures are better.
—A 1950s seven-year-old

no uniqueness and no novelty. Primary process thinking, by itself, has no way of distinguishing whether perceived patterns are real or imagined, nor of determining if they have any utility. Each of these two thinking processes has its own strengths and its own weaknesses—and increased proficiency in one is often accompanied by a comparable deficiency in the other.

In adults, Arieti points out, the occurrence of primary process thinking by itself can be quite problematic—it is associated with the diagnostic label of "Schizophrenia," among others. When appropriately modulated by secondary process thinking, however, it becomes the stuff of genius, creativity and other exceptional abilities. He speaks of the effective coupling of the two processes as "tertiary process thinking." Tertiary process thinking is the theoretical ideal. In tertiary process thinking the full range of human intelligences can manifest in a useful and productive form.

129

In cases of Autism, unmodulated primary process thinking is often found and the combination of heightened sensitivities and sensory processing deficits can lead to synesthesias that result in exceptionally vivid, impactful and memorable imagery. Paradoxically, there is a certain amount of creative giftedness among autistics—and among their biological relatives as well. Joseph Chilton Pearce in *The Crack In The Cosmic Egg* describes this type of thinking clearly and does so without pathologizing it:

> [Autistic thinking] involves using a mode of mind strongly suggestive of early childhood…[It] is an unstructured, non-logical (but not necessarily illogical), whimsical thinking that is the key to creativity. It involves "unconscious processes" but is not necessarily unconscious. Autistic thinking is indulged in, or in some cases, *happens to* one in ordinary conscious states. The autistic is a kind of dream-world mode of thinking. This left-handed thinking is nevertheless a functional part of reality formation…[It is] an autonomous, self-contained kind of thinking that makes no adjustment to the world of other things or other thinkers, but it must have its materials *from* this other source. A[utistic] thinking includes conscious imagination and apparently unconscious processes and so offers a label for a wide range of similar phenomena.…
>
> The creative aspect of A[utistic] thinking is not controllable and cannot be duplicated by a computer, for the autistic mode *adds something* not in the given context. There is a catalystic quality in A[utistic] thinking that gives *more than* the sum of the parts,

suggesting and bringing about the new possibility. This A[utistic] thinking catalyst is not one's *personal* thinking. Rather it happens to a person. …Autistic thinking is unambiguous…To the mind in this state, all things are possible, all postulates are true. *[Italics in original, brackets mine]*

From: Pearce, J.C. 1971. *The Crack in the Cosmic Egg.* New York. Julian. Reproduced with permission from the current rights holder, Park Street Press.

Since most people's thinking, most of the time, is secondary process thinking, that is what is considered normal. Primary process thinking is not. Whether primary process thinking is viewed as madness or as genius depends largely on the degree to which it is tempered by secondary process thinking—in other words, the degree to which it is converted to tertiary process thinking. The insane person directs her/his life according to the unusual tenets of primary process thinking; the creative genius uses those tenets in a controlled manner, generally modifying them according to more conventional norms.

People whose tertiary process thinking is especially well developed can be found among the ranks of mathematicians, physicists, architects, chess players, musical composers, writers, artists and the like. Some names that come to mind are: Michael Faraday, Frank Lloyd Wright, Ludwig von Beethoven, Frederic Chopin, Aldous Huxley, Walt Disney and Andy Warhol.

The fact remains, however, that tertiary process thinkers (especially if they are creative geniuses) are different from the norm and, no matter how important their contribution to society might be, there exists a tendency to label them as "eccentrics." Many of history's creative geniuses have, indeed, had notable eccentricities. Consider, for example, the "absent-minded professor" manner of Sir Isaac Newton or Albert Einstein, the social inappropriateness of Wolfgang Amadeus Mozart or Bobby Fisher and the obsessive-compulsive behavior of Howard Hughes.

> *The creative person*
> *is both more primitive and more cultured,*
> *more destructive and more constructive,*
> *crazier and saner*
> *than the average person.*
> —*Frank Barron*

"Creativity" is extremely difficult to define and almost impossible to quantify. As the term is generally used, it has to do with inventiveness, with imagination and with combining old things in new ways. I abandoned my attempts to develop a creativity scale in early versions of the HISS when it became clear that the creative process involves all of the sensitivities measured by the second-level HISS scales—Physiological sensitivities (of the Sensory sort), Cognitive sensitivities (having to do with tertiary process thinking), Emotional sensitivities (both Intrapersonal and Interpersonal), Altered States of Consciousness sensitivities (especially Association) and Transpersonal Experiences sensitivities (artistic muses being one form of spirit guide).

131

In any event, in this age of specialization—of separation and fragmentation—creative impulses, arising out of tertiary process thinking, are the basis for people's motivation to cross the boundaries of disparate domains and to find similarities between elements in seemingly dissimilar fields. By so doing, they are able to make substantive, unique contributions to society.

> *Unless you know what it is,*
> *I ain't never going to be able*
> *to explain it to you.*
> *—Louis Armstrong*

A number of writers have offered lists of the traits and characteristics common to creative people. Each list has its strengths and each has its weaknesses. The list presented below is a synthesis of the lists suggested by others. Creative people exhibit:

> *We need to make the world safe*
> *for creativity and intuition,*
> *for it is creativity and intuition*
> *that will make the world safe for us.*
> *—Edgar Mitchell*

- Sensitivity—perceptiveness; awareness of and responsiveness to subtle stimuli; emotional acuity; ability to transcend the content and meaning of perceptions.
- Independence—ego strength; an internal locus of evaluation (the ability to shape personal beliefs and values without reference to consensual norms); a subjective sense of psychological freedom; a willingness to take risks.

- Cognitive Complexity—fluency, flexibility and rapidity of thought; the ability to hold numerous ideas simultaneously; the ability to toy with, analyze and reorganize multiple concepts.
- Openness—flexible, permeable boundaries in concepts, beliefs and hypotheses; receptivity to the original, the novel and the unfamiliar; ability to tolerate conceptual ambiguity without forcing closure.
- Non-rationality—holistic, aggregative, visual style of thinking; facility at accessing Altered States of Consciousness; ability to transcend self/not-self differentiation; ability to access primary process motivations and imagery; intuitive and spiritual orientation.

132

Earlier in this chapter, it was stated that the language function is apparently of such overriding importance that, in brains Less Strongly Lateralized (LSL) than the norm, the language function is likely to co-opt neuronal structures normally used for visuo-spatial functions. This co-opting can then lead to a degradation of visuo-spatial abilities that often results in poor eye-hand coordination and general awkwardness or clumsiness.

> *Our creativity is limited only by our beliefs.*
> *—Willis Harmon*

This presents another paradox. While left-handers (who presumably have LSL brains) generally do worse than right-handers on tests of visuo-spatial skills, artists and athletes (both of whom need superior visuo-spatial skills) have an elevated incidence of left-handedness. Apparently, the anomalous neuronal connections in LSL brains are such as to create two groups of individuals—one whose visuo-spatial skills are degraded and the other whose visuo-spatial skills are enhanced. The resolution to this paradox may involve the way in which the self/not-self differentiation strategy of those with LSL brains differs from the norm—specifically their use of the incorporation style, as opposed to the separation style, of perception.

Support for this explanation is found in anecdotal data from studies of baseball players that show brown-eyed players to be better batters than blue-eyed players. ("Blue-eyed" suggests hypopigmentation and, it will be remembered, hypopigmentation is associated with ACL, which suggests a LSL brain.) On the other hand, the eye color finding does not hold true for baseball pitching—and the strengths of Non-Right-Handed pitchers are legendary.

What might be going on is this: In batting, the action required is one of response and in order precisely to locate and respond to a moving object in space, one must be able to perceive that object as being entirely separate from one's self. It is not enough to think: "We (the object and I) are here." One must be able to think: "I am here and that object, which is entirely separate and distinct from me, is there"—and one must be able to specify what "here" and "there" mean. In pitching (and similarly in art), the action required is not one of response, but rather one of initiation. Batting requires a quick response (with fine eye-hand coordination) to the stimulus of an action (the throwing of a ball) initiated by another. Not so with pitching (and art). A pitcher (artist) has time to incorporate the stimulus (ball or artistic medium) into her/his perception of self before initiating an act (throwing or creating). This suggests that the pitcher (artist) uses a holistic (as opposed to sequential) approach to motor control, one that results in a fluid, generalized, intuitive attunement to bodily movements—and that this strategy might be less effective when a quick response to a rapidly moving external stimulus is required. This picture can be completed with the observation that pitchers tend to be notoriously poor batters.

Most of the paradoxes that appear in the course of this study of sensitivities appear to be attributable to the two different types of cognitive processing that arise out of the two different cerebral hemispheres. Emotional sensitivities, which will be discussed in the next chapter, are also related to cerebral laterality, but appear to be considerably more straightforward.

133

CHAPTER SUMMARY

⟹ The symptoms of developmental learning disorders associated with Anomalous Cerebral Laterality (ACL) (and hence with ASPness) include: perceptual impairments, disorders of speech and communication, disorders of thought processes, academic difficulties and disorders of attention and concentration.

⟹ In Less Strongly Lateralized (LSL) brains, the spreading of the language function into the right hemisphere co-opts neuronal structures normally used for visuo-spatial functions and can result in degraded eye-hand coordination.

⟹ While learning disorders can accompany a LSL brain, so too can genius; while attention deficits can accompany a LSL brain, so too can the ability to hyper-focus; while forgetfulness can accompany a LSL brain, so too can extraordinary memory abilities; and while poor eye-hand coordination can accompany a LSL brain, so too can athletic and artistic giftedness.

⟹ People with ACL tend to be emotional and emotions play an important role in shaping learning and mnemonic styles.

⟹ Traditional I.Q. tests, in measuring cortical strengths associated with the left hemisphere, measure the weaknesses of Anomalously Sensitive Persons (ASPs). The cognitive strengths of ASPs involve the right hemisphere and subcortical structures.

⟹ Left hemisphere thinking uses a strategy of separation and differentiation and is spoken of as "secondary-process thinking." Right hemisphere thinking uses a strategy of incorporation and unification and is spoken of as "primary-process thinking." When the two processes are combined in "tertiary-process thinking" the full range of human intelligences can manifest in a useful and productive form.

⟹ The creative process utilizes tertiary process thinking and involves the full spectrum of sensitivities.

⟹ Characteristics of creative people include: sensitivity, independence, cognitive complexity, openness and non-rationality.

CHAPTER 9

Emotional
Indicators Of Sensitivities

Intellect is to emotion as our clothes are to our bodies;
we could not very well
have civilized life without clothes,
but we would be in a poor way
if we had only clothes without bodies.
—*Alfred North Whitehead*

There can be no transforming of darkness into light,
of apathy into movement, without emotion.
—*Carl Jung*

An anomalously high scorer on the HISS Emotional (EMO) indicators scale is likely to report a high level of sensitivities in both the Intrapersonal and the Interpersonal realms. Intrapersonal sensitivities, on the downside, can result in strong mood swings with a tendency toward depression, as well as the likelihood of being easily hurt or upset; on the upside they can lead to significant breadth and depth of affect (feeling), to subtle and nuanced emotional responsiveness and to enhanced self-awareness. Interpersonal sensitivities, on the downside, can result in over-identification and enmeshment with others; on the upside they can contribute to good people skills and humanitarian tendencies.

Claire is emotionally very responsive, easily hurt and highly subject to psychological stress. She experiences a wide range of feelings, is inclined toward anxiety/panic attacks, can feel happy and sad at the same time and is vulnerable to feelings of depression. Sometimes, for no apparent reason, she experiences sudden feelings of ecstasy, bliss, peace, joy and love. She is highly empathic, but being attuned to the thoughts and feelings of others can result in her becoming emotionally overwhelmed in groups. Knowing, at a distance, when someone she cares about is upset, hurt, or in danger is a common experience for her.

She told me that she has put a lot of time and energy into learning how to deal with her emotions. Apparently she has had positive results.

> For many years, I didn't share my emotions with others. I was very well defended. I'm not so private anymore, not feeling the need to defend myself so thoroughly. Learning how to be ambivalent was helpful. No longer do I feel I have to have *an* emotion —I can have several of them simultaneously, or I can have one emotion ambivalently and ambiguously… and still feel that emotion strongly.
>
> Having those strong defenses in place didn't seem to interfere with my effective functioning as a psychotherapist, perhaps because I was highly sensitive to other people's emotions—I could read them accurately and quickly. I don't think I used other people's emotions vicariously as a way of avoiding my own—I was attuned to my own feelings, but just wasn't willing to expose them.
>
> My greatest strength in the emotional realm is definitely empathy. I'm very empathic and can literally "feel with" another person. This ability has served me especially well with animals, with babies, with students and with clients. I'm even learning to

be empathic with people I previously would have considered jerks—and thus am becoming considerably less judgmental.

EMOTIONALITY AND EMOTIONAL ACUITY

With respect to Intrapersonal Emotional sensitivity, an important distinction needs to be made between emotionality and emotional acuity. "Emotionality" implies a tendency to be markedly aroused, agitated, or dominated by emotions. "Emotional acuity" suggests the ability to experience many elements in a subtle emotional palette of which less sensitive people might have no awareness. The downside of Intrapersonal Emotional sensitivity has its genesis in emotionality; the upside arises from emotional acuity. Emotionality will be addressed here first.

137

Where there is a greater than normal involvement of the right cerebral hemisphere in mental processes (i.e., where the brain is Less Strongly Lateralized [LSL] than the norm), an increased level of emotionality is likely to result —and that emotionality has significant downside implications. Studies have shown that, whereas activation of certain regions in the left hemisphere of the brain can result in elation, activation of corresponding regions in the right hemisphere can result in depression. Other studies have shown that:

- Individuals suffering from depression exhibit three times the normal rate of left-handedness and, curiously, their children exhibit six times the normal rate of left-handedness.
- Low serotonin levels (see Chapter 4) are associated with depression, anxiety, violent ideation and aggression.
- Left-handers, by self-description, are more introverted, aloof, cold and quarrelsome than are right-handers.
- Left nostril breathers (there appears to be a contralateral connection between the nostril being used for breathing and the brain hemisphere that is more activated) are more prone to stress related illnesses than are right nostril breathers.
- Hypopigmented children are more introverted and shy, more reactive to sensory stimuli and have higher levels of immuno-suppressive stress hormones than the norm.

Bipolar Disorder,[†] an extreme instance of emotionality, is considered to be a right hemisphere dysfunction in that it frequently accompanies lesions on the right temporal lobe. It is characterized by a cycling of moods (usually with a periodicity of months) between manic episodes and depressive episodes. Individuals suffering from Bipolar Disorder have an increased sensitivity to light and their symptoms may be exacerbated by changes in their sleep/wake cycle. While the causes of Bipolar Disorder are poorly understood, its cyclical nature suggests that the biological clock (with the pineal/hypothalamus/suprachiasmatic nucleus link) is involved —and, in those with Less Strongly Lateralized (LSL) brains, the biological clock is likely to be more sensitive than the norm.

138

The introduction of emotion moves this discussion out of the realm of "thought" alone and into the realm of "cognition." Thought has to do with reason, logic and judgment —processes that are considered to be antithetical to emotion. Cognition, on the other hand, involves both thought (judgment) and awareness (perception). Emotion, at its root level, has much more to do with awareness or perception than it does with thought or judgment. While one might think about one's emotions after they arise (and those thoughts might, in turn, engender other emotions), an emotional *perception* invariably precedes the judgments that are made about that perception. Emotional acuity and affect linking (to be discussed shortly) underlie primary process *cognition* and primary process *cognition,* in its pure form, has to do with awareness —just as secondary process *cognition,* in its pure form, has to do with thought. That being so, then tertiary process *cognition* has to do with a cycling between (or coupling of) awareness and thought.

Emotions are not just cognitive luxuries for those who can afford them. They are a fundamental part of what it means to be human. Without emotion, without primary process cognition, all that remains of the mind is rational, logical, analytical secondary process cognition —and to identify that with humanness is patently absurd. To know oneself, or to know that which lies beyond oneself, one needs ready access to emotion, to primary process cognition. Secondary process cognition is cold, sterile and numb; it is literally unfeeling —and because it is unfeeling, it excludes from its repertoire both creative experiences and Transpersonal Experiences (TPEs).

[†] Formerly called "Manic-Depressive Disorder."

David Gelernter, in *The Muse in the Machine,* discusses in depth the role of emotional acuity in both those types of experiences. The language he uses is rather academic and inaccessible so, in what follows, I have taken the liberty of incorporating a paraphrasing of his ideas into my own.

Emotional acuity sets the stage for affect linking. Affect linking is the establishing of a connection between two or more (perhaps seemingly very dissimilar) stimuli, specifically because each of those stimuli engender the same emotion in the perceiver. Affect linking is the basis for metaphor, for analogy, for intuition, for insight and for the perception of similarities.

139

A man becomes creative, whether he is an artist or a scientist, when he finds a new unity in nature. He does so by finding a likeness.
— *Jacob Brownoski*

Awareness grounded in emotional acuity (and without the intercession of thought)—that is, pure primary process cognition—is able, via affect linking, to transcend both the content and the meaning of the stimuli that it perceives. With that transcendence, it is only the similarities, not the differences among the stimuli that are registered by the mind of the perceiver. In essence, the stimuli all become one.

This ability to perceive similarities among seemingly disparate stimuli by way of primary process cognition is the hallmark of the creative process. A person who is having a creative experience, upon discovering such an unexpected connection, then comes (perhaps is startled) back to secondary process cognition and is thus able to make constructive use of the creatively perceived connection. This coupling of the awareness of primary process cognition with the thought of secondary process cognition is what constitutes tertiary process cognition and the realization of creative potentials.

Transpersonal Experiences (TPEs) are closely linked with creative experiences because they have in common the dynamics that arise out of emotional acuity and affect linking. When primary process cognition is maintained for an extended period of time without the intervention of secondary process cognition, the chain of perceived connections can become so inclusive as to result in the sensation of connectedness among all things—all life, all objects and all events in the outside world, as well as connectedness between the outside world and the inner world of the experiencer. This is the essence of TPEs, the definition of which merits restatement here. Transpersonal Experiences are: "Experiences that occur beyond the ordinary differentiated boundaries of ego, space and time; experiences that suggest the essential interconnectedness (and/or absolute unity) of all that ever was, is, or will be; experiences that imply the existence of mind (as distinct from brain), of spirit, of soul."

140

The difference between Intrapersonal and Interpersonal emotional sensitivity is not always obvious and it is especially important to note that Interpersonal Emotional sensitivity also has many characteristics in common with Transpersonal Experiences sensitivity. An Interpersonal Emotional experience occurs beyond the ordinary differentiated boundaries of the ego (and, perhaps, of space and time as well) and thus suggests interconnectedness with another person, as well as the existence of mind (as distinct from brain).

The association of mind with brain is generally accepted, but if an argument is to be made for a situational or provisional differentiation between mind and brain, it is necessary to look at the brain from a broader perspective than that of just the two hemispheres of the cerebral cortex. What is at issue here is that while the right cerebral hemisphere is, indeed, associated with emotions, contemporary research indicates that emotions arise in the limbic system —an older or deeper brain structure —and it is the right cerebral hemisphere that brings those emotions into awareness by way of the strong neurological connections between the limbic system and the right temporal lobe.

THE TRIUNE BRAIN

Prior to the second half of the 20th century, most discussions of mind and consciousness revolved around the assumption that the cerebral cortex was the only really important component of the human brain. This belief was largely the result of conceptual anthropocentricism grounded in the belief that it was the cortex and the functions of the cortex that made humans superior to the "less evolved" species. According to this view, information flow in the brain (by way of neural impulses) was linear; physical and mental functions could be localized to discrete areas of the cortex; and a hierarchy existed in which the cortex stood supreme, dominating all other parts of the brain.

In 1949, Dr. Paul Maclean at the National Institute of Mental Health proposed the concept of the "triune brain" —a more balanced way of looking at the interconnectedness of the brain's various parts. His position was that, while the brain indeed has three distinct components, each of which *can* be viewed as separate brains (see Figure 9.1, below), those brains are intimately interconnected and they reflect humans' fully incorporated evolutionary heritage from reptiles, early mammals and later mammals:

141

- The ancient brain (the reptilian brain or central core), is an extension of the upper brain stem. It deals with self-preservation and preservation of the species through impulsive reflexes.
- The old brain (the paleomammalian brain or limbic system), exists in other mammals as well as in humans. It deals with emotions that guide behavior.
- The new brain (the neomammalian brain or cortex), is most highly developed in humans. It deals with memory and problem solving, with language, reason, symbols and culture.

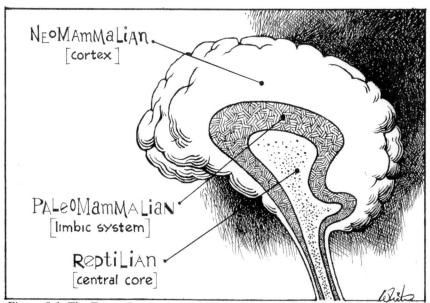

Figure 9.1. The Triune Brain

Each of these three brains can be thought of as having its own form of cognition, each of those forms having a different relationship with the self. At the level of the central core, cognition deals only with sensorimotor experiences; for it, the body and the environment are one and the same. At the level of the limbic system, cognition deals with both externally stimulated perceptions and internally generated imagery, both by way of the same neuronal mechanisms; it is unable to distinguish between them. At the level of the cortex, physical objects become clearly recognizable as belonging to the external world. It is only at the cortical level, then, that the brain is able to separate, to differentiate and to make clear distinctions between that which is self and that which is not-self.

Maclean's work rendered the earlier view of the brain obsolete and led to a more accurate contemporary view that involves five main points:

- The flow of information-carrying neural impulses is parallel and multiplex, not linear—thus invalidating the concept of brain hierarchy.
- Information is distributed, not localized. A given region of the brain serves many functions. Conversely, a given function of the brain is associated with more than one of its regions.
- While the cortex may contain an individual's model of reality and make self/not-self distinctions, it is the limbic system, not the cortex, that determines the relevance of that model and those distinctions.
- Subjective, emotional evaluations—not objective, rational ones—guide and direct an individual's behavior.
- It is emotion, more than reason, that makes people distinctly human; individuality is more non-verbal than it is verbal.

Contemporary holistic researchers are beginning to think of the brain not so much as a creator of consciousness, but as a filtering mechanism that allows only a small part of a larger reality to find its way into cognition. Rather than having access only to its own constructs, the brain is seen as being able to access information from a much broader realm. The efficacy and selectivity of this filtration process is said to depend on what is called the "serotonin screening mechanism," its modulation being a function of the melatonin/serotonin relationship (see Chapter 4). Current thinking holds that serotonin is released in order to dampen the brain's reaction to incoming stimuli whenever it is necessary to protect the brain from excessive perturbation. As previously mentioned, the melatonin/serotonin relationship is influenced by the pineal gland and the pineal gland has connections with the thalamus, the hypothalamus, the hippocampus and the amygdala —the major components of the limbic system. Moreover, the limbic system functions as the conduit through which information from the central core is channeled to the cortex. What is being suggested, then, is that the limbic system functions as the regulator of the cortex.

143

Inclusion of the limbic system moves this discourse beyond the left hemisphere/right hemisphere dichotomy, beyond the constraints of ordinary thought and perhaps even beyond the boundaries of what has been spoken of here as "cognition." It leads to the concept of consciousness and, most importantly for the purposes of this book, to issues having to do with Altered States of Consciousness (ASCs). These matters will be dealt with in the next chapter.

CHAPTER SUMMARY

⇒ Relative to the norm, people with Less Strongly Lateralized (LSL) brains are likely to have heightened levels of both emotionality and emotional acuity.

⇒ Emotional acuity and affect linking (establishing a connection between two or more stimuli because they engender the same emotion) underlie primary process cognition. Primary process cognition has to do with awareness; secondary process cognition has to do with thought; tertiary process cognition has to do with both awareness and thought.

⇒ The ability to perceive similarities among seemingly disparate stimuli by way of primary process cognition is the hallmark of the creative process.

⇒ Transpersonal Experiences (TPEs) can occur when the experiencer maintains primary process cognition over an extended period of time—thus resulting in a perceived connectedness among all things.

⇒ The concept of the "triune brain" suggests that while the three distinct components of the human brain *can* be viewed as separate brains, they are intimately interconnected. The components are: (1) the ancient brain (the reptilian brain or central core), (2) the old brain (the paleomammalian brain or limbic system) and (3) the new brain (the neomammalian brain or cortex).

⇒ While the cortex may contain an individual's model of reality and make self/not-self distinctions, it is the limbic system, not the cortex, that determines the relevance of that model and those distinctions.

⇒ Contemporary research suggests that the brain is not so much a creator of consciousness as it is a filtering mechanism that allows only a small part of a larger reality to find its way into cognition. The limbic system appears to control the efficacy and selectivity of this filtration process.

CHAPTER 10

Altered States Of Consciousness Indicators Of Sensitivities

Science's biggest mystery
is the nature of consciousness.
About all we know about consciousness
is that it has something to do with the head,
rather than the foot.

—*Nick Herbert*

Consciousness
is a fascinating but elusive phenomenon.
It is impossible to specify
what it is, what it does, or why it evolved.
Nothing worth reading has been written about it.

—*Stuart Sutherland*

An anomalously high scorer on the HISS Altered States of Consciousness (ASC) indicators scale is likely to report a high level of sensitivities in the realms of Dissociation, Hallucination, Sleep/ Wake Overlap, Association and Suggestion. As will be shown, ASC sensitivities appear to underlie all the other major sensitivities—

Physiological, Cognitive, Emotional and Transpersonal Experiences—so it is impractical to provide a brief synopsis of their upside and downside manifestations. Suffice it to say that in conventional psychiatric thinking, Altered States of Consciousness are generally considered to be evidence of psychopathology. While it is true that ASCs *can* be associated with psychopathology, it is also true that ASCs *can* be associated with giftedness. Both sides of the issue deserve to be given equal attention.

146

In responding to the HISS questionnaire, Claire reported that she sometimes had experiences of blank spells or missing time, including finding herself in some situation, but not knowing how she got there. These experiences were disconcerting, as were others in which she felt that either she, or people/places/things around her had become changed, distorted, or transformed.

She reported often experiencing, in a nominal waking State Of Consciousness, the feeling that her mind had left her body. She also reported sometimes being distracted by internal voices or other sounds and having experienced other perceptions for which there were no corresponding stimuli in consensus reality—most notably, strong unpleasant tastes and odors.

Her frequently recalled dreams are extremely vivid. The transition from the sleeping state to the waking state is, for her, quite lengthy and she has regularly experienced hypnogogic perceptions (further discussed later in this chapter)—chief among which are the feeling of flying through the air and waking up paralyzed while feeling the sense of a presence.

She is a very imaginative daydreamer and often enters a state of reverie. At such times, she experiences her subjective perceptions as being "more real than real," and finds her inner reality to be virtually indistinguishable from outer reality. Incidents of this sort are the springboard for creative undertakings, such as inspirational writing, in which she feels that it is not she who is doing the creating.

Claire had some difficulty in talking about her Altered States of Consciousness (ASC) sensitivities—not because of any particular reticence on her part (although she did say she found it stressful), but because it was hard for her, during our discussions, to bring to mind any specifics. Presumably this was an example of state-dependent memory in operation. While talking with me, she was most likely in a State of Consciousness (SOC) that differed from the SOCs she had been in during her ASC experiences—so the specific material from those events was not readily accessible to recall and her comments were quite general.

I'm not sure what an "Altered State of Consciousness" is, because I couldn't begin to say what a "non-Altered State of Consciousness" is. In my experience, my States of Consciousness are constantly changing, so at any given moment I am in what might be spoken of as an "idiosyncratic" or "anomalous" State of Consciousness.

Staying with the conventional term, however, I would have to say that I am almost always in some sort of Altered State of Consciousness. Most of the time, the "altered" quality is minimal, but sometimes I go "way out there" and am only aware of having been in an Altered State of Consciousness when I come back to a more ordinary state.

Sometimes I'm aware that I am not aware and sometimes I'm not. Increasingly, I can be aware and not aware at the same time. Perhaps it has something to do with parallel States of Consciousness—the boundaries are very permeable, the states are not separate and distinct. I can be aware that I am not aware that I'm aware. When I'm "way out there," the minute I become aware of being in an Altered State of Consciousness, I come right back.

When I'm in an Altered State of Consciousness, my awareness is both very heightened and very focused. What I'm aware of, I'm incredibly aware of and everything else I'm completely oblivious to. I notice things that other people don't notice, but I miss things that are obvious to everyone else.

When I'm "way out there," it seems that I am regularly operating under the influence of post-hypnotic suggestions. I have no awareness of specific suggestions having been given, but I take everything that is said by others extremely literally. It's as if whoever happens to be speaking when I'm in an Altered State of Consciousness becomes an archetype.

Consciousness

When considered at a very simple level, "consciousness" can be equated with "cognition." From that perspective, it can be seen as being not so much a "thing" as it is a "process"—or set of mind activities, perhaps involving awareness and/or thought—that is associated with the brain. These "Mind Activities" can be compared and contrasted with two other sets of activities associated with the brain, namely "Environmental Interaction Activities" and "Regulation of Bodily Function Activities." Table 10.1., below, helps to clarify the distinctions.

Environmental Interaction Activities	Regulation of Bodily Functions Activities	Mind Activities		
Seeing	Hormones	Alerting	Choosing	Thinking
Listening	Blood Pressure	Attending	Willing	Learning
Feeling	Temperature	Observing	Imagining	Remembering
Tasting	Reflexes	Emoting	Creating	Reading
Smelling	Body Positions	Dreaming	Discovering	Writing
Speaking	Movement	Sleeping		Calculating
	Breathing			Drawing
	Drinking			
	Eating			

Table 10.1 Representative List of Activities Associated with the Brain

Discussions of consciousness, however, seldom take place at a simple level. Once engaged in, they rapidly become exceedingly complex. A 1976 book by Julian Jaynes, entitled *The Origin of Consciousness in the Breakdown of the Bicameral Mind,* is a case in point. Jaynes set out to develop an unassailable definition for consciousness and simultaneously attempted to explain how consciousness originally came into being.

He defined consciousness as subjectivity, self-awareness, having an awareness of one's own awareness (i.e., "reflexive" self-awareness), or having an internal mind-space to introspect upon—and postulated that consciousness requires thought, thought requires language and, given that only humans are capable of producing and/or comprehending language, only humans can be considered to be capable of attaining consciousness.† A logical corollary to his theory would be this: Since the language center, Wernicke's area, is located in the left temporal lobe and, since language, like other left-hemisphere functions, is a logical, linear, rational process, consciousness itself must be considered to be a logical, linear, rational process.

Based on his review of ancient literature, Jaynes argued that consciousness, as we know it, was unavailable to primitive humans until the second millennium BC—a time of enormous social chaos in which the development of consciousness as a means of social control became necessary for human survival. Early humans, he stated, had no subjectivity or self-awareness and no consciousness. Volition, planning and initiative were organized outside conscious awareness in the right hemisphere's analog of the left hemisphere's Wernicke's area. The left hemisphere was then "told" what to do by auditory hallucinations developed in the right hemisphere—these hallucinations being perceived as the voices of gods. Jaynes asserted that this type of mental activity was associated with what he called a "bicameral mind"—that is, a mind having two separate and distinct "houses" (or parts), each corresponding to a different hemisphere of the brain and each having its own specific identity and role.

Evidence supporting this hypothesis, he argued, was provided by the following observations:

- Both cerebral hemispheres are able to understand language, but only the left is normally able to speak.
- There remains today, some vestigial functioning of the right hemisphere that is reminiscent of the voices of the bicameral gods.
- The two cerebral hemispheres, under certain conditions, are able to function independently of one another, almost as if they were two separate individuals. Their relationship reflects the human/god relationship of primitive times.

149

---

† Note that a person can be "unconscious" — that is, can exist in a State of Consciousness such as deep sleep or coma that involves neither awareness nor thought (as far as medical science knows) — but still be capable of attaining consciousness. Note too that a person who is engaged in "conscious" activities will most assuredly be simultaneously engaged in a host of "subconscious" (not readily available to the conscious mind) and "unconscious" (unavailable to the conscious mind) activities.

- The cognitive functional differences between the two hemispheres, as determined by contemporary neuroscience, reflect the functional differences between human and god seen in the early literature.
- The brain has considerably more plasticity than has been previously supposed. It could have undergone a rapid change from bicamerality to consciousness, almost exclusively on the basis of learning and culture.

150

There is a strong parallel, Jaynes stated, between the "voices of the gods" when human minds were bicameral and the auditory hallucinations of contemporary schizophrenics. Stress caused bicameral humans to hear those voices. In today's world, stress can cause schizophrenic decompensation. In modern "normals," the stress threshold for the release of hallucinations is very high. In psychosis-prone persons, it is somewhat lower— schizophrenics are quite susceptible to being overloaded by stimuli. During bicameral times, the hallucinatory stress threshold was extremely low—any novel situation requiring a behavioral change was sufficient to cause auditory hallucinations.

A number of significant cerebral laterality effects associated with Schizophrenia reinforce the perception of its paralleling the processes of the bicameral mind. Among them are:

- Over time, there is greater ElectroEncephaloGram (EEG) brainwave activity in the right hemisphere of schizophrenic brains than there is in the left hemisphere. The normal pattern is one of greater left-hemisphere activity.
- After sensory deprivation (which can cause hallucinations in almost anybody) right hemisphere brainwave activity in schizophrenics is much more pronounced than it is in other people.
- Switching of predominant hemispheric activity occurs less frequently in schizophrenics (about once every four minutes) than the norm (about once every minute).
- In schizophrenics, the corpus callosum is larger than the norm. Its increased size is, perhaps, responsible for the slowing in the switching of predominant hemispheric activity.
- In cases of Temporal Lobe Epilepsy resulting from a lesion on the left temporal lobe (with a presumed accompanying

release of the right from its normal inhibitions), 90% of patients develop Paranoid Schizophrenia. With right temporal lobe lesions, fewer than 10% of patients develop such symptoms—most exhibit Manic-Depressive psychosis instead.

This focus on Schizophrenia may be somewhat misdirected. Bicamerality, as described, seems more closely to parallel what is today spoken of as "Dissociative Identity Disorder (DID)."[†] Note that the primary *DSM-IV* diagnostic criterion for DID is: "The presence of two or more distinct identities or personality states (each with its own relatively enduring pattern of perceiving, relating to and thinking about the environment and self)." In Jaynes' defense, however, it must be stated that Multiple Personality Disorder (as DID was then called) was, in the middle 1970s, an extremely rare diagnosis. Moreover, he did point to a number of parallels between bicamerality and various dissociative phenomena including: possession states, trance states, hypnosis and Tourette's Disorder. Dissociation being an Altered State of Consciousness, it is noteworthy that the terms used by Jaynes—"enhanced functioning of the right cerebral hemisphere," "Wernicke's area," "neuronal plasticity," "enlarged corpus callosum," "stimulus sensitivity," "increased responsiveness to sensory deprivation," "stress-induced hallucinations," "dissociation proneness," and "a high level of hypnotizability"—all apply to the Less Strongly Lateralized (LSL) brain, thereby suggesting a correspondence between ASPness and bicamerality.

151

[†] Louis Tinnen, in a 1990 article entitled "Mental Unity, Altered States of Consciousness and Dissociation," offered a somewhat different take on all this. He suggested that all humans are born with a dual (i.e., bicameral) brain and that for the first few years of life the two hemispheres maintain a cooperative partnership. As the brain develops, a (language based) "governing mental system" begins to emerge in one temporal lobe, normally the left. Sometime during the third year of life, the corpus callosum matures to the point of making an effective connection between the two hemispheres. The verbal, generally left, hemisphere becomes the dominant speaking self and suppresses the expression of the non-verbal, generally right, hemisphere.

Because of the functional plasticity of the nervous system in the early years, premature formation of a governing mental system in one hemisphere results in a parallel governing mental system being formed in the other. This leads, then, to two governing mental systems, both poised to assume cerebral dominance upon final maturation of the corpus callosum. Since only one can be dominant, the other eventually becomes latent. With ultimate left hemisphere dominance, the person is generally right handed; with ultimate right hemisphere dominance, the person is generally left-handed. In either case, a latent mental system continues to exist and, under certain (generally stress-related) circumstances, finds an opportunity to express itself. This theory implies that all humans are born with the potential for multiple personalities. In most cases, however, during the course of normal development, consolidation into a single, unified, sense of self is achieved.

Jaynes' work provides a vitally important foundation for discussions of consciousness. With more than twenty years of hindsight to draw on, however, some modifications are in order:

152

- Bicamerality, as previously mentioned, more closely parallels Dissociative Identity Disorder than it does Schizophrenia.
- The dismissal, as hallucinations, of the right hemisphere's god-voices, is a bit too facile. "God" may simply be a metaphor for the clear and compelling voice of intuition.
- It is unlikely that primitive humans were completely lacking in self-awareness. While changes in the nature of human thinking surely have occurred over time, the nature of those changes has most likely had to do with a reduction in the breadth of consciousness. As a result of the developing emphasis on rational empiricism in the last four eons, humans have simply learned to suppress awareness of information arising in the right hemisphere. The ready and possibly universal access that primitive humans presumably had to what Carl Jung called the "collective unconscious" was driven underground.
- The fluid communication that early humans apparently had between the two hemispheres resulted in a mind that was single, unitary and interconnected—they were able to think with their whole brain, not just with the left hemisphere's cerebral cortex. It is modern humans, then, whose brains are divided into two separate and distinct cortical compartments—who are separated from themselves—and who, therefore, can be thought of as being bicameral. Early humans, by contrast, are more appropriately thought of as being unicameral.
- The "thought" that is said to be required for "consciousness" is no better understood than is "consciousness," itself. It is through the use of the reductionistic approach—claiming that consciousness requires thought, thought requires language and only humans employ language—that the basis for the argument of consciousness being exclusive to humans is established. What, in lower mammals, appears to involve thought, is dismissed as "instinct" (defined as "the ability to make a complex and specific response to environmental

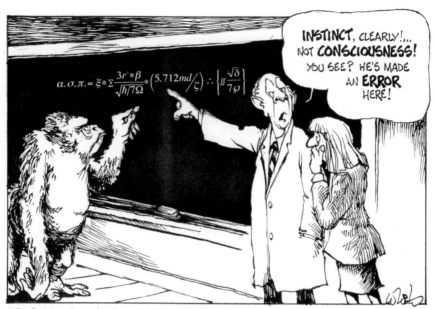

"Definitive Proof" that only Humans Can Attain Consciousness

stimuli without involving reason [or thought]"). Thus, by way of circular reasoning, other species become definitionally incapable of thought and the proof that they are incapable of thought is said to lie in their being incapable of producing and/or comprehending language. What is generally overlooked, however, is that contemporary researchers, using dolphins, whales, gorillas, chimpanzees, dogs and parrots as subjects, have shown that language capabilities are not exclusive to humans.

• Finally, there's the question of whether or not language is truly required for thought. Temple Grandin, a woman with Asperger's Syndrome, in *Thinking in Pictures,* addresses this issue: "...I would be denied the ability to think by scientists who maintain that language is essential for thinking. ...[They cannot] imagine thinking in pictures, nor assign it the validity of real thought. Mine is a world of thinking that many language-based thinkers do not comprehend."

Since this book deals only with the Anomalously Sensitive *Person,* the question of whether or not other species are capable of attaining consciousness is rendered moot. Moreover, the avoidance of theoretical irrelevancies requires postulating that all functional human beings have a mind and are therefore theoretically capable of attaining consciousness. Additionally, to facilitate discussion, the issues of whether or not the awareness involved in consciousness need be reflexive self-awareness and whether or not the thought involved in consciousness need be language-based thought, can also be considered immaterial. Finally, there's the question of whether or not both awareness and thought need be *simultaneously* involved in a specific State of Consciousness at a specific moment in time—and the answer to that is postulated as "no."

154

Three "ordinary" States of Consciousness are generally recognized. They are waking consciousness, dreaming consciousness and sleeping consciousness. Only waking consciousness involves both awareness and thought, the others do not. Dreaming consciousness involves thought but not awareness; sleeping consciousness involves neither. Table 10.2., below, illustrates the relationships among these states.

		THOUGHT	
		NO	**YES**
A W A R E **Y E S**			WAKING CONSCIOUSNESS
N E S S **N O**		SLEEPING CONSCIOUSNESS	DREAMING CONSCIOUSNESS

Table 10.2 Relationships Among Waking, Dreaming and Sleeping Consciousness

For the purposes of this book, then, "consciousness" will be defined as: "a process arising out of one or more mind activities involving awareness and/or thought, or neither."[†] Note that this definition allows for the possibility that in a specific State of Consciousness at a specific moment in time, either awareness, or thought, or both may be absent. Note too that this definition is consonant with the list of "Mind Activities" presented earlier in Table 10.1.

ALTERED STATES OF CONSCIOUSNESS   155

The three "ordinary" States of Consciousness (SOCs) having been specified, it remains to do the same with the various "Altered" States of Consciousness (ASCs). It is, however, impossible to do so—the reason being that *most* SOCs must be considered to be ASCs if the term "altered" is taken to mean "different from ordinary SOCs." The three supposedly discrete and differentiated ordinary SOCs are simply theoretical constructs and seldom (if ever) appear in their pure form. Most SOCs are admixtures of the waking, dreaming and sleeping states—and because they can mix in any proportions, the number of possible combinations is infinite. A rational exploration of ASCs requires that this point simply be acknowledged and set aside.

As it is used in this book, the term "Altered State of Consciousness (ASC)" is intended to mean: "Any State of Consciousness (SOC) that differs substantively from the three ordinary States of Consciousness (i.e., waking, dreaming and sleeping consciousness)." Since the meaning of the word "substantively" is unspecified, both qualitatively and quantitatively, a State of Consciousness can qualify as an Altered State of Consciousness even if it is not able to be recognized as such, either subjectively by the experiencer, or objectively by an observer.

The three ordinary SOCs are usually defined by their characteristic brainwave patterns. Simplistically, the waking state is said to correspond to an ElectroEncephaloGram (EEG) "beta" pattern (that is, brainwaves with a frequency of 14–22 cycles per second), the dreaming state to an EEG "theta" pattern (4–8 cps)

[†] A careful analysis of this definition will reveal that "consciousness" requires nothing more than having a "mind" that engages in "activities." The question of whether or not it is necessary to have a brain (neomammalian, paleomammalian, reptialian, or other) in order to have a mind is not addressed. Further discussion of this issue (with no *definitive* answer) will be found in Chapter 11.

and the sleeping state to a "delta" pattern (0.5–4 cps). Other patterns frequently mentioned in the EEG literature include the "high beta" pattern (22 cps and up), said to correspond to anxiety or hyperactivity and the "alpha" pattern (8–14 cps), said to correspond to relaxed, meditative awareness.†

Most intermixings of SOCs involve an overlapping of one state onto another that is so minor as to be unnoticeable and asymptomatic. A complete collapse of boundaries between states with a major overlapping of one state onto another, however, can have some very interesting consequences. For example, when a waking SOC overlaps onto a prevailing sleeping SOC, sleepwalking or sleep talking can occur. Also, when a waking SOC overlaps onto a prevailing dreaming SOC, lucid (aware) dreaming is likely to be experienced.

Of particular import relative to this discussion is when a dreaming SOC overlaps onto a prevailing waking SOC. That results in a condition known as "hypnogogia." Hypnogogia is characterized by theta-predominant brainwave frequency patterns, synesthesias, muscle atonia, myoclonic jerks, a loosening of ego boundaries, extremely vivid imagery and perceptual intermixing of stimuli from different sources. In the hypnogogic condition, the mind is not able to maintain meta-cognitions (i.e., it is incapable of thinking about its own thinking—it is not reflexively self-aware) and dream stimuli cannot be differentiated from environmental stimuli. The hypnogogic experiencer is incapable of thinking, "this is not happening" or "that is not real." S/he becomes completely

---

† While all of this seems to be pretty clear-cut and simple, there's a problem—it is a less than accurate, highly simplistic description of a very complex situation. Most basic discussions of brainwave frequency patterns treat the brain as if it were a monolithic structure within which, at any given time, every location manifests the same conditions. This simply is not so. Consider the following points, for example: (1) EEGs measure brainwave frequencies from the surface of the brain only, not from the deeper (older) brain structures; (2) EEGs measure brainwave frequencies from specific, discrete locations on the cortex, not from the entire cortex; (3) the patterns of brainwave frequencies exhibited by each of the two cerebral hemispheres can differ markedly from one another at any specific moment; (4) within each hemisphere, the patterns of brainwave frequencies exhibited by each of the lobes can differ markedly from one another at any specific moment; (5) brainwave coherence (brainwaves from different parts of the brain operating in concert) is an important and often overlooked factor in ASCs; (6) when a person is said to be exhibiting a specific brainwave pattern (e.g., when they are said to be "in beta"), the reference is to a predominant frequency—other frequencies are always exhibited as well; (7) the predominant brainwave frequency in the waking state varies with age, infants being delta predominant, young children being theta predominant, older children being alpha predominant and adolescents and adults being beta predominant; (8) research is just beginning into the implications of anomalously high brainwave frequency patterns (40 cps and up), spoken of as "gamma," and; (9) brainwave frequency patterns that differ from the norm, even markedly so, are not necessarily indicative of neuropathology.

absorbed in internally generated imagery and activities, loses her/
his reality testing ability, is generally unable to distinguish that
which is self from that which is not-self and may experience her/
his consciousness as free-floating and not connected to the brain/
body. While it was previously believed that hypnogogia was
invariably
followed by
sleep, that
turns out to
be untrue—
hypnogogia
followed by
w a k i n g

The conscious mind
allows itself to be trained like a parrot,
but the unconscious does not.
Thank God for not making [us] responsible
for [our] dreams.
—Carl Jung

(technically spoken of as "hypnopompia") can also occur.
Moreover, some individuals are capable of deliberately accessing
the hypnogogic state, maintaining it for an extended period of
time and then returning to an ordinary waking State of
Consciousness.

Ernest Hartmann speaks of such people as having "thin
boundaries" between waking, dreaming and sleeping States Of
Consciousness and asserts that they have a number of (ASP-
related) characteristics in common. They are likely to:

- have atypical lifestyles and be particularly artistic/creative;
- be especially open, trusting and vulnerable;
- have a difficult time dealing with stress;
- exhibit unusual sensitivities involving light, sound, emotions
  and empathy;
- have a history of ill health;
- be highly hypnotizable; and
- have a history of Transpersonal Experiences.

Hypnogogia results from the *simultaneous* occurrence of
primary process cognition and secondary process cognition. It is,
therefore, a variant of tertiary process cognition, which normally
involves a *cycling* between primary process cognition and secondary
process cognition. Because hypnogogia involves not only both
hemispheres of the cerebral cortex, but the limbic system as well, it
is appropriate to speak of it and other cognitive processes similar to
it, as "whole brain cognition."

Whole brain cognition clearly qualifies as being an **Altered State of Consciousness** and, to reiterate, it is characterized by slow (theta-predominant) cortical brainwave patterns, especially in the temporal lobes. Brainwave frequency patterns of this sort are associated with such things as early childhood, Attention-Deficit/Hyperactivity Disorder, Temporo-Limbic Epilepsy, dissociation, intrusive sleep disorders, creativity, meditation, hypnosis and psi.

158   Another brainwave factor involved in anomalous sensitivities—one that is every bit as important as predominant brainwave frequencies—is brainwave coherence. Brainwave coherence has to do with brainwaves from different parts of the brain exhibiting the same frequency and amplitude and being mutually entrained so that they operate together in a smooth continuous pattern. The more focused one's awareness is, the more coherent one's brainwaves tend to be. In the ordinary sleeping **SOC**, there is very little coherence; in the ordinary waking **SOC**, there is more; in imaginative involvement in a creative endeavor, there is still more; and in advanced meditation, there is a very high level of coherence.

Interestingly, EEG studies of Albert Einstein's brain showed a highly coherent pattern of alpha brainwaves most of the time. Hans Seyle wrote that every important scientific discovery of which he was aware had occurred in an **Altered State of Consciousness**—Einstein's formulation of his theory of relativity while imagining himself riding on a beam of light being one example. Another example would be that of August Kekulé's conceptualization of the benzene ring while daydreaming about a snake swallowing its own tail.

The greater the communication between different parts of the brain, the greater is the opportunity for brainwave coherence to occur. The **Less Strongly Lateralized (LSL)** brain, with a larger corpus callosum, increased symmetry and greater general interconnectedness relative to the standard brain, permits an elevated level of inter-hemispheric communication. This enhanced communication sets the stage for brainwave coherence and brainwave coherence, in turn, facilitates whole brain cognition. The concept of whole brain cognition gets around the problem of inappropriate emphasis on the cortex, avoids the outdated left-brain/right-brain dichotomization and elevates the limbic system to its rightful place as an integral part of all cognition.

HALLUCINATIONS

When cortical brainwaves are slowed (the limbic system, perhaps, initiating that slowing) and when they become coherent, the cortex can be thought of as idling. When it is idling, the cortex's functions, including its filtering function (see Chapter 9), becomes less effective—thus allowing for greater two-way interaction, or communication, between the limbic system and the environment. Not only can environmental stimuli more readily impress themselves upon the limbic system, the limbic system can also more readily explore and express itself in the external world—a role that is normally reserved for the cortex.

With cortical idling, the limbic system is free to create vivid imagery in all sensory modalities and to project that imagery out into the environment. In the absence of cortical reality judgment, these extremely vivid images are perceived as "more real than real"—they assume the status of perception, not just that of imagination or fantasy—and are powerfully impressed upon awareness. This process, called the "Perky Effect," is named for psychologist C. W. Perky who performed experiments along such lines in 1910. Perky's work demonstrated not only that human brains construct perceptions, but also that perceptions and internally generated images both utilize the same mental mechanisms. Thus, the differentiation of imagery as an internal event, from perception as an internal representation of an external event, becomes confounded—and the consolidation process for memory does not distinguish between them. Absent effective cortical reality judgment, perception and imagery are remembered as being equally real.

When extremely vivid images of this sort occur in the hypnogogic state, they are spoken of as "hypnogogic hallucinations." Since such hallucinations result from the overlapping of a dreaming SOC onto a prevailing waking SOC, it can be seen that the only substantive difference between dreams and hallucinations is the particular set of prevailing brainwave patterns in which each appears. Perceptions such as these are considered to be entirely normal during that portion of a person's life spent in a dreaming SOC, but are considered to be distinctly abnormal during the two-thirds of a person's life spent in a nominal waking SOC. This reasoning supports the argument for the existence of a neurological mechanism (the serotonin screening mechanism discussed in Chapter 9) that normally blocks such imagery in the waking state, but does so less effectively in those who are prone to hypnogogia (i.e., those who have a Less Strongly Lateralized brain). A reduction in serotonin levels in a nominal waking SOC can inactivate inhibitory mechanisms, permit increased activity of dopamine (another neurotransmitter, elevated levels of which are associated with Schizophrenia) and lead to the emergence of hallucinatory symptoms.

REALITY

IS FOR THOSE WHO LACK

IMAGINATION.

—*Bumper Sticker*

160

There are some very interesting corollaries to this hypothesis. Consider these, for example:

- A decrease in cortical activity does not necessarily result in a decrease in awareness; it results only in a decrease in the specificity of awareness—specificity related to sequential-temporal and spatial relationships.
- Realness—meaning the sense of reality, as opposed to the judgment of reality—may be a function of decreased cortical activity accompanied by increased subcortical activity.
- The perceptions of subcortical awareness are subjective, synesthetic and flexible; the perceptions of cortical awareness are objective, discrete and stabilized.
- Hallucinogenic drugs evidently achieve their effect by inhibiting the production of serotonin (with an accompanying surfeit of dopamine)—thereby reducing cortical awareness and enhancing subcortical awareness.
- When melatonin (which is complementary to serotonin) is metabolized in the pineal gland, it is converted to 5-methoxy-tryptamine. Tryptamines are abundantly present in certain hallucinogenic tropical plants.
- The deficit of serotonin (with an accompanying surfeit of dopamine) that apparently underlies the schizophrenic's

experience of being overloaded/hyperagitated by stimuli may, to a lesser extent, be an operative factor in anyone with a brain that is Less Strongly Lateralized than the norm.

The subject of hallucinations is a tricky one. While it is generally assumed that hallucinations (absent the ingestion of hallucinogenic substances) are evidence of significant psychopathology, that is not necessarily true—as shown by the discussion of hypnogogic hallucinations above. In order further to explore this subject, a definition of the term "hallucinations" is in order and the one provided by Ghasi Asaad in, *Hallucinations in Clinical Psychiatry* provides a starting point: "Hallucinations are…perceptions that occur in the absence of corresponding external stimuli."

On the surface, this definition appears to be clear-cut and simple, but since one of the central issues in this discussion is whether or not Transpersonal Experiences are "really real," it warrants closer examination. At issue is the question of what is meant by "external stimuli."

Most people would agree that "external stimuli" are those stimuli that are said to exist in the world of objective reality. Most people would also agree that the "objective reality" status of such stimuli is a function of their being able to be quantified and/or qualified by objective scientific methodologies. The assumption underlying such thinking, however, implies that "reality" (as such) does not exist beyond the boundaries of *current* scientific thinking. It wasn't too long ago that germs, viruses and atoms (let alone such things as quarks, gluons and mesons) would not have qualified for "objective reality" status.

Carrying this line of thinking a step further, one has to wonder about the current reality status of something as simple as the feeling of love. From a scientific perspective, love is neither quantifiable nor qualifiable, yet

One must not mistake majority for truth.
—Jean Cocteau

most reasonable people would agree that love is "really real"—that it is not a hallucination. In practice, reality status is generally determined by consensus—if the majority of people agree that something is real (whether objectively so or not), then it is real; if the majority agrees that it is not real, then it is not. For the purposes of this book, then, a more useful definition of "hallucinations" would be: "Perceptions that occur in the *apparent* absence of corresponding stimuli in *consensus* reality."

Most thinking about reality is focused on "consensus reality," and consensus reality is determined by the majority (Science, as society's dominant belief-shaping institution, has not yet formalized this process with a duly appointed commission, but …) in accordance with their subjective perceptions and their subjective cortical reality judgments (i.e., in accordance with the tenets of secondary process cognition). In other words, the empirical basis for distinguishing reality from hallucination, at a specific moment in time, is the consensus of the majority of people drawing on their subjective experience while in an ordinary waking State of Consciousness.

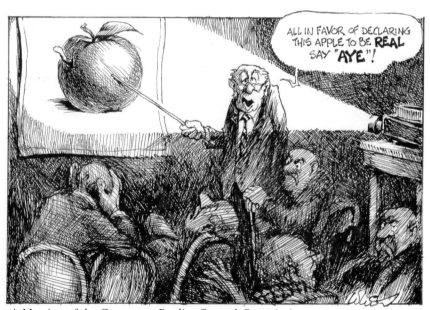

A Meeting of the Consensus Reality Control Commission

Since hallucinations are generally agreed to arise out of impaired sensory input coupled with impaired cortical reality judgment, what is to be made of *enhanced* sensory input coupled with *enhanced* subcortical reality sense—as might be the case with somebody having a brain that is Less Strongly Lateralized than the norm? Consider, for example, the (simplistically overstated) case of an individual whose olfactory acuity is equivalent to that of a dog—with corresponding emotional and behavioral responsiveness to olfactory stimuli. Such a person might well be perceived, not as having an exceptional ability, but as suffering from hallucinations (and goodness

WARNING:
I brake for Hallucinations!
—Bumper Sticker

163

knows what else), as being mentally ill and as requiring medical intervention. Presumably that is an unrealistically extreme example, but it may perhaps also be an appropriate parody of something that happens in the mental health field with distressing regularity.

If judgments about reality—and therefore about sanity—are to be made by reference to the consensus of those who are in an ordinary waking SOC, some other questions arise for consideration:

- How "altered" does an individual's Altered State of Consciousness have to be and for what duration, before it is considered to be evidentiary of mental illness?
- What if the majority of people, even for a moment, were to be in the same Altered State of Consciousness? Would reality then be redefined as a function of that particular State of Consciousness?
- Might there be as many different realities as there are different States of Consciousness—presumably an infinite number of them?
- Might "reality" be nothing more than a different label for "State of Consciousness?"

The point here is that a person who is in an ASC is simply functioning in a SOC that is positioned on the continua of awareness and thought somewhere other than the positions of the three ordinary SOCs (see Table 10.2., presented earlier in this chapter). In other words, her/his State of Consciousness is such that s/he will perceive things differently and will judge (the reality status of) things differently from the consensual norm—but there is nothing inherently pathological about that.

Dissociation, Association and Hypnosis

Altered States of Consciousness can be deliberately induced under laboratory conditions through the use of hypnotic techniques—and have been studied in some depth by Ernest Hilgard and others. For the purposes of this discussion, it is especially noteworthy that Hilgard identified two seemingly very different pathways by which ASCs are accessed in everyday life.

One of those pathways has already been encountered in the earlier discussion of Trauma and Abuse (see Chapter 5) and can be thought of as the "dissociative pathway" for accessing ASCs. It has to do with avoiding aversive stimuli and involves the separation and fragmentation of consciousness. Dissociation is an involuntary (automatic) response to significant stressors and, being a useful survival strategy, can rapidly become over-learned and inappropriately utilized—hence its characterization as pathological.

The other pathway can be thought of as the "associative pathway" for accessing ASCs. It has to do with approaching attractive stimuli and involves incorporation into and unification within, consciousness. Association is a voluntary response to significant attractors and is a process that plays a role in such things as daydreams and fantasies, creativity and invention, intuitive insight and transcendent experiences. Table 10.3., below, sums up the differences in these two pathways for accessing ASCs.

	Pathways for Accessing ASCs	
	Dissociative	**Associative**
A Process of	Avoidance	Approach
Characterized By	Pathologies	Abilities
Associated With	Stressors	Attractors
Degree of Control	Involuntary	Voluntary

Table 10.3 The Dissociative and Associative Pathways to ASCs.

Dissociative pathologies and associative abilities can manifest on continua of degrees from the mild to the extreme. Table 10.4., below, illustrates some examples.

Dissociative Pathologies	Degree	Associative Abilities
Over-learned Behaviors	**Mild**	Psychological Absorption
Simple Amnesias	⇓	Creative Immersion
Hysterical Amnesias	**Moderate**	Deep Meditation
Functional Paralyses	⇓	Psychic Attunement
Post-Traumatic Stress Disorder	**Extreme**	Out-Of-Body Experiences
Dissociative Identity Disorder		Mediumship (Trance Channeling)

Table 10.4. Continua of Dissociative Pathologies and Associative Abilities

The key element in contrasting dissociation and association has to do with the way in which differentiation between that which is self and that which is not-self is handled in these two different approaches to ASCs. The dissociative pathology involved in Dissociative Identity Disorder and the associative ability involved in trance channeling are representative. In Dissociative Identity Disorder, one mind (or State of Consciousness) is separated from an other mind (or State of Consciousness) in such a way that fragmentation into two or more apparently separate and distinct modes of cognition (identities or personalities) results. Conversely, in trance channeling, one mind (or State of Consciousness) is incorporated into another mind (or State of Consciousness) in such a way that unification of two apparently separate and distinct modes of cognition (identities or personalities) results.

While there is utility in thinking of dissociation as involving separation and fragmentation and of association as involving incorporation and unification, there is also an inherent contradiction in doing so. In dissociation, when various aspects of experience become separated, fragmented, or split off from the mainstream of ordinary waking consciousness, they lose their attachment to normal points of reference and become free-floating.

165

They are then able to recombine, fuse, or associate with each other in new, different and unusual ways. In other words, while the dissociative and associative pathways for *accessing* Altered States of Consciousness (ASCs) might be quite different, under certain circumstances, the ASCs so accessed and the ways in which those ASCs manifest, might be quite similar.

Dissociation and association, separation and incorporation, fragmentation and unification are two different sides of the same coin—and that coin is apparently the currency of the realm in the entire spectrum of sensitivities. Consider, for example, that it was noted:

- in the discussion of the cerebral cortex (Chapter 8), that one of its roles was to *separate* self from the environment;
- in the discussion of the bicameral mind (Chapter 10), that communications generated by the right hemisphere equivalent of Wernicke's area were *separated* from self and perceived as not-self;
- in the discussion of Braun's BASK model of dissociation (Chapter 5), that behavior, affect, sensation and knowledge can all be *separated* from self in the appropriate State of Consciousness;
- in the discussion of immune system dysfunctions (Chapter 7), that autoimmune disorders were caused by *separation* of self from self and that cancer was caused by *incorporation* of not-self into self;
- in the discussion of sensory sensitivity (Chapter 7), that overloading from *incorporation* of external stimuli can be a result of the suppression of cortical filtering;
- in the discussion of hypnogogia (Chapter 10), that meta-cognition becomes unavailable and the environment is *incorporated* into self;
- in the discussion of synesthesias (Chapter 7), that they involve the *incorporation* of one sensation into another sensation being activated by an external stimulus;
- in the discussion of creativity (Chapter 9), that the *incorporation* of seemingly disparate stimuli into a single perception can result in a useful new synthesis; and
- in the discussion of emotional acuity and affect linking (Chapter 9), that the *incorporation* and *unification* of all things into one's inner world is the basis for Transpersonal Experiences.

These observations, collectively, direct our attention to the point that is central to this entire discussion of Altered States of Consciousness—that Transpersonal Experiences are characterized by the mind's incorporation and unification of a broad variety of stimuli as a result of enhanced subcortical awareness and suppressed cortical thought. It follows then, that awareness without thought is a fourth theoretically discrete State of Consciousness complementary to the three ordinary states—waking, dreaming and sleeping consciousness. It finds its rightful place in the upper left cell of Table 10.2. (presented earlier in this chapter) and is appropriately spoken of as "Transpersonal Consciousness (TPC)." That table, in its completed form, is reproduced as Table 10.5., below.

167

		THOUGHT	
		NO	YES
A W A R E N E S S	Y E S	TRANSPERSONAL CONSCIOUSNESS	WAKING CONSCIOUSNESS
	N O	SLEEPING CONSCIOUSNESS	DREAMING CONSCIOUSNESS

Table 10.5. The Place of Transpersonal Consciousness

From the perspective of brainwave patterns, Transpersonal Consciousness (TPC) appears to involve:

- a very high level of brainwave coherence;
- just enough beta to maintain alertness;
- strong alpha and theta, the amplitude of alpha being greater than that of theta; and
- a level of delta considerably greater than that which normally appears in any State of Consciousness not presenting as deep sleep.

Because of the strong alpha patterns involved in TPC (and because of conceptual symmetry with the strong beta, theta and delta patterns involved in the waking, dreaming and sleeping states, respectively), one might be inclined to think of Transpersonal Consciousness as an "alpha" State of Consciousness—but that could be misleading. The most important brainwave characteristics of TPC are its high level of brainwave coherence and its *anomalously* high level of delta brainwaves, not its *absolutely* high level of alpha (and theta) brainwaves.

Anna Wise, in *The High-Performance Mind,* refers to this anomalously high level of delta brainwaves as "the radar of the unconscious mind," and suggests that it is indicative of a mind searching for information of a different kind from that which normally registers in cortical (beta) thinking. The high amplitude coherent alpha (and to a lesser extent theta) waves, she says, primarily serve to maintain alertness and awareness. They function as a bridge or conduit by which information gathered by the "radar of delta" can be made available to the cortex for processing and recall. People who exhibit this pattern of brainwaves (which she calls "the awakened mind") are, she says, extremely sensitive and highly prone to being overwhelmed by a variety of stimuli.

All indications are that the brainwave pattern of Transpersonal Consciousness—because it inactivates cortical filters—sets the stage for anomalously high levels of sensitivities in all of the realms (i.e., Physiological, Cognitive, Emotional, Altered States of Consciousness and Transpersonal Experiences).[†] Moreover, as its name suggests, Transpersonal Consciousness appears to be the key to understanding the dynamics involved in all Transpersonal Experiences—and that is where this discussion will head in the next chapter.

[†] Given that Transpersonal Consciousness appears to have its genesis in the limbic system (paleomammalian brain) and to involve suppression of neuronal activity in the cortex (neomammalian brain), it follows that Transpersonal Experiences can be considered a "primitive" mind activity rather than an "advanced" mind activity. Transpersonal Consciousness is inhibited (possibly as a result of cultural conditioning), not enhanced, by reflexive self-awareness and language-based thought. This could well account for the elevated frequency of Transpersonal Experiences among those who are less acculturated than the norm (i.e., children and indigenous peoples). Were this line of reasoning to be extended further, it might well lead to the conclusion that Transpersonal Consciousness is the "normal" state for the "lower" mammals—but then what dog (or cat) owner doesn't already know that?

CHAPTER SUMMARY

⇒ Julian Jaynes defined "consciousness" as "reflexive self-awareness" (i.e., having an awareness of one's own awareness) and postulated that consciousness requires thought, thought requires language and, given that only humans are capable of producing and/or comprehending language, only humans are capable of attaining consciousness.

⇒ For the purposes of this book, a broader definition of consciousness will be used, specifically: "a process arising out of one or more types of mind activities involving awareness and/or thought, or neither." In a specific State of Consciousness (SOC), either awareness, or thought, or both may be absent.

169

⇒ The three "ordinary" SOCs—waking, dreaming and sleeping consciousness—seldom appear in their pure form. Most SOCs are admixtures of them.

⇒ As it is used in this book, the term "Altered State of Consciousness (ASC)" is intended to mean: "Any State of Consciousness that differs substantively from the three ordinary States of Consciousness." An SOC can qualify as an ASC even if it cannot be recognized as such, either subjectively by the experiencer, or objectively by an observer.

⇒ Hypnogogia and other cognitive processes similar to it, qualify as ASCs that can be spoken of as "whole brain cognition."

⇒ In addition to predominant brainwave frequencies, brainwave coherence is another important factor involved in anomalous sensitivities. Brainwave coherence has to do with brainwaves from different parts of the brain having the same frequency and amplitude and being mutually entrained so that they operate in a smooth continuous pattern.

⇒ The enhanced inter-hemispheric communication of Less Strongly Lateralized (LSL) brains sets the stage for brainwave coherence that, in turn, facilitates whole brain cognition.

⇒ When cortical brainwaves are slowed, the filtering function of the cortex becomes less effective and the limbic system can more readily interact with the environment. Images arising in the limbic system, in the absence of cortical reality judgment, assume the status of perceptions—and are spoken of as "hallucinations."

⇒ "Hallucinations" are usually defined as "perceptions that occur in the absence of corresponding external stimuli." In practice, the reality status of a stimulus is generally determined by consensus of those who are functioning in an ordinary waking SOC (and thus making subjective judgments in accordance with the tenets of secondary process cognition). For the purposes of this book, a more useful definition of "hallucinations" is: "Perceptions that occur in the *apparent* absence of corresponding stimuli in *consensus* reality."

⇒ A person in an ASC will perceive things differently and will judge (the reality status of) things differently from the consensual norm—and there is nothing inherently pathological about that. "Reality" might be nothing more than a different label for "State of Consciousness."

⇒ There are two seemingly different pathways by which ASCs are accessed in everyday life. The dissociative pathway has to do with avoiding aversive stimuli and involves separation and fragmentation of consciousness. The associative pathway has to do with approaching attractive stimuli and involves incorporation into and unification within consciousness. The key element in contrasting dissociation and association has to do with the way in which self/not-self differentiation is handled.

⇒ Transpersonal Experiences (TPEs) are characterized by the mind's incorporation and unification of a broad variety of stimuli as a result of enhanced subcortical awareness and suppressed cortical thought.

⇒ "Transpersonal Consciousness (TPC)" is a fourth theoretically discrete SOC that is complementary to the three ordinary states—waking, dreaming and sleeping consciousness—and involves awareness without thought.

CHAPTER 11

Transpersonal Experiences Indicators Of Sensitivities

> The greatest pleasure in life is
> doing what people say you cannot do.
> —*Walter Bagehot*

> The only way to discover the limits of the possible
> is to go beyond them to the impossible.
> —*Arthur C. Clarke*

An anomalously high scorer on the HISS Transpersonal Experiences (TPE) indicators scale is likely to report frequent TPEs of both the verifiable psi (perception and influence) and unverifiable psi-related (manifestation of mind) varieties. Experiences of transpersonal perception and transpersonal influence, as anomalous abilities, have considerable inherent upside potential. Their downside lies in the potential for their misuse and for their being perceived by others as evidence of psychopathology. As for experiences of transpersonal manifestation of mind—with the possible exception of the spirit possession experience (which is almost universally perceived as being negative) and the Near-Death Experience

Transpersonal Abilities Often Accompany Non-Right-Handedness

(with its associated trauma)—it seems that their upsides and downsides are primarily a function of the experiencer's interpretation.

It is noteworthy that Claire, while reporting a high level of frequency in all three categories of Transpersonal Experiences (TPEs), also reported a low level of belief in the reality of TPEs in general. In our discussions, she gave the impression that she takes her experiences of transpersonal perception for granted. Despite indicating on the HISS that she often or regularly has experiences of déjà vu, synchronicity, telepathy, precognition, psychic dreams and clairvoyance/clairaudience/clairsentience, she had little to add, stating, "That's just the way things work for me." Similarly, she had little to say about her experiences of transpersonal influence. Despite having indicated that she frequently performed psychic healings, she said, "it's just little stuff, nothing especially grand or dramatic." Moreover, notwithstanding her telling me that she often influences light bulbs and electrical/electronic equipment, she indicated on the HISS that she experienced electrical PsychoKinesis only rarely. "That's not something I do," she said, "it's just something that happens when I'm around." She also reported that she experiences (non-electrical) PsychoKinesis only rarely.

Some of her experiences of transpersonal manifestation of mind, however, were sufficiently anomalous to get her attention. She told me:

> As I child and into my twenties, I was able to observe things from locations outside my body. From those locations, I could see both my body and other things elsewhere—things that were unobservable from the position of my body. It was like having a special kind of periscope. These experiences weren't necessarily related to stressful situations. They were more likely to be driven by curiosity than anything else.
>
> Also as a child, I frequently thought I was making myself invisible. I would just "go somewhere else" and, as long as I stayed there, I believed I couldn't be seen. I have no objective evidence of truly becoming invisible, but from my subjective point of view, that certainly seemed to be the case.
>
> Spirit guides were a regular part of my childhood. I usually encountered them in the woods—sometimes they were people, sometimes they were animals. When I was eighteen, a well-known psychic told me that I was very psychic and that I had spirit guides with me all the time. While I was somewhat surprised to hear that I was psychic, I wasn't the least bit surprised to hear about the spirit guides. They were just a part of my ordinary, everyday reality. In a way, that's still the case. It's hard to put into words, but there is a sense of people at a distance, or people who are no longer alive, or people who have yet to be born, being a part of my "perceptual field." It's always people, never anything like extra-terrestrials, ancient entities, or the other forms of spirit guides that are currently in vogue. There's no real sense of separateness from these spirit guides—there's more a sense of there being one big collective spirit that expresses through different people, different animals, or different imaginary companions. The nature of the communication, of that which is expressed, can vary. Sometimes it's insight, sometimes it's information, sometimes it's suggestions and sometimes it's a feeling of being supported.

173

There have also been times when I have experienced apparitions, or spirits that were distinctly separate from me—the most memorable being Emma Doyle.[†] Emma was the daughter of the man who originally built the house I lived in when I was a young mother. Shortly after moving into the house, I began seeing the figure of a woman near the fireplace. When I mentioned it to an elderly neighbor who had known the Doyles, she said, "Oh, yes, that's Emma. She always appears next to the fireplace." Also, the proprietress of my daughter's nursery school told me that the woman who lived there before me had likewise reported seeing the image of a woman near the fireplace.

A teen-aged boy, who was then living with us, said he saw the figure regularly. One day, when he was walking up the stairs, she appeared and he said, "Emma, I don't believe you're real"—then something tripped him. Also, my son, who was about five years old at the time, would sometimes reach out as if to take Emma by the hand and say, "let's go upstairs now."

THE TRANSPERSONAL REALM

In the taxonomy of Transpersonal Experiences (TPEs) developed in Chapter 1, eighteen of the most representative experiences were defined and grouped into three general categories. Table 1.1., which illustrated this categorical breakout, is reproduced, next page, as Table 11.1., to facilitate further discussion.

An orderly classification of this sort suggests clear boundaries and distinctions, both between the categories and between the individual experiences themselves—but those distinctions are mostly illusory. The reasons for this should become clear in what follows.

Early exploration into Transpersonal Experiences focused primarily on the possibility of post-mortem survival. The most common approach was that of utilizing experiences of mediumship to contact spirit guides. It didn't take long for investigators to recognize that such a method did not lend itself to replication using scientific methods and that most results could be explained as instances of telepathy.

This realization then led to studies, using scientific methods, that were designed to explore evidence for the existence of telepathy. Many of

_____

[†] Pseudonym

Experiences of Transpersonal Perception	Experiences of Transpersonal Influence	Experiences of Transpersonal Manifestation of Mind
Déjà Vu Synchronicity Telepathy Precognition Psychic Dream Clairvoyance	Psychic Healing Electrical PsychoKinesis PsychoKinesis	Contact With Spirit Guides Out-Of-Body Experience Past-Life Recall Apparition Mediumistic Episode UFO Sighting Near-Death Experience Spirit Possession Alien Contact

Table 11.1. Three Categories of Transpersonal Experiences.

those experiments involved the use of a specially designed deck of cards, from which a card was drawn at random by a telepathic sender, who would then attempt to transmit the image on the card to a telepathic receiver. It was soon determined that similar results could be obtained without the involvement of the telepathic sender, thus suggesting clairvoyance rather than telepathy as the operative mode of perception. No experimental design has yet been developed that will unequivocally differentiate pure telepathy from pure clairvoyance.

One tentative approach to making that differentiation involved the use of purely mental targets. The problem was that the target eventually had to become objectively known upon recording of the results of the trial. As soon as that happened, the possibility then arose of precognition being the operative mode of perception. No experimental design has yet been developed that will unequivocally differentiate pure clairvoyance from pure precognition.

Theoretically, it can be argued that in instances of pure clairvoyance, the boundaries of space become blurred, whereas in instances of pure precognition the boundaries of time become blurred. Practically, however, the differences between telepathy, real-time clairvoyance and precognition are purely semantic and have nothing to do with the fundamental properties of transpersonal perception. It was by way of acknowledging the artificiality of the distinctions that J. B. Rhine, of Duke University, coined the umbrella term "Extra-Sensory Perception (ESP)" to refer to instances of perception that are bounded by *neither* space *nor* time.

The primary difference between a telepathic/clairvoyant/ precognitive experience and a psychic dream experience is the prevailing State Of Consciousness (SOC) in which the respective experiences occur. The former presumably occurs in a prevailing waking SOC; the later presumably occurs in a prevailing dreaming SOC. Other than that, it appears that in both cases the experiences are characterized by the overlapping of waking and dreaming SOCs, with the accompanying occurrence of a slow, coherent pattern of brainwaves.

176   More than half of all reported spontaneous ESP experiences occur while the experiencer is in what is nominally a prevailing dreaming SOC, thus supporting claims that the likelihood of occurrence of TPEs is enhanced by a condition of quiet mind. A quiet mind can also be fostered by hypnosis, meditation, sensory deprivation and other similar techniques. The apparent paradox of Anomalously Sensitive Persons (ASPs) being especially facile at accessing quiet mind, while also being especially sensitive to all types of stressors, can be resolved by recognizing that ASPs have learned to enter Altered States of Consciousness (ASCs) as a way of coping with situations that might otherwise overwhelm them.

Another interesting point relative to experiences of ESP is this: Despite experiments (involving distance, shielding, etc.) having demonstrated that while ESP is not, itself, an Electro-Magnetic Radiation (EMR) event, a high level of activity in the Earth's field of EMR (e.g., solar, lunar, tectonic, thunderstorm activity) can interfere with ESP abilities. It appears, however, that such EMR activity tends to increase the frequency of occurrence of other Transpersonal Experiences (e.g., *spontaneous* PsychoKinesis, apparition, UFO sighting, alien contact). The precise neurological mechanisms involved are unclear, but it all apparently has something to do with "Electro-Magnetic Sensitivity (EMS)," which will be discussed shortly.

There is some difficulty in determining the appropriate taxonomic placement for synchronicity. Some people might claim that synchronicities are experiences of transpersonal influence rather than of transpersonal perception, but synchronicities are, by definition, apparently acausal and thus, at least semantically, seem to belong in the category of experiences of transpersonal perception. What appears to be most important about synchronicities is the experiencer's perception of the meaningfulness of the relationships among the events.

In thinking about the items in the category of experiences of transpersonal influence, it becomes apparent that both psychic healing and electrical PsychoKinesis can be considered to be subsets of "ordinary"

PsychoKinesis (PK)—it's all a matter of what it is that is being influenced. Technically, psychic healing involves the influencing of living objects, electrical PK involves the influencing of electrical or electronic non-living objects and ordinary PK involves the influencing of other non-living objects.

To date, most formal laboratory experiments dealing with PK have employed unstable random systems (dice, random number generators, etc.). There are anecdotal examples of what appear to be pure cases of PK involving stable objects that do not fluctuate spontaneously—the bending of spoons, or the moving of individual small objects, for example— but no systematically controlled replications by multiple investigators have yet been conducted. While PK experiences appear to involve an active intention, in contrast to the passive perception of ESP, it may be that the experiencer actually precognitively perceives the results of the event that s/he is supposedly influencing (i.e., simply selecting a favorable moment for interacting with the system through passive perception). Once again, no experimental design has yet been developed that will unequivocally differentiate pure precognition from pure PsychoKinesis. 177

As will be discussed shortly, the subset of electrical PK is especially relevant to this discussion because Electro-Magnetic Sensitivity (EMS) may be a key factor in *all* Transpersonal Experiences and also because ASPs appear to exhibit anomalously high levels of EMS. Of note for the moment is that electrical PK occurs considerably more frequently than does PK involving non-electrical objects—most likely because electrical and electronic equipment are inherently unstable systems.

The subset of psychic healing is another issue entirely because it involves living objects and, at least in the case of humans, the possibility for the occurrence of the placebo effect. It can, nevertheless, still be considered a subset of PsychoKinesis. Moreover, the qualifier "living" implies at least the possibility of awareness and, where awareness is involved, telepathy might also be involved. As has already been shown, however, telepathy might not be telepathy at all, but rather clairvoyance…and clairvoyance might not be clairvoyance at all, but rather precognition…and precognition ...Well, the point is that there is much more to be gained by exploring the similarities among psi experiences (ESP and PK collectively) than there is by emphasizing their differences.

Because psi experiences can be independently verified, over the years an immense amount of scientific evidence has been accumulated that affirms their legitimacy. The question no longer is one of whether or not there is adequate evidence of the existence of psi; it is now one of how to evaluate the abundance of evidence that is on hand. The authenticity of these experiences is so well established that many psi researchers no longer conduct experiments of the proof-oriented variety. Their focus has shifted to process-oriented experiments that are designed to determine what factors influence psi performance and how psi works.

Meta-analysis of data from a multitude of psi experiments shows that the odds against the observed results occurring by chance alone are generally greater than a million to one. Such odds don't actually *prove* the genuineness of psi, but they do make it clear that chance definitely can be ruled out as an explanation for whatever it is that is happening. Disagreements over what "it" is continue to exist, but there is no question that an interesting effect has been scientifically demonstrated beyond any reasonable doubt.

The story with respect to experiences of transpersonal manifestation of mind is somewhat different. Unlike psi experiences, these psi-related experiences cannot be independently verified. They do not lend themselves to laboratory research using standard scientific methods and they have been studied mostly on an anecdotal

> *There are no unnatural or supernatural phenomena, only very large gaps in our knowledge of what is natural, particularly regarding relatively rare occurrences.*
> *—Edgar Mitchell*

basis. They are, however, sufficiently "far out" that they make for great tales, provoke considerable controversy and sell lots of books.

From an experiential perspective, the most important difference between psi experiences and psi-related experiences is the different way in which mind *appears* to manifest in the two contexts. In psi experiences (experiences of transpersonal perception and transpersonal influence), it appears that there is only one mind (that of the experiencer) involved in the perceiving or the influencing. In psi-related experiences (experiences of transpersonal manifestation of mind), it appears that there are other minds involved as well.

As is implied by the meaning of the term "Transpersonal Experiences"—"...experiences that suggest the essential interconnectedness [and/or absolute unity] of all that ever was, is, or will be..."—the idea of "other" minds in the transpersonal realm is oxymoronic. From a theoretical perspective, the transpersonal concept renders the idea of "other" meaningless. A pure experience of the transpersonal realm, however, is dependent on the experiencer being in a pure state of Transpersonal Consciousness—and, as was stated in Chapter 10, Transpersonal Consciousness is, itself, only a theoretical construct and seldom (if ever) occurs in its pure form. Practically speaking, then, from the perspective of a specific experiencer's perception, appearances would lead to the belief that other minds are much more a part of experiences of transpersonal manifestation of mind than they are of experiences of transpersonal perception or experiences of transpersonal influence. Since the experiencer's perception is of utmost importance in understanding experiences (as opposed to phenomena), the ensuing discussion of experiences of transpersonal manifestation of mind will be framed in terms of the appearance of "otherness."

179

Simply put, appearances shape perceptions, perceptions shape thinking and the appearance of there being more than one mind involved shapes thinking about experiences of transpersonal manifestation of mind. That having been said, it can then be seen that the only substantive difference between psi experiences and psi-related experiences has to do with the consciousness status of that which is being perceived and/or influenced. Consider that:

- psi/psi-related experiences involve the appearance of the experiencer's mind being able to perceive and/or influence from a perspective that is bounded by neither space nor time;
- if there can be one experiencer, there can be other experiencers simultaneously having similar psi/psi-related experiences;
- if the one experiencer's mind can transpersonally perceive and/ or influence, so too can the other experiencers' minds;
- each of those *apparently* differentiated minds can perceive and/ or influence the others; and thus
- in a state of Transpersonal Consciousness, mind not only can perceive and/or influence transpersonally, it can also be perceived and/or be influenced transpersonally.

From this perspective, then, those minds that are perceived and/ or influenced by an experiencer in a nominal state of Transpersonal Consciousness assume the same reality status as the mind of the experiencer. What this implies is that ghosts, apparitions, poltergeists, spirits, demons and the like—often collectively referred to as "entities"—are other minds that also happen to be functioning in a state of TPC. Whether or not those minds are human minds is quite irrelevant. What is important is

It is an absurd prejudice to suppose
that existence can only be physical.
As a matter of fact, the only form of existence
of which we have immediate knowledge
is psychic [i.e., in the mind].
We might as well say, on the contrary,
that physical evidence is mere inference,
since we know of matter only in so far as we perceive
psychic images mediated by the senses.

—Carl Jung

that the experiencer's mind perceives another mind and assigns to the appearance of that other mind a subjective interpretation, which then becomes a linguistic label serving to separate and differentiate that specific Transpersonal Experience from other possible TPEs. An experience of this sort is classified as a psi-related experience of transpersonal manifestation of mind, rather than as a psi experience of transpersonal perception, specifically because it appears to involve entities (that is, other minds). Because such entities are generally considered to be purely subjective constructs of the experiencer's individual mind and because, as such, they are said to be not a part of consensus reality, such experiences are held to be unverifiable.

Different types of entities are perceived in different ways. Apparitions are generally perceived through the visual sensory modality; spirit guides are generally perceived through the auditory sensory modality; poltergeists are generally perceived through the ...well, poltergeists ("noisy ghosts") are a special case. Poltergeists *do* things—they make noise, they move objects, they generally wreak havoc. Poltergeist experiences have a lot in common with PsychoKinesis experiences (experiences of transpersonal influence)—spontaneous and unwitting PK, admittedly, but PK, nonetheless. This explanation is so commonly accepted by researchers that the poltergeist experience is often referred to as "Recurring Spontaneous PsychoKinesis (RSPK)." Poltergeist activity has been found to be associated with individuals—primarily adolescent females—who are experiencing significant stress. The poltergeist experience thoroughly confounds the categories of Transpersonal Experiences (it wasn't even included in the taxonomy). It also is centered on two key elements that relate to anomalous sensitivities—femaleness and stress.

The entities involved in mediumistic experiences seem to be much more closely associated with the experiencer's mind than are the entities involved in apparitional experiences. Great trance mediums have much in common with great artists. Just as many of art's finest masters have a seemingly differentiated "creative self" to whom they attribute their abilities, so too do mediums have a seemingly differentiated "knower" to whom they ascribe their talents. In both cases, sensitivity to Altered States of Consciousness (involving either dissociation, association, or both) appears to be operative. In the context of highly hypnotizable individuals, Ernest Hilgard called this second self the "Hidden Observer;" in the context of Multiple Personality Disorder patients, Ralph Allison called it the "Inner Self Helper." According to Allison, this second self is characterized by:

181

- having no identifiable time or purpose of origin;
- being all-knowing and capable of predicting the future;
- being pure intellect yet still projecting love and acceptance;
- being genderless;
- affirming the existence of reincarnation, of God and sometimes of the devil; and
- being able to communicate with entities beyond conventional physical boundaries.

The definitions of "mediumistic episode" ("...a 'spirit' using the voice...or hand...of the experiencer...") and "spirit possession" ("...another mind...attempting to take [or having taken]...over control of the experiencer's body or will") are quite similar.[†] A mediumistic episode is generally voluntary and short-lived, whereas a spirit possession experience is neither—but both experiences (as well as most other experiences of transpersonal manifestation of mind) involve the experiencer's mind interacting transpersonally with other minds. The theoretical distinction between possession and other experiences of transpersonal manifestation of mind might be framed this way: If an other mind appears to have been incorporated within the apparent boundaries of the mind of the experiencer, that qualifies as possession; if it hasn't, then it doesn't. That distinction, however, is mostly semantic and the notion of possession is key to any

---

[†] There are those who would argue that the experiences are very different— that mediumistic entities are non-invasive (and therefore "good") and that possessing entities are invasive (and therefore "bad"). While such may be the case, an individual in a state of Transpersonal Consciousness by definition loses the ability to differentiate and is therefore extremely vulnerable to disruptive psychological influences. Moreover, possessing entities are infamous for their disingenuousness. Anna Wickland, one of the all-time great trance mediums, spent the later years of her life in a mental institution.

thinking about experiences of transpersonal manifestation of mind because of its implications vis-à-vis personal boundaries, free will and such.

Allison, in his cutting-edge Multiple Personality Disorder work during the 1970s, took the position that the concept of possession had considerable theoretical and therapeutic utility. As a result, he was driven out of the profession by his colleagues. In *Minds in Many Pieces,* he identified five grades of possession:

- Grade I Possession—can be thought of in purely psychiatric terms as obsessive-compulsive neurosis. In this type of possession, the individual is controlled or dominated by such things as obsessions, compulsions, ideas, involuntary acts, or addictions.
- Grade II Possession—is caused by a negative alter personality in individuals with Multiple Personality Disorder. In many cultures, this alter personality would be viewed as a classic example of an evil spirit that has breached the boundaries of the individual's psyche. Deep hypnosis, however, is able to reveal the psychosocial roots and mental splitting involved in such cases.
- Grade III Possession—occurs when the controlling influence is the mind of another human being who is currently living. Witchcraft and voodoo are examples of this type of possession. Under certain psychosocial conditions, hex death can result.
- Grade IV Possession—is control by the mind of another human being who is currently deceased.
- Grade V Possession—is control by a mind that has never had a physically embodied life of its own and identifies itself as an agent of evil. Cases of this sort represent the classical form of demonic possession.

Adam Crabtree, in *Multiple Man,* offers another set of useful distinctions relative to possession. Possessing entities, he says, may be either personal or non-personal; they also may be either human or non-human. Personal entities are those that have an existence in their own right and are not the product of anyone or anything else. Because they have a spirit core, they have free will and are able to initiate actions. Personal and human entities that have possessing potential may be either living or dead (depending on whether or not they still have an extant physical body). Personal and non-human entities that have possessing potential include not only demons, devils and Satan himself, but gods, muses and spirit guides. Non-personal entities are those that are created either by intelligent beings or by nature itself. Such entities may appear to behave intelligently, but they do not have independently existing minds—they are the product of concentrated thought and their strength and lasting power depends completely on the energy being focused on them by their creator(s). Such entities are sometimes called "thought-forms."

> *From ghoulies and ghosties*
> *and long-leggety beasties,*
> *And things that go bump in the night;*
> *Good Lord, deliver us!*
> —*Cornish prayer*

183

There are some experiences in which the mind appears to separate itself completely (or almost completely) from the brain—the "conventional" death experience, the Near-Death Experience and the Out-Of-Body Experience, for example. While none of these experiences necessarily involves the manifestation of an other mind, they often do.

After-the-fact reports on the characteristics of the conventional death experience are hard to come by, but the recollection of a death in a previous lifetime offers the opportunity for some insight. If the past-life recall experience is truly the recollection of a former life (and death)—one that was specific and exclusive to the experiencer—then other minds need not necessarily be involved (except, perhaps, in supporting roles). Such an explanation implies the veridicality of reincarnation and can thus account for many of the phenomena (birthmarks, memories, unusual behaviors, phobias and exceptional abilities) associated with past-life recall. Absent other minds, however, such an experience could be accounted for by retrocognition (the temporal mirror image of precognition) and would thus be an experience of transpersonal perception rather than of transpersonal manifestation of mind.

There is, on the other hand, an alternative explanation—one that implies that the terms "past-life" and "recall" are being used erroneously. Perhaps, rather than recalling one's own past life, the experiencer is transpersonally perceiving a very real life of a very real (other) person that occurred during a time frame that, by convention, is said to be "in the past." As an experience that clearly involves an other mind, it would appropriately be categorized as an experience of transpersonal manifestation of mind and the question of reincarnation would then be rendered moot.

Similarly Out-Of-Body Experiences and Near-Death Experiences do not necessarily involve the manifestation of other minds. They can and frequently do, but they don't have to. When they do not, such experiences can be accounted for by clairvoyance (again, an experience of transpersonal perception rather than of transpersonal manifestation of mind)—even though that which is perceived clairvoyantly may have little in common with consensus reality.

Experiences of "aliens," "grays," "space brothers," "extraterrestrials," "UFOnauts"—and their mode of transportation, "Unidentified Flying Objects"—probably generate more controversy than do all the other Transpersonal Experiences combined. Most likely that's because so many people argue that these *subjective experiences* qualify as *objective phenomena.* In keeping with the standard approach throughout this book, however, the ensuing discussion of Unidentified Flying Object Experiences (UFOEs) is experientially rather than phenomenologically based.[†]

184

From the perspective of experiences of transpersonal manifestation of mind, it can be argued that a UFOE is an experience in which the mind of the experiencer transpersonally perceives another mind (not necessarily Earth-based or human)—and that something about the appearance of that other mind causes the experiencer to ascribe to it the interpretation of "UFO" (whether vehicle, or occupant, or both). In other words, "UFOs" need not be saucer-shaped (indeed, many reports suggest otherwise) structured craft of extraterrestrial

> *UFOs ARE REAL*
> *THE U.S. AIR FORCE IS*
> *A PRODUCT OF MASS HYSTERIA.*
> *—Bumper Sticker*

origin—they may simply be a conditioned perception that arises out of cultural suggestion. Further illustrating the ways in which the supposedly discrete TPEs overlap one another are findings of UFOs (specifically their occupants) functioning as possessing entities. William Baldwin, in *CE-VI: Close Encounters of the Possession Kind,* describes numerous clinical cases in which possessing entities were found to be alien or extraterrestrial in nature.

Also meriting consideration relative to the UFO experience are the following points:

[†] For the sake of verbal economy, experiences of UFO sightings and experiences of alien contact will be collectively spoken of as "Unidentified Flying Object Experiences (UFOEs)," the people who have such experiences will be spoken of as "UFOEers," and that which is experienced— both the vehicle and its occupants— will be spoken of as "UFOs."

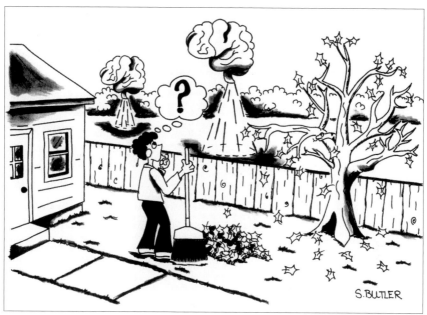

Another Way of Looking at UFOs.

- UFOEers frequently report that they begin to have the full spectrum of Transpersonal Experiences following their UFO experience;
- UFOEs have many marked similarities to OOBEs (Out-Of-Body-Experiences) and NDEs (Near-Death-Experiences);
- Many reports of UFOEs and NDEs indicate that both frequently involve significant electrical, magnetic and light radiation components, thus suggesting that Electro-Magnetic Sensitivity may play an important role in such experiences;
- In a study of the "vanishing twin phenomenon" (the disappearance of one of a set of twins while in utero—said to be associated with UFOEs), 12 out of 100 surviving twins were determined by CAT scan/MRI to have double pineal glands (the pineal gland, as discussed in Chapter 4, has an important biochemical role in anomalous sensitivities); and
- Various studies of UFOEers have shown that, as a group, they have many of the same traits that characterize Anomalously Sensitive Persons (ASPs)—sleep disorders, vivid and frequent dream recall, amnesia and hypermnesia, creativity, active imaginations, tertiary process cognitive style, iNtuitive perception abilities, emotional acuity, a high level of hypnotizability and a history of childhood abuse, among them.

The preceding material is intended to bring to light the similarities among the supposedly differentiated Transpersonal Experiences and to suggest that *all* TPEs (both psi and psi-related) should perhaps be considered to be different facets of a single meta-experience. It's not that some people are especially sensitive to ESP experiences, others to PK experiences and others to mediumship experiences, UFO experiences, or past-life experiences; it's that some people are especially sensitive to the entire spectrum of Transpersonal Experiences—and those are the people being identified here as Anomalously Sensitive Persons (ASPs).

186

The primary point here is that all TPEs are equal—but the HISS data does reveal that some TPEs are "more equal" than others. By that I mean that if an individual reported having one or more of certain "major" TPEs—specifically the PsychoKinesis, mediumship, alien contact, spirit possession, or Near-Death Experiences—s/he almost assuredly reported having most other TPEs as well. Conversely, if an individual reported having certain "minor" TPEs—specifically

> *All knowledge of reality*
> *starts from experience,*
> *and ends in it.*
> *—Albert Einstein*

the telepathy or synchronicity experiences (both of which are relatively commonplace)—s/he was considerably less likely to report having other Transpersonal Experiences. The remaining eleven TPEs fall somewhere in between the major ones and the minor ones with respect to their relative importance.[†] In the HISS data, notwithstanding this use of "major" and "minor" terminology, correlations among frequencies of occurrence for *all* of the individual TPEs are quite robust.

In Chapter 10, two very important questions were raised. Those questions were:

- Might there be as many different realities as there are different States of Consciousness?
- Might "reality" be nothing more than a different label for "State of Consciousness?"

Given that Transpersonal Experiences appear to be markers for alternate realities and given that TPEs appear to arise out of Altered States of Consciousness, indications are that those questions can now

---

[†] See Chapter 14, "The Findings," for the statistical methodology used in making these determinations.

be appropriately answered in the affirmative. What remains is to take a look at some of the possible explanations for the connections between those Altered States of Consciousness and those alternate realities.

ELECTRO-MAGNETIC RADIATION

Patterns of electrical, magnetic and light radiation are a normal part of nature. Anywhere on Earth, these patterns are continuously changing and all living creatures, including humans, are subject to the effects of those changes. The day/night and seasonally changing patterns of light radiation are quite obvious and the effects of light, by way of the pineal gland, on the limbic system's hypothalamus, as well as light's modulation of the biological clock, are well known (see Chapter 4). The focus in the ensuing discussion will be on the effects of electrical and magnetic fields.[†]

187

The changes in the radiation patterns of the electric and magnetic fields surrounding the Earth are quite subtle. It has been known for some time that the hypothalamus is extremely sensitive to electrical fields and recent research has revealed a similar sensitivity to magnetic fields (thought to be caused by deposits of magnetite located near the pineal and pituitary glands). The mechanisms by which such sensitivities operate are not well understood.

Most humans have adapted smoothly to the changing patterns of natural Electro-Magnetic Radiation (EMR), but those who are especially sensitive to EMR—people who are Electro-Magnetically Sensitive (EMS)—often experience significant reactions to such changes. The natural EMR changes to which an EMS individual might be unusually reactive include such things as seasonal variations, solar storms, phases of the moon, approaching thunderstorms and Santa Ana type winds. Illustratively, studies have shown that the number of people signed into psychiatric wards with diagnoses of Schizophrenia and Bipolar Disorder, increases markedly shortly after major disturbances in the Earth's magnetic field.

In recent years, the possible effects of man-made EMR on humans have become a highly controversial subject. Reputations, positions, fortunes and progress are all at stake. While most researchers would agree that direct electrical stimulation of the brain can lead to anomalous neuronal activity, anomalous perceptions and anomalous behaviors, it is over the

---

[†] Early HISS data revealed that sensitivities to electrical, magnetic and light radiation were strongly correlated with each other, but that sensitivity to light radiation was less useful than were the others in predicting ASPness. Indications were that this was a result of sensitivity to light radiation being considerably more commonplace than were sensitivities to the others. In the version of the HISS used for this study, no direct inquiries were made about sensitivity to light radiation.

issue of indirect or subtle stimulation and the possible link to immune system dysfunctions, that most of the conflicts arise. Those who debunk Electro-Magnetic Sensitivity point out that the vast majority of people *apparently* are not affected by exposure to man-made EMR and suggest that those who claim to experience problems are hypochondriacs, alarmists, or attention seekers. Studies have shown, however, that regular exposure to man-made EMR is associated with an increased incidence of hormone dependent cancers, allergies, mood disorders and suicide. Moreover, other studies have shown that in a setting of partial sensory deprivation, indirect exposure to EMR commonly results in dizziness, "pins and needles," psychological dissociation, the sense of a presence and psi/psi-related experiences

188

Norman Shealey, the founder of the American Holistic Medical Association, speaks of the condition that can result from chronic exposure to man-made EMR as "Electro-Magnetic Dysthymia (EMD)." EMD, he states, is characterized by adrenal exhaustion as well as liver and heart muscle dysfunction. Its symptoms include:

- chronic fatigue;
- disrupted immune system functioning;
- depression;
- biochemical deficiencies—including DHEA, intracellular magnesium and essential amino acids; and
- EEG brainwave pattern abnormalities—including, in extreme cases, all the symptomatology of Temporal Lobe Epilepsy (TLE).

There are a number of other points about Electro-Magnetic Sensitivity (EMS) that are especially relevant to ASPness, including:

- EMS is associated with a history of medical trauma.
- The illnesses associated with chronic EMR exposure do not involve a specific pathogen, but rather are characterized by a generalized disruption of immune system functioning. The negative consequences of such exposure are, therefore, likely to be very subtle and elusive.
- Having experienced a major electrical event (such as being rendered unconscious by electrical shock) apparently is associated with an individual being Electro-Magnetically Sensitive.
- Some people with EMS are purported to be "electrical disrupters," that is, their presence appears to interfere with the operation of

electrical and electronic equipment. This phenomenon (a spontaneous form of electrical PsychoKinesis) is not well understood, but it has been suggested that, by some unknown mechanism, such people generate within their bodies brief charges of high voltage electricity that have significant disruptive potential.

- Many symptoms of EMS are identical to symptoms related to low melatonin levels (discussed in Chapter 4)—thus suggesting both a pineal/endocrine/immune system connection and a pineal/hypothalamus/limbic system connection in the etiology of EMS.

189

- Women are considerably more likely than men to report EMS symptoms. This would follow naturally from their having a greater degree of interconnectedness (by way of a larger corpus callosum and other pathways), than do men, between the different parts of the brain.

- The mechanism by which EMS operates appears to be this: Chronic EMR exposure leads to entrainment of neuronal discharges, entrainment of neuronal discharges leads to neuronal hypersynchrony (neuronal connections that operate faster and with greater sensitivity than the norm) and neuronal hypersynchrony results in a heightened sensitivity to a wide variety of stressors.

Some authors claim that certain TPEs—notably the Near-Death Experience and the alien contact experience—are, in and of themselves, electro-magnetic *phenomena* and that, as such, they can *cause* an individual to become Electro-Magnetically Sensitive. There is, however, no evidence in the HISS data to support this contention (see Chapter 14 for further discussion).

Other authors explain away TPEs as nothing more than idiosyncratic symptoms of EMS. Their arguments appear to be grounded in the presupposition that Transpersonal Experiences are not "really real," and must therefore simply be hallucinations resulting from anomalous neurological activity. What is overlooked in such reasoning is that *all* experiences arise out of neurological activity and the fact that some experiences arise out of *anomalous* (i.e., other than secondary process cognition) neurological activity does not necessarily render those experiences invalid. In other words, the mechanism by which an individual is able to have *any* conscious experience—whether transpersonal or otherwise—is that of electrical and chemical activity occurring in the neurons and synapses of the brain. Thus, while "normal" experiences arise out of "normal" neurological activity, "anomalous" experiences (TPEs) arise out of "anomalous" (perhaps engendered by fields of Electro-Magnetic Radiation) neurological activity (which results in Altered States of Consciousness)—and the term "anomalous" addresses issues of commonness, not issues of veridicality.

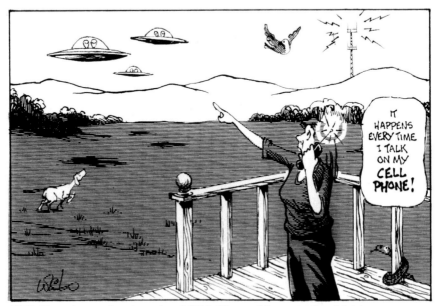

UFO Experiences Are Associated With Electro-Magnetic Sensitivities

Claire's report of her own EMS experiences proves to be an excellent vehicle for getting a better sense of what Electro-Magnetic Sensitivity is all about:

> Thunderstorms...I get really frightened during thunderstorms, but *before* the storm breaks, I experience heightened awareness and feel very alive and alert. All external stimuli, especially colors and sounds, are extremely vivid. Once a thunderstorm starts, however, I find both the thunder and lightning to be very unnerving.
>
> My response to moving water is very similar to what happens *before* a thunderstorm. Everything is vivid; I'm hyper-alert. It's a very positive experience—especially since it's not followed by thunder and lightning. I really like waterfalls, bubbling brooks and ocean waves.

I hate fluorescent lights! When I'm around them, I go a bit nuts. I get headaches, I become very tired, I have bad moods, I experience trouble concentrating, ...and my stockings run—really, my stockings run.

I don't have a problem with incandescent lights, but they apparently have a problem with me. Light bulbs seem to last for me about one-tenth as long as they last for other people. The situation is improved now, but in the past I was constantly changing light bulbs. I could walk into a room, wouldn't touch a thing and a light bulb would blow. Also, the lights in a room could be off, I'd walk in and one or more of them would turn on without my doing anything.

Power lines—the big transmission lines—I stay away from them. I go out of my way to avoid them. I don't like them! And those boxes in a cage, those transformers or whatever they are...when I'm driving by one, I get tingling sensations, unusual metallic tastes and strong feelings of anxiety.

Electrical and electronic machines tend to malfunction in my presence...except for those times when I seem somehow to fix them. A man who tried to repair my broken VCR said he couldn't understand how it got so messed up inside, just by my pushing the buttons. I've also inadvertently destroyed cell phones, radios, televisions and computers.

But it works both ways. I can fix things as well as break them. When I worked in an office, it was sort of a joke—if a machine wasn't working, somebody would come get me, I'd go look at it and it would start working again. Given that I don't understand anything about machines, that's pretty funny.

My computer used to crash all the time—then I reached some kind of agreement with it. Now it works fine. The difference between my breaking things and my fixing things seems to be a matter of intentionality. I don't mess things up intentionally—that happens spontaneously—but to get things not to break, or to get things that are broken to work again, I have to concentrate on positive intentions.

EPILEPSY AND KUNDALINI

Exposure to Electro-Magnetic Radiation can, in EMS individuals, lead to all of the symptomatology of Temporal Lobe Epilepsy (TLE). Michael Persinger appropriately suggests that Temporal Lobe Epilepsy be spoken of as "Temporo-Limbic Epilepsy (TLE)" because it involves the limbic system as well as the temporal lobes of the brain.

The components of the limbic system are extremely sensitive to stressors—and neuronal hypersynchrony in the limbic system, in addition to being stimulated by Electro-Magnetic Radiation, can also be stimulated by a number of other factors such as hyperventilation, sleep deprivation, physiological imbalances, simple sensory overload, trauma, drugs and toxins. Repeated exposure to stressors can lead to alterations of limbic system structuring such that the threshold for TLE is progressively lowered (a process known as "kindling") and sensitivity extends to ever more subtle stimuli.

In full-blown Temporo-Limbic Epilepsy (often called "complex partial seizures," "psychic seizures," or "psychomotor epilepsy"), the actual seizures are spoken of as the "ictal" stage and the period between seizures is spoken of as the "interictal" stage. The ictal stage is often, but not always, characterized by slow (theta) temporal lobe EEG brainwave patterns. In the seizures of TLE, there are no convulsions of the sort exhibited in classical grand mal seizures. The symptoms, which are more subtle, can be grouped into six categories:

- hallucinatory symptoms—visions, sounds (including voices), tastes, smells;
- emotional symptoms—depression, euphoria, anger, anxiety;
- physical symptoms—heartbeat irregularities, breathing difficulties, dizziness, flushing, vomiting;
- motor symptoms—tremors, twitching, transient paralysis, lip smacking, staring;
- sensory symptoms—pain (or insensitivity to pain), "pins and needles," "bugs crawling" under the skin, sensation of a limb having been lost; and
- experiential symptoms—dreaminess or trance, flashbacks, automatisms, memory distortions, time distortions, sense of a presence and psychological dissociation.

The interictal symptoms are even more subtle and appear as part of the individual's ongoing personality. Norman Geschwind identified five

192

especially salient traits (after his death in 1984, they have been spoken of collectively as the "Geschwind Syndrome") as: hypergraphia (excessive writing or drawing), hyperreligiosity, "stickiness" (hypersociability), aggression and altered sexuality (hypo-, hyper-, or non-traditional). Later work by Bear and Fedio added 13 more traits to the list: elation, sadness, anger, guilt, emotionality, hypermoralism, obsessionalism, "circumstantiality" (loquacious, pedantic, overly detailed), "viscosity" (tendency to repetition), sense of personal meaning and destiny, dependence, humorlessness and paranoia. Of the total of 18 traits, a group of six—obsessionalism, circumstantiality, hyperreligiosity (or hyperphilosophicality), anger, emotionality and sadness—is said to provide a solid basis for identifying people likely to be prone to TLE.

Some people, it turns out, while exhibiting many of the interictal symptoms, never develop the full-blown ictal symptoms and therefore cannot be appropriately diagnosed as having TLE. In other words, while not experiencing seizures, they nevertheless have neuronal hypersynchrony in the temporal lobes and limbic system of the brain. Such neuronal hypersynchrony is associated with emotionality, vivid imagery and memory, a proneness to hypnotic susceptibility and psychological dissociation, unusual beliefs and a history of psi/psi-related experiences.

While the literature in the field of transpersonal psychology argues for a childhood sexual abuse/psychological dissociation/Transpersonal Experiences connection, the literature in the field of neurology suggests a childhood sexual abuse/Temporo-Limbic Epilepsy connection. Consider, for example, a 1993 study by Teicher, et. al. using a paper-and-pencil test instrument entitled the "Limbic System Checklist (LSCL-33)." High scores on this instrument were likely to be accompanied by EEG-confirmed temporo-limbic abnormalities. As compared to those subjects who reported no childhood abuse, scores for those who reported sexual abuse, but not physical abuse, were 49% higher; scores for those who reported physical abuse, but not sexual abuse, were 38% higher; scores for those who reported both sexual and physical abuse were 113% higher. Of those who were either sexually abused or physically abused, but not both, abuse before age 18 had a greater effect than abuse at a later age; for those who were both sexually and physically abused, the age at which the first abuse occurred apparently made no difference. Another referenced study demonstrated that, of 22 patients who had been involved as the child (or younger member) in an incestuous relationship, 77% had EEG abnormalities and 36% had full-blown clinical seizures.

The way in which the brain responds to childhood abuse and other stressors need not be held as an either/or ("Temporo-Limbic Epilepsy"/"Dissociative Disorder") diagnostic conflict. Many of the symptoms associated with the two different labels are quite similar. People with TLE frequently report episodes of disorientation, amnesia and behavioral/emotional changes (all characteristic of dissociation); people with Dissociative Disorders are often found to have EEG abnormalities and increased incidence of TLE and other seizure disorders. In the absence of *proven* brain damage (the presence of slow brainwaves in the temporal lobes does not constitute proof), it may be that the differences between some Temporo-Limbic Epilepsies and some Dissociative Disorders are mostly semantic. With respect to a certain set of symptoms, neurologists will tend to use the former term and psychiatrists will be inclined to use the latter.

Further complications with respect to diagnostic specificity arise when it is recognized that considerable similarity exists between those symptoms diagnosed as Temporo-Limbic Epilepsy and those diagnosed as Bipolar Disorder. Both are cyclical in nature, both involve significant mood swings and Altered States of Consciousness and both can manifest with a variety of psychotic, neurotic and physiologic symptoms. Absent definitive proof of brain damage, the most marked difference lies in the rapidity of cycling. Bipolar cycling generally occurs over a period of months, or occasionally years; Temporo-Limbic Epilepsy cycling generally occurs over a period of hours, days, or occasionally weeks. When the specifier "With Rapid Cycling" is added on to the *DSM-IV* "Bipolar Disorder" diagnosis, however, this distinction is effectively eliminated. Many patients diagnosed as having "Bipolar Disorder With Rapid Cycling," while not responding to lithium (the drug of choice for treating Bipolar Disorder), do respond to Tegretol (the drug of choice for treating TLE).

Finally, to completely confound the issue, there is another interpretation of these symptoms that has nothing whatsoever to do with the diagnostic labels of psychopathology or neuropathology. It is that of "kundalini arousal." Kundalini, in the Hindu tradition, is said to be a subtle form of bioenergy lying dormant, coiled up like a sleeping serpent, at the base of the spine. When the energy of kundalini is aroused, it moves upward along the spine, in a special channel and activates certain energy centers (called "chakras") along the way. The arousal of kundalini is purported to have the potential for transforming the central nervous system in such a way as to lead to genius, creativity, higher states of consciousness, psi/psi-related experiences, mystical experiences and spiritual enlightenment.

194

The path, however, is often a difficult and dangerous one. Explosive and destabilizing energy transformations can occur and these are experienced both physiologically and psychologically. Symptoms said to be associated with kundalini arousal include:

- intense involuntary body movements—shaking, vibrating, jerking and twitching;
- involuntary yogic phenomena—body postures, hand movements, mental images, chants, words and tones;
- physiological problems—activation of latent illnesses, immune and autoimmune disorders, apparent heart problems, gastrointestinal problems and intense pains (especially in the head and along the spine);
- psychological/emotional turbulence—intensification of unresolved issues, fear of insanity or death, extreme mood swings involving anxiety, anger, guilt and depression or, conversely, compassion, empathy and unconditional love;
- non-sensory perceptions—visual perceptions (lights, symbols, visions, entities), auditory perceptions (tones, music, voices), kinesthetic perceptions (electricity, tingling, rushes of energy), olfactory perceptions (perfume, incense) and gustatory perceptions;
- psi experiences—ESP, PK and synchronicities; and
- mystical experiences—states of unity, peace, love, joy, light and energy.

195

The symptoms associated with kundalini arousal are almost identical to the seizure symptoms of classical TLE—hallucinatory symptoms, emotional symptoms, physical symptoms, motor symptoms, sensory symptoms and experiential symptoms. It is noteworthy that the symptoms of both TLE and kundalini arousal cover the entire spectrum of sensitivities—Physiological, Cognitive, Emotional, Altered States of Consciousness and Transpersonal Experiences— explored in the HISS. Also noteworthy is that most of those symptoms can be elicited through the use of classical hypnosis techniques. The central operative factor in both, it appears, is Altered States of Consciousness characterized by slow, coherent cortical brainwaves (especially in the temporal lobes) and an anomalously high level of limbic system involvement in cognitive processes. The endless arguments over whether such symptoms should be pathologized as

Temporo-Limbic Epilepsy or extolled as kundalini arousal definitely appear to be counter-productive. If TPEs are going to be understood, it will be through an ongoing, open-minded observation of the processes involved, not through the application of labels that inhibit further questioning.

By this point in the discussion, it should be quite clear that the argument being developed here centers on neurophysiological differences playing a major role in the occurrence of Transpersonal Experiences. Simply stated, the process involved seems to be this: Anomalous neurological structuring (a brain that is Less Strongly Lateralized than the norm) permits anomalous neurological functioning (Altered States of Consciousness including Transpersonal Consciousness) which, in turn, permits the occurrence of anomalous (Transpersonal) Experiences. It is during the occurrence of Transpersonal Experiences that the mind appears to be least brain-like and most spirit-like or soul-like in its manifestation.

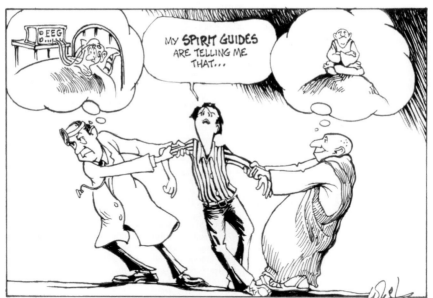

The Symptoms of "Temporo-Limbic Epilepsy" and "Kundalini Arousal" Can Be Virtually Indistinguishable

In thinking about the Less Strongly Lateralized brain and the *appearance* of the mind, it is noteworthy that, over the years, different thinkers have posited the "seat of the soul" as being located in the right temporal lobe (sometimes specifically the right Sylvian fissure), or in the pineal gland, or in the thalamus, or in the hypothalamus (the latter having been called "the man in the machine"). The ACL/LSL/ASC/TPE/ASP connections explicated in Chapters 4 through 11 should now be making themselves clear.

There is yet another link to the Eastern traditions and it has to do with what is spoken of as the "third eye," the organ of spiritual vision. According to this tradition, spiritual (transpersonal) vision, which used to be readily accessible to humans, has been temporarily (for eons) lost due to an evolutionarily necessary descent into matter, but it will be regained at some time in the future. The hypothesized location of this third eye appears to correspond precisely to the anatomical location of the pineal gland— and the pineal gland (as was discussed in Chapter 4 and elsewhere) plays a central role in the LSL brain's creating the conditions necessary for the emergence of Transpersonal Consciousness and the occurrence of Transpersonal Experiences. Research by the Russians has shown that the pineal gland is relatively larger in children than it is in adults and more developed in women than it is in men—and children and women appear to be more sensitive to TPEs than do men.

197

We have looked at the "what" of Transpersonal Experiences— Altered States of Consciousness, specifically Transpersonal Consciousness. We have also looked at the "why" of Transpersonal Experiences—the unconscious mind's enlisting of the limbic system in support of its search for information of a new and different sort. Now it is time to turn our attention to the "how" of Transpersonal Experiences. Insight will be offered from both a philosophical ("imaginal realm") and a scientific ("quantum realm") perspective.

The Imaginal Realm

As has been previously stated, it is commonly assumed that there are only two ways of looking at the possible veridicality of Transpersonal Experiences: Either they are "really real," or they are the product of fantasy, delusion, hallucination, or hoax. Such thinking may appeal to common sense, but it is simplistic, reductionistic and probably wrong—there's a lot of unexplored territory between the two extremes.

> *Common sense is the collection of prejudices acquired by age eighteen.*
> *—Albert Einstein*

Polarized thinking of this sort is the result of contemporary Western scientific thought still being dominated by Cartesian dualism. The postulate that something is either mind or it is matter, is a legacy from the French philosopher René Descartes, best known for his statement *"Cogito ergo sum"* ("I think, therefore I am").

There is another option that allows one to move beyond this seemingly all-encompassing, dichotomous approach to TPEs. It is the concept of the "imaginal realm." Note the use of the word "imaginal" as opposed to the word "imaginary." This distinction, introduced in 1972 by the French Islamic scholar Henry Corbin, is crucial. The word "imaginary," as it is generally used today is equated with the unreal, with something that is outside the framework of being and existing. In the case of things "imaginal," however, the allusion is not to the stuff of fantasy, but to imagination as a creative power, as an organ of perception in its own right. This concept merits some explanation.

> *René Descartes*
> *was sitting in a sidewalk cafe in Paris.*
> *The waitress asked*
> *if he would like more tea.*
> *"I think not," he responded*
> *and promptly disappeared.*
> —*Anonymous*

198

Most people would agree that there is a physical realm that we infer on the basis of ordinary sensory data interpreted by our brain. Likewise, most would agree that there is a realm composed exclusively of "mind stuff"—fantasies, dreams, fabrications and inventions—and that it has no substance beyond that of its being in the mind of its creator. Corbin argued for the existence of a third realm, the imaginal realm, access to which is dependent neither on ordinary sensory perception nor on ordinary cognition (including fantasy), but on the experiencer's being in an Altered State of Consciousness—one that destabilizes the ordinary perceptual modalities and cognitive systems.

The most important characteristic of the imaginal realm is that it is ontologically real—it has form, it has dimension, it has color, it has objects (both inanimate and animate). In short, it has equivalents for everything that exists in the world of the ordinary senses. Its features, however, cannot be perceived by the ordinary senses as if they were properties of physical bodies—they can be perceived only by the psycho-spiritual (or mind) senses. While the imaginal realm might be thought of as the cumulative product of human imaginative thought, it is also something that is objectively self-existent. Corbin asserted that, despite the imaginal realm's having no location in either time or space (and thus being an alternate reality), "its reality is more irrefutable and more coherent than that of the empirical world where reality is perceived by the senses." Experiences of the imaginal realm are, in some respects, doubly real, because they combine the substance of objectivity with the impact of immediate experience.

The imaginal realm is an intermediate realm—a realm that exists, conceptually, somewhere between what is called "mind" and what is called "matter." As such, it may be regarded as the source of events that simultaneously seem to belong both to an alternate reality and to consensus reality. These imaginal realm experiences, which are undifferentiable from Transpersonal Experiences (TPEs), can involve the manipulation of physical reality (e.g., movement of objects), defiance of the laws of science (e.g., nullification of the effects of gravity) and the generation of dynamic resonances within the human psyche (psi/psi-related experiences). While such experiences can show up in the conventional space/time continuum (something fantasies cannot do), their origins are in the imaginal, not in the physical, realm—and their medium of expression is the human mind. Such physical manifestations wreak havoc with conventional categories of existence. Since the appropriate framework and terminology for this third realm are lacking (the experiences are non-temporal and non-spatial, while ordinary language is structured in terms of temporal and spatial concepts), there is a natural tendency to attempt to assimilate imaginal realm experiences (TPEs) into conceptualizations of physical reality—thus resulting in dichotomous Cartesian thinking.

Experiences of stigmata (discussed in Chapter 7) provide a relatively straightforward example of the imaginal realm intruding into the physical realm. Stigmata are real, verifiable *phenomena* —they occur in the physical realm (consensus reality) and can be reliably and objectively witnessed, photographed, measured, analyzed, etc.—yet, having no discernible physical cause, their origins are clearly not in the physical realm.

There is also the issue of pattern consistency. One stigmatic experience is very much like another. Such is also the case with Out-Of-Body Experiences, Near-Death Experiences, UFO Experiences and all the other Transpersonal Experiences. Unlike fantasies, which tend to be idiosyncratic and ephemeral, each specific type of imaginal realm experience (TPE) seems to be characterized by a consistently repeating pattern, even when the experiencer has no prior knowledge of that pattern. Also, unlike fantasies, these experiences have powerful aftereffects that may be traumatizing and/or transforming.

The patterns of the specific experiences appear to exist within an "experiential matrix" (Stanislav Grof's term) that provides structure and coherence and to be "archetypal" (Carl Jung's term) in nature—that is, they are "primordial constellations of images based on cumulative, collective human experience that can nevertheless express themselves in forms conditioned by the times." Moreover (as mentioned in Chapter 3 and further elaborated upon earlier in this chapter), my own work with hypnotherapy clients suggests that the (supposedly differentiated) patterns which might, on the surface, appear to be specific to each of the (supposedly differentiated) TPEs, have much in common with each other and might appropriately be thought of as different aspects of a single meta-experience.

200

Corbin's imaginal realm explanation for Transpersonal Experiences is a brilliant theoretical construct. It is, however, presented in the language of philosophy and for many people, philosophy has very little to do with reality. There is, however, another way of explaining the same principles in the language of modern physical science—specifically quantum mechanics.

THE QUANTUM REALM

It has long been a tenet of Eastern philosophies that time, space, separateness and causality are merely mental constructs linked to particular States Of Consciousness (SOCs) and have little relevance in accurately describing reality. Only in the 20th Century has this idea begun to make some inroads into Western thinking—interestingly, primarily by way of the work of physicists. Perhaps the two most important concepts in contemporary theoretical physics are the theories of relativity (both general and special) and the theory of quantum mechanics. Relativity deals with the large-scale structures of the universe; quantum mechanics deals with the small-scale structures of subatomic particles.[†]

Einstein's general theory of relativity posits that space is curved and that the influence of mass bends space in proportion to the amount of the mass's gravitational field. His special theory of relativity suggests that the traditional notions of space and time are inadequate and that space and time together form a static four-dimensional space-time continuum in which space and time are integral functions of one another. What pertains in the special theory also pertains in the general theory, so it follows from the positing of the space-time continuum that a curvature of space implies a curvature of time.

[†] Relativity theory and quantum theory are both complementary and contradictory to one another. Each is useful in its own realm, but not in the realm of the other. Scientists are continuing their efforts to reconcile the two and to develop a "Unified Field Theory (UFT)," or a "Theory of Everything (TOE)."

Kurt Godel, a colleague of Einstein's, went so far as to suggest that there is sufficient mass in the universe to curve space-time completely around on itself. Such a picture of time implies that everything that ever was or will be now is, that m o v e m e n t through time,

Nothing puzzles me more than time and space; and yet nothing troubles me less, as I never think about them.
—Charles Lamb

201

both forward and backward, is possible and that the future is every bit as determinable as the past. Besides showing that the space-time continuum is affected by the presence of matter, Einstein's theories also indicate that matter has nothing to do with substance but is, rather, a form of energy. In other words, there is nothing but space-time and energy and they are the same thing!

Quantum theory suggests that a search for the ultimate "stuff" of the universe is fruitless, because there isn't any. Primary reality, in quantum theory, is conceived of as nothing more than a conglomeration of frequencies, waveforms, or interference patterns. From this perspective, the objective world ceases to exist and what remains is an insubstantial universe consisting solely of waves and frequencies—matter (subatomic particles) coming into being only as the result of instantaneous interactions between energy fields at a specific locale.

What this implies is that "particle" is simply one way of describing the behavior of that which is called "matter," and that "particles," as such, do not exist. Under a different set of circumstances, the behavior of that which is called "matter" would more appropriately be described by the word "wave." Paradoxically, at the quantum level, matter is both particle-like and wave-like simultaneously. Each way of describing matter complements the other (the quantum "Principle of Complementarity") and only with simultaneous inclusion of both possibilities can a complete picture be presented. The particle-like aspects and the wave-like aspects of matter are equally fundamental. Both, together, are what matter really is—but only one aspect can manifest at any given instant since the different manifestations are mutually exclusive. The position of something like an electron can be measured when it manifests as a particle, or its momentum can be measured when it manifests as a wave, but an exact simultaneous measurement of both manifestations can never be made (the quantum "Uncertainty Principle").

The whole situation becomes curiouser and curiouser when it is recognized that a specific manifestation apparently is determined (or created) by the act of measurement. Thus, for an observer measuring particle-like characteristics, matter will behave in a particle-like fashion, but for an observer measuring wave-like characteristics, matter will behave in a wave-like fashion. Both potential manifestations exist together until an observer

Why, sometimes I've believed as many as six impossible things before breakfast.
—Lewis Carroll
(Alice's Adventures in Wonderland)

202

makes a measurement. At the moment of measurement, since the two behaviors preclude one another, one manifestation is realized and the other ceases to exist (or, according to the "Many Worlds" interpretation of quantum theory, manifests in an alternate reality).

Another major piece of this puzzle is Bell's theorem (ultimately proven in 1982[†]), which states that two particles, originally in a unitary state, retain their interconnectedness no matter how far they are separated in space (the quantum "Principle of Nonlocality") and such particles are able to communicate with each other instantaneously. Instantaneous communication means one of two things: (1) either objective, differentiated reality does not exist and it is meaningless to speak of matter as having any reality beyond the mind of the observer, or (2) instantaneous (not just faster-than-light) communication with the past and the future is possible. These are not just hypothetical assertions. The confirmation of Bell's theorem has proven that one or the other of these statements must be true. The weight of the evidence points toward the first option being the more likely, thus leaving one to struggle with the implications of all reality being a function of mind. What is more, since all of this occurs in transcendence of the ordinary differentiated boundaries of space and time, any notion of causality in the process is rendered meaningless (the quantum "Principle of Synchronicity").

This may seem odd, but that's not my fault.
—Bertrand Russell

[†] Alain Aspect and others from the Institute of Optics at the University of Paris produced a series of twin photons by heating calcium atoms with lasers. They then measured the polarization of the photons as they traveled through space in opposite directions. After ruling out the possibility of communication between the photons by any known physical process, the correlations they found in the results were such as to confirm Bell's Theorem.

In light of the definition of Transpersonal Experiences—
"Experiences that occur beyond the ordinary differentiated boundaries of
ego, space and time; experiences that suggest the essential
interconnectedness (and/or absolute unity) of all that ever was, is, or will
be; experiences that
imply the existence of
mind (as distinct from
brain), of spirit, of
soul"—it can be seen
that the implications of

What is mind? No matter.
What is matter? Never mind.
—Thomas Hewitt Key

the above material are central to everything this book is about. These
findings, in hard physical science, point to an intimate interconnectedness
between mind and matter, the observer's mind having a fundamental role
in the manifestation of matter.

In quantum theory, then, the physical world is not a structure built
out of independent entities. It is, rather, an interconnected web of
probabilities of relationships between entities (which are, themselves,
interactions between energy fields) whose meanings arise solely as a result
of their relationship to the whole. Everything in the universe that appears
to exist independently is actually part of a single all-encompassing organic
pattern and nothing is separate from that pattern or from anything else. In
other words, if the universe is non-local at a sub-quantum level, then reality
is seamless and unitary and any attempt to partition it into discrete entities
is based on false premises. There is no longer a clear distinction between
what is and what happens, between the observer and the observed,
because they are all part of an interconnected whole. In the microcosm of
the atom, location, separateness and causality simply have no meaning
whatsoever.

Another central point to be considered is that in a quantum
universe, reality is organized holographically. Holography is a type of lensless
photography that uses laser light and is based on interference patterns (the
patterns generated when two or more waves ripple through each other).
Any part of a holographic image, no matter how small, includes all the
information (albeit with reduced resolution) necessary to create a complete
image of the original subject. It can therefore be said that the information
in a hologram is distributed non-locally—thereby rendering the concept
of location meaningless—and by extension, information in
any holographically organized environment is also distributed non-locally.

In order to perceive and interpret a reality that is holographically
organized, the brain itself must be able to function holographically. Karl

203

Pribram, a Stanford University neurophysiologist, reasoned that brains mathematically construct objective reality by analyzing the interference patterns of waves generated (in response to a stimulus) at the ends of neurons, overlapping with waves generated at the ends of other neurons and breaking down those complex interference patterns into their component parts. Those parts are then converted into perceptions of familiar consensus reality by a process analogous to the laser illumination of a piece of holographic film. Despite the constituents of primary reality being nothing more than the momentary interaction of energy fields and despite space and time having no real meaning, the mind, drawing on representations arising from a holographically organized brain, is able to read out from this reality, in a variety of coordinates, what is occurring. Space and time just happen to be two sets of coordinates that are especially useful in constructing a functional representation of consensus reality.

> *REALITY*
> *is a fiction invented by those*
> *who feel insecure without*
> *a solid ground to stand on.*
> *—Anonymous*

204

While there is, as yet, no definitive proof that what applies in the microscopic world of quantum mechanics also applies in the macroscopic world of psychology and neurology, the evidence for non-locality in one realm is definitely suggestive of its possibility in another. Moreover, there are a number of capabilities of the brain that have not been explainable by the conventional neuroanatomical model, but which make sense within the context of a holographic model. Among these are:

> *The psyche's attachment to the brain,*
> *i.e., its space-time limitation, is no longer*
> *as self-evident and incontrovertible*
> *as we have hitherto been led to believe.*
> *It is not only permissible to doubt the*
> *absolute validity of space-time perception,*
> *it is, in view of the available facts,*
> *even imperative to do so.*
> *—Carl Jung*

- Distribution of memories—A specific memory appears to be stored throughout the brain rather than in one location. When brain damage occurs, any resulting loss of memory seems to be related to the amount of damage done rather than to the location of that damage.

- Vastness and speed of memories—It has been calculated that during an average human lifetime, the brain stores something on the order of 2.8×10^{20} (280,000,000,000,000,000,000) bits of information.[†] Additionally, if only one bit of information were processed per second, the neuroanatomical model would require the generation of 3×10^{10} (30,000,000,000) nerve impulses per second. That is an inconceivable amount of neural activity.

- Associative memory—All memories are linked by a multiplicity of associative connections. When two things are mnemonically associated and an individual thinks of one of them, the other tends to automatically spring to mind.

- Eidetic imagery—Those who are capable of eidetic imagery (photographic memory) are able to scan a scene they wish to memorize and later "project" its image, either with their eyes closed or while staring at a blank surface. Such a projection occurs with a high degree of detail and accuracy.

- Recognition of the familiar—When one recognizes, say, a familiar face in a crowd, the recognition process takes place with extraordinary speed and generally with a very high degree of certainty.

- State-dependent memory—That which is learned in a particular State Of Consciousness (SOC) often can be recalled only when the individual is again in that same SOC. Similarly, re-creation of initial conditions and context is necessary for the generation of a holographic image.

- Transference of learned skills—The ability to transfer a skill learned by one part of the body to another part (drawing a simple picture with one's foot, for example), without establishing neural pathways through repetitive learning, cannot be adequately explained by the neuroanatomical model.

- Phantom limb sensations and body boundaries—Phantom limb sensations, the auras that extend beyond the physical body (as seen in Kirlian photographs) and the ability to interpret perceptions as being of things beyond the boundaries of the body, all raise questions about the storage of body image and what constitutes its physical boundaries.

[†] To put all of those zeros into perspective, consider that it would require one hundred and forty trillion high-density computer floppy disks to store that much information.

- Synesthesia—The activation of a sense other than the one being directly stimulated (e.g., perceiving colors in association with sounds) suggests the layering and overlapping, rather than the specific localization, of the senses.
- Mechanics of consciousness—The ability of the brain to reflect upon itself, to have self-awareness, has eluded understanding within the neuroanatomical model.
- Transpersonal Experiences—Need anything more be said about this?

206

Physicist David Bohm of the University of London has suggested that the frequencies which the holographically organized brain analyzes in order to construct consensus reality are ultimately projections from another dimension, a deeper order of reality—one that is beyond both space and time. He refers to that order of reality as the "enfolded" or "implicate order" while referring to consensus reality as the "unfolded" or "explicate order." The explicate order, he says—that which is perceived through the ordinary senses or with the aid of scientific instruments—represents only a small fragment of the whole of reality. It is a special form of—contained within and emerging from, a more generalized totality of existence—the implicate order. In the implicate order, all that which is extant is intimately and meaningfully inter-related in such a way as to render meaningless all boundaries, including those of space and time.

Many other researchers have presented models of reality that are harmonious with Bohm's "Implicate Order" model. Rupert Sheldrake speaks of "Morphic Fields," Henry Morgenau of "Universal Mind," Erwin Schrodinger of "One Mind," Carl Jung of the "Collective Unconscious," and, of course, Henry Corbin of the "Imaginal Realm." While Bohm's and Corbin's models are presented with very different terminology, both are nevertheless describing essentially the same thing—the domain from which Transpersonal Experiences (TPEs) arise.

Central to Corbin's model, as previously discussed, is the assertion that imaginal realm experiences (synonymous with TPEs) are accessible only when the experiencer is in an Altered State of Consciousness (nominally Transpersonal Consciousness [TPC]). That being the case, it follows that implicate order experiences (also synonymous with TPEs) are also accessible only when the experiencer is in an ASC (nominally TPC). In Chapter 10 and elsewhere, it has been shown that Anomalously Sensitive Persons (ASPs) are likely to be more sensitive than the norm to ASCs in general and to TPC in particular—so it follows that ASPs are more likely than the norm to have Transpersonal Experiences, imaginal realm experiences or implicate order experiences.

The quantum scientific explanation for the ASP's facility at accessing TPEs relates directly to the coherent brainwave patterns that occur in TPC. Wave patterns are central to quantum theory and, by extension, to implicate order experiences (TPEs). As stated previously, any coherent wave-like phenomenon, not just light, can create the interference patterns that are involved in holographic organization and holographic perception. Brainwaves are wave patterns of Electro-Magnetic Radiation and specific States Of Consciousness (SOCs) are characterized by specific brainwave patterns. The predominant brainwaves frequencies of TPC, especially in the temporal lobes, are on the order of eight cycles per second (the alpha/theta boundary) and this pattern has been demonstrated to be associated with extremely vivid and realistic imagery, with creativity and with psi/psi-related experiences. Research by Winifred Lucas also points to the presence of strong flares of delta (0–4 cps) during the recollection of certain TPEs, thus providing supporting evidence for Anna Wise's profile of the "awakened mind" (see Chapter 10) and its role in TPEs.

When the accessing of TPEs is looked at from the perspective of brainwave patterns and energy fields, additional explanatory information comes to light. Surrounding the Earth, between the Earth's surface and the bottom of the ionosphere, there is a cavity with dimensions such that energy having a frequency of about 7.8 cycles per second is able to travel vast distances without significant attenuation. This fundamental frequency of the Earth, called the "Schumann Resonance Frequency," is in the same frequency range as the alpha/theta brainwave boundary and suggests the existence of a tuned resonant system. An individual in TPC, having an abundance of coherent brainwaves with a predominant frequency of approximately 7.8 cps, may be in resonance with the planetary system in such a way that a mutual exchange of energy occurs and information accessed by delta brainwaves (Wise's "radar of the unconscious") becomes available to conscious awareness. In other words, the energy required to support TPEs already exists within the environment and is able to be accessed when an individual is in a state of Transpersonal Consciousness.

Additional circumstantial evidence for the holographic organization of implicate order experiences (TPEs) is provided by the observation that there is a high level of coherence in the brainwave patterns of TPC. The concept of brainwave coherence parallels that of quantum wave function coherence and also that of light wave coherence in holography—and coherence appears to be a necessary condition for the effective transmittal of information by such waves. Danah Zohar suggests that there are a number of other similarities between mind processes and quantum mechanical processes that cannot easily be dismissed as mere coincidence. Among these are:

208

- It is impossible to pin down a quantum event with great precision because the act of observation changes the event (the "Quantum Uncertainty Principle"). Similarly, if a person attempts to observe what s/he is thinking about while the thought is occurring, the act of observation changes the way the thinking proceeds thereafter.
- The non-local relationships associated with the Quantum Uncertainty Principle imply that an entire system must be perceived on the basis of its indivisible interconnectedness, rather than attempting to break it down into separate parts affecting each other causally. Each "piece" has relevance only in terms of its context within the whole. Again, the same is true of thoughts. If an individual attempts to analyze her/his thoughts with greater and greater precision, eventually the point is reached where further analysis loses all meaning. Much of the significance of each element of thought apparently has to do with its connectedness with the other elements in the thought process.
- A parallel exists between the role of classical Newtonian concepts in permitting people to describe the consensus world of separate objects and causal connections (which are the limits of quantum processes) and the role of logical concepts in the structuring of free-flowing thought (primary process cognition). Just as everyday life would be impossible without the present classical limits to quantum mechanics, so too would be everyday thought without the ability to express its results in logical terms (secondary process cognition).

In the implicate order model, moments of form, thought and behavior are projected from the implicate order, an order of existence beyond both space and time, into the explicate order (consensus reality). The implicate order provides a medium through which, in Larry Dossey's words, communication is unmediated, unmitigated and immediate—the three main features of non-locality. The implicate order is the theoretical underpinning for the non-local, the transpersonal, the universal mind (spirit, or soul). Transpersonal Experiences, as defined, imply the existence of universal mind and, conversely, the existence of universal mind (operating within the implicate order) provides an explanation for the occurrence of Transpersonal Experiences. The primary characteristics of mind-based TPEs are essentially the same as the characteristics of Bohm's implicate order model. Most relevant are:

- the interconnectedness of all things;
- the transcendence of time, space and causality; and
- the non-differentiation between matter, energy and consciousness, between the part and the whole, between self and not-self, between thought and not-thought.

209

Restating the Perky Effect (discussed in Chapter 10) from a quantum perspective, it can be said that it is because of the essential unity, the essential oneness of all things, that the brain is not always able to distinguish between reality and imaginality, between what is consensually agreed to be "out there" and what is subjectively perceived to be "out there." In a quantum reality, not only is there no difference between the way perceptions and mental images are processed by the brain, there is no inherent difference between the perceptions and the images themselves. All

*Time and space
are modes by which we think,
and are not conditions
in which we live.*
—Albert Einstein

experiences, whether "consensual" or "imaginal," are reduced to the same common language of holographically organized waveforms. The only reason some realities are experienced as external and others are experienced as internal is because that is where the mind (perhaps in part as a result of cultural conditioning) happens to locate them when it generates the internal hologram that is experienced and referred to as "reality." Ultimately, that which is thought (self) and that which is not-thought (not-self) cannot be separated. For the purposes of practical functioning in consensus reality, however, it is necessary for the brain to make at least a provisional differentiation. Some brains, namely those that are Less Strongly Lateralized (LSL) than the norm, do this less effectively than other brains. Both the weaknesses and the strengths inherent in the anomalous perceptual style of ASPs arise out of their brains (and hence the interpretation of perceptions by their minds) being less differentiative—

and thus less oriented to ego, space and time—than the norm.

Using the language of quantum mechanics metaphorically, when cognitive processes are looked at from the perspective of the particle/wave duality, it can be seen that in ordinary waking consciousness, mind appears to be particle-like and localized in time and space. Conversely in a state of Transpersonal Consciousness (TPC), mind appears to be wavelike and neither temporally nor spatially localized. The apparent localization of mind in ordinary waking consciousness is within the brain. In TPC, while mind can appear to be localized in another corner of the room, another corner of the earth, or another corner of the universe, since everything in a holographic reality is non-local, mind is actually everywhere, nowhere and elsewhere. Access to implicate order experiences (TPEs) can occur only when the mind is in an ASC (nominally TPC) and is thus released from the limitations of spatio-temporal localization that results from a close association with the physical brain.

Given that mind can range throughout the totality of all that is and can influence, as well as be influenced by, everything else, it is presumably not only possible for it to experience all manifestations of the holographic reality, but also to play a part in changing those manifestations, including the manifestations of physical (consensus) reality. In short, mind is involved in the process of bringing physical realities into existence. Because the experiential matrices of all realities are holographic in nature, Transpersonal Experiences are available to mind and mind participates in shaping the realm of appearances in which physical existence is organized.

Quantum theory can be seen to allow for the presence of mind, at least in some elementary form, in the most fundamental entities of creation. On that basis, experiences of transpersonal perception and experiences of transpersonal influence can appropriately be considered to be experiences of transpersonal manifestation of mind. There is, then, no inherent difference, vis-à-vis consciousness, between psi experiences and psi-related experiences, because (seemingly) "other" minds are present in *all* experiences of both types. In other words, mind is present in

> *Physical concepts are free creations of the human mind, and are not, however it may seem, uniquely determined by the external world.*
> *—Albert Einstein*

everything and just as minds that are normally manifest in the explicate order may, under the appropriate conditions, be able to range into the implicate order, so too may minds that are normally manifest in the implicate order be able to range into the explicate order—and because of the essential interconnectedness and/or absolute unity of all minds, this "ranging" is not something that "happens," it is, rather, simply a manifestation of what "is."

Quantum physics provides solid scientific support for the assertion (made earlier) that there are likely to be as many different realities as there are different States Of Consciousness (SOCs). It all has to do with waves and interference patterns:

211

- According to the tenets of the holographic model, reality is nothing more than a conglomeration of frequencies, waveforms, or interference patterns.
- States Of Consciousness are, by definition, patterns of brainwaves.
- A specific SOC (pattern of brainwaves) is associated with a specific reality.
- There are as many realities as there are SOCs—presumably an infinite number.
- Because mind can shift from one SOC to another, it can also shift from one reality to another.
- Mind participates in establishing the rules that govern each reality with which it is associated and thus can be considered to be involved in the creation of those realities.

Observing, as does Freeman Dyson, that the universe shows evidence of mind on three levels can complete this scenario:

- The first level is that of elementary quantum mechanical physical processes in which matter is an active agent of choice, constantly making selections among alternate possibilities according to the laws of probability. As demonstrated by quantum experiments, there appears to be an element of mind inherent in every subatomic particle and mind is undifferentiable from matter.
- The second level is that of direct human experience in which the brain apparently serves as a device that filters, amplifies and concretizes the mental component of quantum choices made by neuronal molecules.

- The third level follows from the first and second—it is mind as a mental component of the universe. Being non-local, mind is without boundaries and without limits; it is timeless, spaceless and immortal—attributes which, in traditional religious thinking, also pertain to God. The implicate order, then, is a domain in which the nature of man and the nature of God overlap, in which humans are truly venturing into the realm of the spirit, the realm of the soul.

Not once in the dim past,
but continuously by conscious mind is
the miracle of the Creation wrought.
—Arthur Eddington

While much of this material dealing with the implicate order, Transpersonal Experiences and mind is hypothetical and has yet to be proven, it has immense explanatory value, at least in metaphorical terms. Quantum theory, as it currently stands, deals with non-living matter and does not address higher-level concepts such as meaning, purpose and significance. By extrapolation, however, the existence can be posited (as Bohm does) of a superimplicate order that stands in relationship to the implicate order much as the implicate order stands in relationship to the explicate order. This superimplicate order would act as a higher-level organizing principle for the implicate order in much the same way that mind acts on the brain. Further extrapolation could be made from the superimplicate order to a super-superimplicate order and from there to a super-super-superimplicate order and so on. Most likely, the current form of quantum theory will ultimately be determined to be a special case (one dealing with the behavior of non-living matter under certain circumstances) of a larger, more encompassing theory—presumably the "Theory of Everything" (mentioned earlier in this chapter).

If we do discover
a complete [unified] theory [of the universe],
then we shall all be able to take part in the discussion
of the question of why it is that we and the universe exist.
If we find the answer to that,
it would be the ultimate triumph of human reasoning—
for then we should know the mind of God.
—Stephen Hawking

THE SHORT VERSION

My objective in undertaking research with the HISS questionnaire and in writing *The H.I.S.S. of the A.S.P.,* was to attempt to develop a way to explain, without pathologizing, why some people have more Transpersonal Experiences than do others. That goal has presumably been achieved in the preceding pages and the explication has, of necessity, been rather extensive and complex. It might be helpful, therefore, to provide a short-form model—one that is presented in a visual format—for those who experienced difficulty in tracking the verbal explanation. This model is presented in Figure 11.5., page 215, along with some brief clarifying comments below.

213

Transpersonal Experiences (TPEs) arise out of Altered States of Consciousness (ASCs) (nominally Transpersonal Consciousness [TPC]). The symptomatology associated with those ASCs that underlie TPEs is spoken of by some as "Temporo-Limbic Epilepsy," and is spoken of by others as "kundalini arousal." For the purposes of this book, those labels can be considered to be red herrings. What is relevant is that certain individuals are more sensitive to ASCs than the norm because they have anomalous neurophysiological structuring (specifically a brain that is Less Strongly Lateralized [LSL] than the norm) that facilitates the emergence of ASCs. A host of factors, both endogenous and exogenous, can influence neurophysiological structuring and/or directly stimulate ASCs. The primary endogenous factors are Biological and Temperament Type Preferences; the primary exogenous factors are Substances, Electro-Magnetic Radiation, Trauma and Abuse, other stressors (mental, emotional and spiritual) and hypnosis, meditation, or training. An individual with the appropriate neurophysiological structuring, who has been subjected to the appropriate combination of influencing factors, will have a high level of Altered States of Consciousness sensitivities and a high level of Transpersonal Experiences sensitivities—as well as accompanying high levels of Physiological, Cognitive and Emotional sensitivities. In short, that individual will be an Anomalously Sensitive Person (ASP).

This non-pathologizing neurophysiologically-based way of explaining Transpersonal Experiences may have raised, for many readers, more questions than it has answered—the most far-reaching of which being "are Transpersonal Experiences 'real'?" The simplest and most direct answer to that question is, "it depends ...on what one means by 'real.'" A review of this and the preceding chapter can stimulate further musings about the nature of reality. After such a review, if you are still confused, or if you take issue with my thinking on this subject, I ask only that you continue to ponder these ideas in a spirit of open-minded inquiry. That will be sufficient for me to feel that I have achieved my objective—especially if your consideration of these matters prompts you to pursue some additional investigation on your own.

The final chapter of this part of the book will be devoted to looking into the future—the future of the HISS and the future of the ASP.

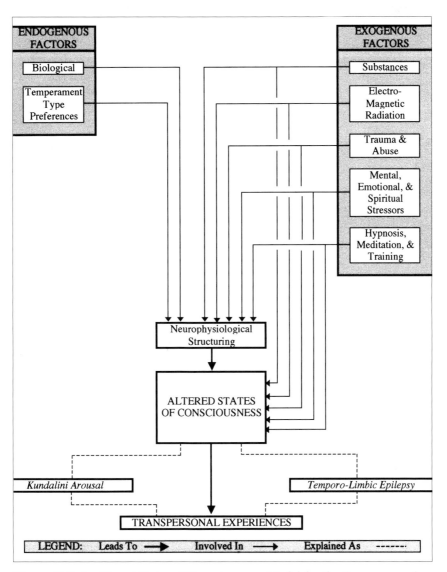

Figure 11.5. An Altered States of Consciousness Model for the Occurrence of Transpersonal Experiences.

CHAPTER SUMMARY

⇒ Transpersonal Experiences (TPEs) can logically be grouped into three general categories: (1) experiences of transpersonal perception, (2) experiences of transpersonal influence and (3) experiences of transpersonal manifestation of mind.

⇒ The distinctions between experiences of transpersonal perception and experiences of transpersonal influence, both categorically and individually, may be more semantic than they are substantive.

⇒ Experiences of transpersonal manifestation of mind appear to involve "other" minds as well as the mind of the experiencer. In the transpersonal realm, the concept of "other" is oxymoronic, so the distinction is one of appearances only.

⇒ In a state of Transpersonal Consciousness (TPC), mind not only can perceive and/or influence transpersonally, it can also be perceived and/or influenced transpersonally.

⇒ All of the supposedly differentiated individual TPEs may simply be different facets of a single meta-experience.

⇒ Anomalously Sensitive Persons (ASPs) are especially sensitive to the entire spectrum of TPEs.

⇒ Given that TPEs appear to be markers for alternate realities and given that TPEs appear to arise out of Altered States of Consciousness (ASCs), it can be argued that: (1) there are as many different realities as there are States of Consciousness (SOCs) and (2) "reality" is nothing more than a different label for "State of Consciousness."

⇒ The components of the limbic system are extremely sensitive to a variety of stressors including Electro-Magnetic Radiation (EMR). Those who are especially sensitive to EMR are said to be "Electro-Magnetically Sensitive (EMS)." EMS can result in neuronal hypersynchrony, which sets the stage for ASCs, which, in turn, open the door to TPEs.

⇒ EMS can result in all of the symptomatology of Temporo-Limbic Epilepsy (TLE). The seizure symptoms of TLE can be grouped into six categories: hallucinatory symptoms, emotional symptoms, physical symptoms, motor symptoms, sensory symptoms and experiential symptoms. The symptoms of kundalini arousal are almost identical to those of TLE. Kundalini arousal, in the Hindu tradition, is said to be a major pathway to enlightenment. The symptoms of both TLE and kundalini arousal include psi/psi-related experiences.

⟹ The concept of the "imaginal realm" offers a third alternative to the usual dichotomous thinking (either they're "really real" or they're fantasy) about TPEs. The imaginal realm, which is accessible only in an ASC, is the source of events that seem to belong simultaneously both to an alternate reality and to consensus reality. Imaginal realm experiences (TPEs) are ontologically real and can manifest in the physical realm.

⟹ Einstein's theories of relativity (both general and special) posit: (1) the existence of a space-time continuum that is affected by matter; (2) that matter is a form of energy; and (3) that there is nothing but space-time and energy—and they are the same thing.

⟹ Quantum theory suggests that primary reality is nothing more than a conglomeration of frequencies, wave forms, or interference patterns and that matter comes into being as a result of instantaneous interactions between energy fields at a specific locale.

⟹ At the quantum level, matter is both particle-like and wave-like simultaneously, but only one aspect can manifest at any given instant. Which aspect manifests is apparently determined by which aspect an observer is measuring—in other words, by the mind of the observer.

⟹ Bell's theorem (proven in 1982) suggests that objective, differentiated reality has no existence beyond the mind of the observer and that the acausal mind/matter relationship transcends the boundaries of both space and time.

⟹ In quantum theory, the physical world is not a structure built out of independent entities. It is, rather, an interconnected web of probabilities of relationships between entities (which are, themselves, interactions between energy fields) whose meanings arise solely as a result of their relationship to the whole.

⟹ In a quantum universe, all reality is holographically organized. In order to perceive and interpret such a reality, the brain itself must be able to function holographically.

⟹ The frequencies analyzed by the holographically organized brain in order to construct consensus reality, are ultimately projections from another dimension, a deeper order of reality that is beyond both space and time. Physicist David Bohm refers to that order of reality as the "implicate order."

217

⇒ Experiences of the implicate order (TPEs) are accessible only when the experiencer is in an ASC. ASPs, because of their facility with ASCs, are more likely to have implicate order experiences (TPEs) than the norm.

⇒ In a quantum reality, there is no difference between perceptions and mental images. All experiences, whether "consensual" or "imaginal," are reduced to the same common language of holographically organized waveforms.

218

⇒ Mind can experience all manifestations of holographic reality and can have a role in changing those manifestations, including the manifestations of physical (consensus) reality. In other words, mind plays a role in bringing physical realities into existence.

⇒ Quantum theory allows for the presence of mind in all that exists, so experiences of transpersonal perception and experiences of transpersonal influence can also be considered to be experiences of transpersonal manifestation of mind.

⇒ Quantum theory lends support to the assertion that there are as many different realities as there are SOCs—presumably an infinite number.

⇒ Being non-local, mind is without boundaries and without limits; it is timeless, spaceless and immortal—attributes which, in traditional religious thinking, pertain to God as well. The implicate order, then, is a domain in which the nature of man and the nature of God overlap, in which humans are truly venturing into the realm of the spirit, the realm of the soul.

CHAPTER 12

The Future

Our deepest fear is not that we are inadequate;
our deepest fear is that
we are powerful beyond measure.
—*Nelson Mandela*

To conquer fear is the beginning of wisdom.
—*Bertrand Russell*

An interesting research project to follow up on the work already done with the HISS would be that of conducting in-depth case studies—similar to the one done with Claire—of individuals who meet the criteria for basic ASPness. While all ASPs, by definition, have very high scores (two or more standard deviations above the mean) on both of the first-level HISS scales—Predispositions toward sensitivities and Indicators of sensitivities (see Chapter 14 for more about the data), they are otherwise quite different from one another.

Illustratively, among the ten ASPs in the HISS Reference Group, scores were less than two standard deviations above the mean on second-level scales for four (including Claire) on Biological predispositions, for three on Trauma and Abuse predispositions, for one on Temperament Type Preferences predispositions, for two on Cognitive indicators, for two on

Emotional indicators, for one on **Altered States of Consciousness** indicators and for two (including Claire) on **Transpersonal Experiences** indicators. It happens that I personally know four of the ten **ASPs** and they definitely do not give the impression of having been cast from the same mold. As different from each other as **ASPs** are, however, they are alike in being *very* different from the population norm.

220

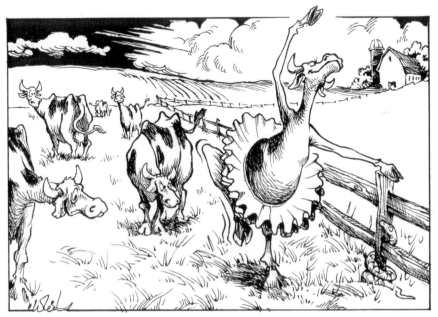

An ASP is Definitely Not "Just One of the Herd."

The study of a single individual's anomalous sensitivity in just one realm—Physiological, Cognitive, Emotional, **Altered States of Consciousness**, or **Transpersonal Experiences**—can be most intriguing and revealing. **Transpersonal Experiences** being my primary interest, the investigations I undertook with Claire went somewhat further in that particular area than they did in the others.

Claire had indicated on the HISS that she regularly experienced clairvoyance (actually claircognizance—"knowing," rather than "seeing"), so I decided to see what she could do. At the time, I was also working on another research project, the subject matter of which was only marginally related to **ASPness** and about which it was clear she knew very little. After developing an extensive list of questions about that issue and introducing her to a few of the structured protocols for Controlled Remote Viewing (further discussed later in this chapter), I spent several days with her (over a period of a few months), finding out what she could tell me, claircognizantly, about the subject under investigation.

My primary goal was the gathering of information relative to the other project, so the methodology employed with Claire did not necessarily meet accepted scientific research standards, but every effort was made to conduct a detached and objective inquiry and to avoid leading her in any way. The first set of questions presented to her were ones to which I already knew the correct answers. She responded to them with a degree of accuracy so extraordinary that it seemed she might have been accessing the information telepathically—in other words, just reading my mind.

The next set of questions pertained to material for which I did not know the correct answers. When follow-up research in the pertinent literature demonstrated that once again she had achieved an extremely high level of accuracy, telepathy had to be ruled out as the operant perceptual modality. There remained, however, the possibility that she was simply demonstrating cryptomnesia (detailed and accurate recall of information that was previously learned, often unconsciously and then forgotten)—she was, after all, extremely well read.

With the third set of questions, not only did I not know the answers, I didn't even know if it would be possible to find them. Many of her responses to the questions she answered initially struck me as patently absurd—but later extensive research in the available literature did not reveal a single instance in which she had answered incorrectly. This is not to say that she was infallible. Of the questions in this set, she declined to answer about one third and I was not able to unearth answers for another third—but her responses to the remaining third were, without exception, later determined to be valid. In one instance, it was six months before I was able to confirm that she had, indeed, provided valid information in response to a specific question.

Cryptomnesia no longer seemed to be a viable explanation for what was going on in that, despite my considerable familiarity with the material, I had a great deal of difficulty locating the correct answers. Surely Claire hadn't just happened to see the information somewhere. All things considered, it turned out that claircognizance did appear to be the most likely interpretation of what it was that she was doing.

221

The Future of the HISS

Much has already been learned from the results of testing with the HISS and the potential exists for learning a lot more—especially through the administration of the questionnaire to sub-populations of particular interest and comparison of their scores with the scores of the Reference Group. Specific sub-populations that come to mind include: familial groups, ethnic groups, age groups, occupation groups, socioeconomic groups, groups with a shared medical diagnosis, groups with a shared psychiatric diagnosis, groups of meditators and/or yoga practitioners and groups of individuals who have a specific type Transpersonal Experience in common.[†]

A few projects of this sort are already underway. The sub-populations of special interest that are currently being studied are:

- NDEers—the New Being Project, of Guerneville, California, has administered the HISS to 68 subjects who meet their preliminary criteria for being Near-Death Experiencers.
- UFOEers—the New Being Project, of Guerneville, California, has administered the HISS to 76 subjects who meet their preliminary criteria for being UFO Experiencers (either UFO sighting or alien contact).
- CRVers—Problems>Solutions>Innovations (P>S>I), of Alamogordo, New Mexico has administered the HISS to 29 subjects, all of whom have been trained in Controlled Remote Viewing.

A preliminary analysis of the CRVers data has been completed and the results are quite thought provoking. Before moving on to a discussion of those findings, however, a bit of history is called for.

In the 1970s, the U. S. military intelligence community established a psi-based intelligence-gathering program using a methodology spoken of as "Controlled Remote Viewing (CRV)." That is another name for clairvoyance (with its various sub-categories) performed under controlled conditions using stringent, structured protocols. When the existence of this program became public knowledge, its sponsors claimed that it had proven to be ineffective and was being disbanded—this after 20 years and the investment of more than $20 million. Well...maybe...but having

---

[†]Serious researchers are invited to submit inquiries and/or proposals to: The ASP Project, c/o Headline Books, Inc., P.O. Box 52, Terra Alta, WV 26764 (email: ASPproject@headlinebooks.com)

trained in CRV, having had first-hand subjective experience doing CRV and having analyzed the statistics on the results of CRV, there is little question in my mind about its efficacy. Most likely, the intelligence community's disclaimer was necessitated by security considerations and/or a desire to avoid the opprobrium of the "giggle factor."

The objective of the HISS CRVer study was to determine in what ways, if any, the collective HISS profile of CRVers differed from the collective HISS profile of the Reference Group. That information could then be used to develop a better understanding of CRVers and of the efficacy of P>S>I's CRV training program. A broad-brush illustration of the results of this study is presented in the FANGS ("Findings—ANomalous Group Sensitivities") chart, Figure 12.2., below and is followed by a brief discussion.

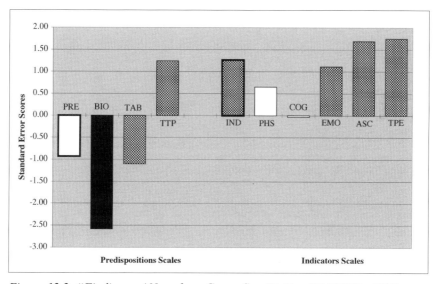

Figure 12.2. "Findings—ANomalous Group Sensitivities (FANGS)"—CRV Group Mean

This chart reflects the relationships between the mean scores of the CRV group and the mean scores of the Reference Group. It is interpreted in the same way as was the individual TAILS chart for

Claire (Figure 3.4).[†] Solidly shaded columns represent CRVers' mean scores that exhibit a very noteworthy (two or more standard errors) difference (either positive or negative) from the Reference Group mean, crosshatched columns represent CRVers' scores that exhibit a noteworthy (one or more, but less than two, standard errors) difference from the Reference Group mean and unshaded columns represent CRVers' scores that exhibit no noteworthy (less than one standard error) difference from the Reference Group mean.

224   Relative to the Reference Group mean, CRVers' mean scores for the first-level Predispositions (toward sensitivities) scale were low (almost to a noteworthy degree), while their scores for the first-level Indicators (of sensitivities) scale were high (to a noteworthy degree). Those two scores would normally be expected to vary from the Reference Group's mean scores in the same direction and by approximately the same amount. The fact that they don't, combined with the degree to which they don't, is very noteworthy.

The CRVers' low mean Predispositions score resulted primarily from their very low mean Biological (BIO) predispositions score (and secondarily from their low mean Trauma and Abuse [TAB] predispositions score), which more than offset their high mean Temperament Type Preferences (TTP) predispositions score. Their high mean TTP score (the factors involved in TTP are discussed in Chapters 6 and 14) resulted from their high mean Introversion (Orientation scale) and iNtuition (Perceiving scale) scores—their mean Feeling (Judging scale) score being somewhat lower than the Reference Group's mean.

The CRVers' high mean Indicators score resulted primarily from their high mean Emotional, Altered States of Consciousness (ASC) and Transpersonal Experiences (TPE) indicators scores. Not surprisingly, their high mean TPE score reflected an elevated incidence of psi experiences (but not of psi-related experiences)— CRV (or clairvoyance) is, after all, a psi experience. Also not particularly surprising was that their high mean Emotional indicators score reflected a high level of Interpersonal (but not Intrapersonal) sensitivity—Interpersonal sensitivity may well involve the experience of telepathy and telepathy is a psi experience.

[†] There is one important difference in the handling of the statistics. Whereas numerical scores on the TAILS for an individual are "standard deviation (s.d.)" scores, numerical scores on the FANGS for a group are "standard error (s.e.)" scores. The "standard error" is the "standard deviation" divided by the square root of the number of subjects in the group. (See Chapter 13, "A Statistical Primer," for more information on the mathematics involved.)

Since CRVers were shown by the HISS to be more sensitive than the norm, but to be less predisposed (especially biologically) toward being sensitive, it holds to reason that some exogenous factor must be responsible—and the most likely factor is, of course, their training in Controlled Remote Viewing. Note that those scales on which they exhibited notably higher levels of sensitivities than the norm—Emotional

> *Training is everything.*
> *The peach was once a bitter almond;*
> *cauliflower is nothing but*
> *cabbage with a college education.*
> *—Mark Twain*

sensitivity (Interpersonal, but not Intrapersonal), Altered States of Consciousness sensitivity and Transpersonal Experiences (psi, but not psi-related) sensitivity—all relate to the efficacy of Controlled Remote Viewing. Note too that while Temperament Type Preferences are technically considered to be Predispositions (toward sensitivities) rather than Indicators (of sensitivities), they are presumably subject to change exogenously—and the two TTP factors for which CRVers showed high mean scores, Introversion and iNtuition, also relate to the efficacy of Controlled Remote Viewing.

Many people who are intrigued by the concept of the ASP, once they have a basic understanding of it, then want to know their own status vis-à-vis ASPness. As has been stated previously, sensitivities are more appropriately thought of as degrees on continua rather than as an anomalous/non-anomalous dichotomy—and understanding the specific individual sensitivities has considerably more utility than does the application of the "ASP" label. Nevertheless, human nature being what it is, this tendency to want a simple, straightforward, dichotomous answer is entirely understandable.

The version of the HISS used in this study was designed primarily for research purposes. With its 50 scored scales (many of them quite subtle), it is too long, it is too complex and its results are too subject to misinterpretation for it to be used in a casual manner. It could, however, be made available to clinicians after they have received a brief training in its use and interpretation

225

If your curiosity has gotten the best of you, don't despair. An abbreviated version of the questionnaire is currently available to the general public.[†] It provides scores for the first- and second- level Predispositions and Indicators scales that very closely parallel those of the full scale version of the HISS. Even if you are one of those people who *must* know *right now* whether or not you are an ASP, there is a reasonably acceptable solution. An individual's score on the "Electro-Magnetic Sensitivities" scale, by itself, has very strong predictive reliability for both Predispositions and Indicators scores—and hence for basic ASPness. If you would like to check it out for yourself, go to Appendix D, "The HISS EMS Scale," answer the six questions that appear there, do the requisite math (it's easy) and your score will provide a fairly good indication of your ASP/not-ASP status.

Many people also want to know if there's a way—based on objective criteria alone—to determine if someone else is an ASP. The answer is "probably not," but there are six questions addressing objective data that, when considered together as a (arbitrary and artificial) scale, have a moderate degree of predictive reliability for sensitivities in general. The questions are:

- Is the person female?
- Is the person hypopigmented?
- Is the person Non-Right-Handed?
- Is the person's occupational category Artistic (fine arts, acting, music, writing, etc.), Investigative (science, legal, higher education, computer, etc.), or Social (human services, teaching, religion, etc.)?
- Was the person born as one of a set of twins/triplets/etc.?
- Does the person have an other-than-conventionally-heterosexual sexual orientation?

If the answers to all, or most, of these questions are affirmative, the person would *probably* score toward the high end of the sensitivities continua. Negative responses to most, or even all, of these questions, however, do not necessarily indicate than an individual would score toward the low end of the sensitivities continua.

[†] Contact: The ASP Project, c/o Headline Books, Inc., P.O. Box 52, Terra Alta, WV 26764, 800-570-5951 (email: ASPproject@headlinebooks.com). The cost for scoring is $15.00—VISA/MC accepted. Your scores and an explanation of their significance will be sent to you in two to three weeks.

There is nothing inherently "good" or "bad" about either high scores or low scores on the HISS. What is important is whether high levels of sensitivities or low levels of sensitivities are more appropriate to an individual's particular life circumstances and, if there is a mismatch, how that mismatch is handled. As previously discussed, high levels of sensitivities can serve an artist, inventor, or humanitarian well, because they can foster insight, intuition, attunement and creativity...but they can also lead to physiological or psychological difficulties. Conversely, low levels of sensitivity can be important to soldiers, law enforcement officers and emergency service personnel because they can serve as a buffer against stimuli that might otherwise be overwhelming...but they can also inhibit the appreciation of all the richness and fullness that life has to offer.

227

Some people say that they would like to be ASPs and some say that they wouldn't. In Western society, ASPs have clearly been underdogs for the last few centuries, but the wheel continues to turn and it appears to be only a matter of time before they come into their own. The potentials inherent in ASPness are significant, but the life of an ASP will, almost assuredly, continue to be a challenging one.

THE FUTURE OF THE ASP

As was discussed in the chapter devoted to each, anomalously heightened sensitivity in all of the realms—Physiological, Cognitive, Emotional, Altered States of Consciousness and Transpersonal Experiences—has both a downside and an upside. There seems to be a widespread tendency, however, to place considerably more emphasis on dealing with the downsides than on unleashing the upside potentials. Illustratively, consider these questions:

- In the Physiological realm—How does the number of specialists dealing with (the downside of) drug dependency compare to the number working to unleash (the upside of) psychogenic healing potential?
- In the Cognitive realm—How does the amount of funding available for dealing with (the downside of) dyslexia compare to that available for unleashing (the upside of) poetic potential?
- In the Emotional realm—How does the time and energy devoted to dealing with (the downside of) depression stack up against that directed toward unleashing (the upside of) empathic potential?

Dealing with the downside is usually done by way of a medical model approach and often involves the administration of drugs to suppress the symptoms of what has been diagnosed as a disorder. In cases of *proven* disorders, especially certain ones involving the immune system, there is certainly a place for such aggressive treatment. The problem is that drugs and such are often used to treat conditions that may be "differences" rather than "disorders"—and are likely to suppress the upside potentials as well as the downside symptoms.

228

Consider the case of Liza (discussed in Chapter 1), for example. It would be difficult to take issue with the prescription of antibiotics (unless over-prescribed) for the treatment of her infections, respiratory problems and Lyme disease, but the list of drugs prescribed for her "occult illnesses" and "psychiatric disorders" was seemingly endless. In the course of just a few years, she was given prescriptions for more than 40 different drugs in a variety of classes—amphetamines, analgesics, antianxietants, anti-ADHD, anticonvulsants, antidepressants, antimigraines, antipsychotics, benezodiazepines, beta blockers, calcium blockers, hypnotics, opoids, muscle relaxants, steroids, and thyroid hormones, among them. In many cases, not only had the effectiveness of the drug in treating the "disorder" for which it was prescribed not been proven, the true nature of the "disorder" was itself unknown. The number of the drugs was astounding, several of them were extremely potent, many had very serious potential side effects and combining two or more of them was often strongly contraindicated.

Whether or not those drugs helped Liza in any way will never be known, but according to her reports she felt like a zombie and her life did not seem to be worth living. Consequently, feeling she had nothing to lose, she

> *An unhatched egg is the greatest challenge in life.*
> *—Elwyn White*

set about discontinuing their use. Self-empowerment was an important issue for her, so she began a program of study in "Reike"—a meditative form of hands-on (self-) healing. She also set about reducing the stress—physical, chemical, electro-magnetic, mental, emotional and spiritual—in her life. She moved to a new environment, changed vocations, restructured her relationships, altered her sleep habits, modified her diet, linked up with alternative health practitioners, began working with a psycho-spiritual counselor and so on. In short, she took personal responsibility for her own physical and psychological health.

Today, Liza is a relaxed, happy, self-confident, successful artist who appears to be well on her way to developing her Transpersonal Experiences sensitivity into extraordinary giftedness. She still has some physical health problems, but they no longer incapacitate her the way they used to—she considers them to be simply another set of challenges to be taken in stride as she proceeds along her life's path.

229

There are many different types of mind-based alternative healing modalities—Reike being just one of them—and it is significant that most have three factors in common: (1) relaxation, (2) focused attention and (3) suggestion. These three factors are all central to Altered States of Consciousness (ASCs) and, as has been shown, ASCs underlie the manifestations of anomalous sensitivities in all of the realms. Chaotic and stressful ASCs are likely to lead to manifestations of the downsides of anomalous sensitivities; organized and peaceful ASCs are likely to lead to manifestations of the upsides of anomalous sensitivities. In other words, effective management of Altered States of Consciousness can result in the realization of the upside potentials of sensitivities— and the downsides get handled simply as a collateral consequence.

The mind is its own place and in itself
Can make a heav'n of hell,
a hell of heav'n.
—*John Milton*

Managing States of Consciousness (SOCs) can be thought of as managing brainwave patterns. It's really not a new idea—for eons people have been doing it by way of techniques such as meditation, drumming, chanting and the like. The problem with these traditional approaches (mind-altering substances aside) is that they require considerable time, dedication and natural ability to achieve any degree of success. Thanks to modern technology, however, there now exists a way—EEG biofeedback—that is not only much faster and more precise, but also lends itself to replication, verification and validation by standard scientific methods.

EEG biofeedback is a training strategy that facilitates an individual's learning to regulate her/his own brainwave patterns by feeding back to her/him real-time objective information about those patterns. It is a non-intrusive procedure using electronic sensors placed on the head. Brainwaves are monitored by those sensors, amplified and analyzed by computer-based instruments and converted to a feedback signal that is either auditory, visual, or both. The trainee is tasked to alter the feedback signal, using only the powers of her/his mind, according to protocols designed to meet the specific objectives of the training. The brain responds to reinforcement cues and a learning of specific brainwave patterns occurs.

230

EEG biofeedback methodologies are still in the developmental stage and training protocols have yet to be developed for unleashing many of the relevant upside potentials of ASPness—but EEG biofeedback, by definition, involves managing States Of Consciousness and that's where the whole process begins. Because of cultural conditioning, most of the work with EEG biofeedback to date has been oriented toward dealing with the downside of things—

A mind that trusts itself
is light on its feet.
—Nathaniel Branden

and considerable promise has been shown in the management of a variety of disorders associated with ASPness including: addictions, anxiety/panic disorders, attention/learning disorders, auto-immune disorders, chronic pain, Chronic Fatigue Syndrome, Epilepsy, migraine, mood disorders, Post-Traumatic Stress Disorder, sleep disorders, Tourette's Disorder and traumatic brain injury. There have, as well, been several studies in which the efficacy of EEG biofeedback has been demonstrated in facilitating peak performance and experiences of psi.

While it is a relatively simple undertaking to locate organizations that will assist an individual in managing the various downsides, finding those that are oriented toward the realization of upside potentials is a different story—they are few and far between. Appendix F, "Resources for the ASP," lists some organizations that might be able to offer guidance and assistance to those who are looking for positive self-empowering approaches.

The potentials inherent in (what I am now speaking of as) ASPness have, for the last few centuries, generally been ignored or even denigrated by Western society. Objective, intellectual, sequential thinking and facility with the manipulation of words, symbols and rules has been rewarded with success; subjective, intuitive, holistic thinking and facility with the imaginative transformation of mental images has (at best) generally been dismissed as being characteristic of eccentricity. As was mentioned previously, whereas the auditory (secondary process, or digital) cognitive style is generally considered to be advanced, the visual (primary process or analog) cognitive style is often considered to be primitive.

It was with the evolution of language into the written word that the current prevailing worldview—so dismissive of the strengths of the ASP—began its rise to dominance. In the early stages of language development, words were used to evoke specific images that enabled one person to share intimately with another, an experience at which the other had not been present. Later, these words served not only to evoke images and experiences, but also to allow people to detach themselves from their experiences—to externalize and to analyze them. Eventually, language became so far removed from experience that it ceased to evoke the images and sensations of the experience to which it referred. In general usage, language has become a sterile tool by which one can label, categorize, or pigeonhole objects and events as either familiar or unfamiliar, benign or threatening, useful or irrelevant—and deal with them as abstractions rather than as a part of oneself.

The societal status of the ASP may now be changing as computer systems are developed—with graphical representations and intuitive modes of operation—that are user-friendly to those who rely more heavily on the visual style than on the auditory style of cognition. In the very near future, ASPs should be able to depend on the strengths of the machine to perform all of those functions in which they, themselves, are weak and they will be freed to direct the entirety of their creative energies toward those areas in which they

> *If you're not on the edge,*
> *you're taking up too much room.*
> *—Anonymous*

excel. Because their strengths lie in the perception of similarities, once they are given the opportunity, they will be able to draw on a variety of different cognitive domains and perform syntheses from which truly new, truly unique, truly transformative changes in worldview can arise.

The implication here is that the next step in the evolution of human cognitive style may be that of returning to the distant past—a time when (those who I am now referring to as) **ASPs** were treated with deference and respect. In primitive societies, even if an **ASP** lacked the aggression, coordination and physical health to join in the hunt (i.e., "to earn a living"), her/his intuitive abilities were recognized as being vital to the survival of the tribe and s/he was cared for accordingly. It was the **ASP** who knew where to find water, how to locate game, what weather to expect and how to attend to the injured and the sick.

232

In early historical times and in various indigenous groups today, those who had special facility at managing **SOCs** were recognized and acknowledged as sorcerers, witches, witch doctors, medicine men and seers. In referring to such individuals, modern anthropologists generally use the term "shaman" to encompass all the other terms, because it lacks their prejudicial overtones and conflicting meanings. "Shaman" comes from the language of the Tungus people in Siberia and can be narrowly defined as: "one who, at will, enters into **Transpersonal Consciousness (TPC)** and experiences her/his mind or spirit journeying to other, normally hidden, realities and interacting with other entities to acquire knowledge and power and to help other people." A broader definition that better serves the purposes of this book, is: "one who, at will, enters into **Altered States of Consciousness (ASCs)** in service of her/his community." The traditional shamans were, first and foremost, healers. They were visionaries and mystics who could communicate with nature, with gods and with spirits. They were able to perceive things that others could not and to make meaningful connections between objects and events separated by both time and space. They were keepers of knowledge, both sacred and secular. They were artists, poets, singers and dancers. They were psychologists, social workers, consultants and mediators. They were masters of ecstasy and masters of death.

Having epilepsy or other nervous disorders was considered to be a definitive indicator of shamanic talent. Often, the circumstances under which the call to a shamanic vocation was revealed involved an acute physical, mental, or emotional crisis. Any close encounter with death, from which the individual emerged with knowledge of what transpired (and perhaps with a specialized immunity as well), was considered to be a clear calling to the role.

Refusal of a call to shamanism was no small matter—it was said to put the individual at great risk for illness, insanity, or even death.

Traditional shamans used a variety of techniques —heat, fasting, sleep deprivation, dancing, monotonous chanting and rhythmic drumming, to name a few—to assist themselves in entering ASCs. It is noteworthy that in the rhythmic drumming technique, the drumbeat frequencies used—and to which the brainwaves of susceptible individuals became entrained—were generally in the range of four-to-eight cycles per second. This frequency range corresponds to the EEG theta brainwave pattern, theta being the bridge between alpha and delta in the brainwave pattern of TPC and "the awakened mind." Theta is also the predominant brainwave pattern in young children—a group that shows a very high level of facility in the TPE realm.

The roots of Western shamanism are said to lie in the practices of the "wise women," the priestesses of early Anglo-Saxon times. As spiritual leaders, they helped their people to understand and to live within, the framework of a worldview that was called *"wyrd"*† and which suggested that:

- all things and all events are intimately interconnected, as if by a seamless web, on all levels of reality;
- objects that are perceptible to human senses are nothing more than local manifestations of larger energy patterns;
- that which is imperceptible to human senses is just as important as that which is perceptible;
- any event, anywhere, affects everything else, everywhere, as a result of vibrations transmitted throughout the web;
- everything, everywhere, is alive—that is, consciousness is all-pervasive;
- body, mind and spirit are all one; and
- the entire universe is sacred and has purpose and meaning.

That worldview, it will be recognized, is essentially undifferentiable from the concepts of the imaginal realm and the implicate order (both discussed in Chapter 11). Those ideas, which today strike us as being strange—in part because they seem so new and different—were actually commonplace many hundreds of years ago.

---

† Pronounced the same as "weird."

233

"Wyrd" now seems "weird"—well, yes, but that's more than just a semantic coincidence. When the Christians came to power in Britain, anything that had important spiritual meaning to those they considered heathens automatically became anathema and every effort was made to eradicate it. "Weird," with its connotations of strange, bizarre, supernatural and unworldly was a deliberate Christian distortion of the concept of *"wyrd."* By 1000 AD, the shamans of the indigenous population had been largely replaced by Christian missionaries, at least in the circles of the ruling elite. Among the general populace, however, the traditional attitudes, methods and values continued to survive for another several hundred years. Eventually, the Church launched its now infamous witch-hunting trials to eliminate the competition presented by the female shamanic practitioners (who had generally been ignored by the original Christian missionaries) and to solidify the Church's domination and control of the people.

234

The "modern" worldview—based on anthropocentrism, humanism, rationalism, mechanism and materialism (see Chapter 2)— authorizes and even encourages, aggression, exploitation and destruction. Grounded in a literal, fundamentalist interpretation of Genesis 1:28, in which humans are said to have been given "dominion over the fish of the sea and over the fowl of the air and over every living thing that moveth upon the face of the earth," its tacit assumption is that the world and everything in it exists for our benefit and that we are free to do with it as we please. Our multitudinous machinations—our fantasies and our fears, our ignorance and our irresponsibility, our enthusiasm and our egocentricity, our possessiveness and our politics—have led to a situation in which the state of the world reflects the state of our minds, in which the conflict without mirrors the conflict within, in which the external chaos echoes the internal chaos.

In short, we tend to perceive ourselves as being separate from and superior to everything else...as well as separate from and superior to each other. As a species, we emphasize separateness over interconnectedness, independence over interdependence and differences over similarities. Such a posture provides few checks and balances against our aggressive tendencies—

> *We have met the enemy and he is us.*
>
> *—Walt Kelly*
> *(1970 Pogo Cartoon)*

and aggress we do...against nature, against each other and against ourselves.

The shamanic worldview of *wyrd,* on the other hand, provides a viable, life-enhancing alternative for human behavior. Taken seriously, experienced directly and lived as if the future of humankind depended on it (which perhaps it does), *wyrd* would permit us to perceive our individual selves as sharing a common identity and a common destiny with all other human beings, to accept all living things as being interconnected and interdependent and to honor the Earth as a living entity vital to our survival. Instead of separation, conflict, alienation and chaos, the human experience would be one of unity, harmony, coop-eration and order. From a psychological perspective, a change such as this would

235

As we let our light shine,
we unconsciously give others
permission to do the same.
As we are liberated from our own fear,
our presence automatically liberates others.
—Nelson Mandela

help people, both individually and collectively, to satisfy one of their deepest needs, that of connectedness and belonging; it would relieve those feelings of aloneness and isolation that lead to anxiety, depression and ill health; it would provide a sense of harmony, of meaning, of purpose and of personal value.

For quite some time, Claire has been an adherent of the shamanic worldview. After having been introduced to the concept of the Anomalously Sensitive Person, she offered some valuable insights about the interrelationship between the shaman and the ASP.

Not all ASPs are shamans, but all true shamans are ASPs. Shamanic abilities arise out of anomalous sensitivities. An ASP can learn to be a shaman, but nobody can learn to be an ASP—one is either born with a high level of sensitivities, or one is not. A person who retains those sensitivities into adulthood can be considered to be "inadequately socialized" because s/he has not taken on the perceptual and cognitive filters that are normally imposed on an individual by society. The ASP does not follow the normal rules about what one is allowed to perceive and how one is allowed to perceive it.

For any individual, *everything* is filtered, either to a greater or to a lesser degree; it is impossible to filter out the negative and take in only the positive. An ASP, having filters that are far more permeable than the norm, will be anomalously sensitive to the entire spectrum of stimuli. In order to function effectively, an ASP needs to learn shamanic strategies for letting go of the negative stimuli. Otherwise s/he will become ill—physically ill, mentally ill, emotionally ill, or spiritually ill.

Other shamans may guide and support an individual during this learning process, but it is essentially a personal, individual undertaking. While the strategies, techniques and philosophies of shamanism can be taught, shamanism itself cannot be—and the idea of a "credentialed shaman" is absurd. A true shaman would never subscribe to a system that involves credentialing by others, let alone attend conferences, conventions and such.

A shaman can be many different things, including philosopher, consultant, guide and teacher, but above all, a shaman is a healer—a healer of individuals, of families, of groups and of institutions. A true shaman, however, will never be found in a traditional leadership position. Such a role would require the acceptance of conventional structures, attitudes and beliefs—at which point, the shaman would cease to be a shaman. Originality and creativity are the shaman's stock-in-trade and s/he can only effect change or transformation by operating outside traditional organizational frameworks. After the changes have come about, the shaman needs to move on—because those changes, no matter how beneficial they might be, will evoke resentment in those who adhere to institutional thinking. The shaman is a solo practitioner who will always be an outsider.

While few are born with the sensitivities necessary to be true shamans, many more might be willing to adopt the shamanic worldview of interconnectedness if they are shown the way. The shamans can be the guides. They can assist us in understanding who we really are, help us to appreciate why it is that we are here and support us in becoming more fully human. Shamans can show us that we have a deeper level of connectedness with each other than that which appears in hierarchies or on organizational charts.

237

Because of the cultural conditioning to which we, as adults, have been subjected over decades and to which we, as a society, have been subjected over centuries, adoption of a shamanic worldview may prove to be a difficult undertaking—one that requires much in the way of introspection, reevaluation and attitudinal shifting. The process can be accelerated, however, by focusing on our children before they have succumbed to the denigration, pathologizing and suppression of things shamanic and transpersonal that has been so much a part of our

> *We cannot solve the problems*
> *we have created*
> *with the same thinking*
> *that created them.*
> *—Albert Einstein*

own experience. If we permit (or actively encourage) our children to do what they know how to do instinctively and naturally, if we listen to what they have to tell us and if we internalize the wisdom inherent in their experiences, the prospects for their future (and perhaps ours as well) might be greatly enhanced. Such a process can be thought of as (borrowing a phrase from Ken Ring) "the shamanizing of modern humanity."

Several years ago, I met a young girl who presented herself in such a way that I could not help but imagine that she would grow up to become the quintessence of a neo-shaman. That encounter resulted in my writing an article

> *Thinkest thyself a puny form when*
> *within thee the universe is folded?*
> *—Ancient Sufi Tradition*
> *(attributed to Ali)*

about her for the *Bulletin of Anomalous Experience*. It is reproduced on the next page.

OF LIZARDS AND WIZARDS

Magic! I've always been entranced by magic. In junior high school I used to perform magic shows at birthday parties for the "little kids." In college I read everything I could find about hypnosis. When Neuro-Linguistic Programming first came on the scene, I knew I had to take the training, if for no other reason than that its developers had written books with titles like *The Structure of Magic* and *Frogs Into Princes*. As a boy, I wanted to grow up to be a magician. Today, in the guise of a hypnotherapist, I've secretly realized that boyhood wish.

It is probably no coincidence that at the medieval faire, presented at my children's grammar school each fall, my role is that of Merlin the magician. Decked out in conical hat and purple robe with gold trim, I make my way through the crowds handing out "magical Merlin stones" (tumbled amethysts) and telling tales of enchantment to the little ones. Boys and girls greet me with cries of "Wizard, Wizard" and quickly form an entourage, following in my wake as I make the rounds. Supported by the full authority of the set and setting, it is easy to perform numerous dramatic feats of "instant therapy" with these young "clients"—healing the hurt of a bee-sting here, improving sibling relationships there and validating the "princes" and "princesses" who seek acknowledgment.

Toward the end of this year's faire, a 2 1/2 year old girl, with baby-sitter in tow, tracked me down because she had something important she wanted to share. After directing me to sit on the grass, she launched into a description of what it had been like when she was "in her mommy's tummy." She reported that it had been dark and wet, but that the wetness had been warm and she had been comfortable and that it wasn't wet anymore when she had come out into the sunshine. With great delight, I listened to her narration of this charming

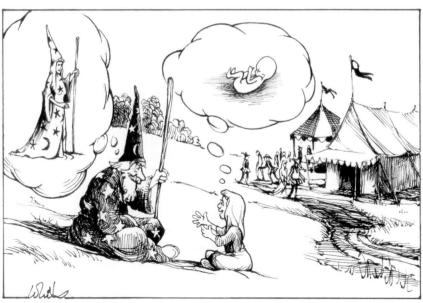

A Shaman in the Making

tale. She also stated that, while inside, she had been visited several times by a "lizard." Being a bit nonplussed by this assertion, I didn't know whether to think of her experience in terms of sensory perceptions or archetypal imagery. In any event, we completed our conversation, introduced ourselves by name and went our separate ways.

After the faire was over, while driving away, I was reflecting on this encounter and then recalled that, whereas the other children had called me "Wizard," she had persisted, despite being given a couple of gentle corrections, in calling me "Lizard"...and she had also talked about being visited by a "lizard" when she was in her mommy's tummy. I wondered if there was something about me that stimulated for her the recall of some in utero experiences. Thinking more about our visit together and recalling her beautiful and unusual name, I was amused by the coincidence of its being the same name as the daughter (whom I had never met) of a former client who had sought assistance in preparing for natural childbirth supported by hypnosis.

Much of my time in those sessions had been spent talking directly to the fetus—offering love, caring, support and guidance. The possibility that the meeting at the faire was something more than mere coincidence was fascinating! Upon arriving home, I rushed to the telephone, called my former client and discovered that her daughter had, indeed, been at the faire with a baby-sitter...and had come home with a glowing report about her conversation with a "lizard." We had a good laugh about the "coincidence," and allowed for the possibility that it might be an example of "synchronicity" at work. After hanging up the telephone and allowing myself some time to mull over the implications of this experience, I concluded that it proved nothing...other than that little children can bring a lot of magic into our adult lives if we allow them to do so.

> *listen:*
> *there's a hell of a good universe next door;*
> *let's go*
> *—e. e. cummings*

While that experience did, indeed, *prove* nothing, it may, perhaps, have suggested a great deal about the way things might be. Through the grapevine, I was able to follow this child's development until she was about five years old—hearing reports of her "chats with angels," of her tales about "the time when she was big and her mommy was little," of her predictions (eventually validated) of future events and of her perceiving and reporting illnesses in others prior to their diagnosis by physicians.

Admittedly, this is just one anecdote—and I don't know if she retained her apparent abilities into adulthood as I had hoped—but it effectively serves to illuminate the potentials inherent in neo-shamanism. Perhaps we are a lot closer to the shamanizing of modern humanity than anyone realizes. Whether we think of Transpersonal Experiences in terms of *wyrd*, the imaginal realm, or the implicate order, maybe, just maybe, a transformation is poised and waiting to happen tomorrow...or the next day...or the day after that.

CHAPTER SUMMARY

⇒ Studies, using the HISS questionnaire, of the following sub-populations of special interest are currently under way: NDEers (Near-Death Experiencers), UFOEers (UFO Experiencers) and CRVers (Controlled Remote Viewers).

⇒ Relative to the Reference Group, the CRV group had high mean scores on the Temperament Type Preferences, Indicators, Emotional, Altered States of Consciousness (ASC) and Transpersonal Experiences (TPE) scales and low mean scores on the Predispositions, Biological and Trauma and Abuse scales. The difference between the CRVers' mean Indicators score and their mean Predispositions score was very noteworthy.

⇒ A determination as to whether or not an individual is an Anomalously Sensitive Person (ASP) can be made, with a reasonable degree of accuracy, from her/his score on the six-question Electro-Magnetic Sensitivities (EMS) scale alone. (See Appendix D.)

⇒ Six objective criteria, when considered collectively, might indicate that an individual would be likely to score toward the high end of the sensitivities continua. Those criteria are: femaleness, hypopigmentation, Non-Right-Handedness, occupation (Artistic, Investigative, or Social), multiple birth and an other-than-conventionally-heterosexual sexual orientation.

⇒ ASCs underlie the manifestations of anomalous sensitivity in all of the realms. Chaotic and stressful ASCs are likely to lead to manifestations of the downsides of anomalous sensitivities; organized and peaceful ASCs are likely to lead to manifestations of the upsides of anomalous sensitivities.

⇒ Management of States of Consciousness (SOCs) has been done for eons by way of techniques such as meditation, drumming, chanting and the like. Today, management of SOCs can be achieved by using EEG biofeedback techniques.

⇒ Modern anthropologists refer to those who, in early historical times, had special facility at managing SOCs as "shamans." Broadly defined, a shaman is: "one who, at will, enters into ASCs in service of her/his community."

⇒ The brainwave patterns of the shamanic SOC are generally in the range of four-to-eight cycles per second. This frequency range corresponds to the EEG theta brainwave pattern, theta being the bridge

241

between alpha and delta in the brainwave pattern of Transpersonal Consciousness (TPC) and the "awakened mind."

⟹ The early Anglo-Saxon shamans helped their people to understand and to live within, the framework of a philosophy they called *"wyrd."* The worldview of *wyrd* is essentially undifferentiable from the concepts of the imaginal realm and the implicate order.

⟹ The "modern" worldview authorizes and even encourages, aggression, exploitation and destruction. We tend to perceive ourselves as separate from and superior to everything else...as well as separate from and superior to each other. The shamanic worldview of *wyrd* provides a viable, life-enhancing alternative. It would permit us to perceive our individual selves as sharing a common identity and a common destiny with all other human beings, to accept all living things as being interconnected and interdependent and to honor the Earth as a living entity vital to our survival.

⟹ Children instinctively understand the philosophy of *wyrd*. If we listen to what they have to tell us, if we internalize the wisdom inherent in their experiences, the prospects for the future might be greatly enhanced.

⟹ Perhaps the shamanizing of modern humanity is poised and waiting to happen tomorrow...or the next day...or the day after that.

242

PART II

The Evidence

CHAPTER 13

A Statistical Primer

There are in fact two things, science and opinion;
the former begets knowledge, the latter ignorance.
—*Hippocrates*

I always find that statistics are hard to swallow
and impossible to digest.
The only one that I can ever remember
is that if all the people who go to sleep in church
were laid end to end,
they would be a lot more comfortable.
—*Mrs. Robert A. Taft*

Two hundred and ninety-five questionnaires, each with 221 responses, generated a lot of data—65,195 data points in all. In order to make sense out of all those data points—to

381% of all statistics are meaningless.
—Anonymous

explore the relationships among them and to transform them into useful information—the use of statistical analysis techniques was required.

Most ASPs (and many other people as well) find statistical studies incomprehensible—yet those are exactly the people for whom the material in this book is likely to prove most valuable. The objective of this chapter is to make the statistics of the HISS research accessible to individuals who have historically shied away from mathematics. Those who are simply not interested in the data can skip this and the following chapter, entirely. Those who already have a working knowledge of basic statistics can bypass this chapter and go directly to Chapter 14.

Thou shalt not sit with statisticians
Nor commit a social science.
—Wystan Hugh Auden

246

PICTURES

There are two basic approaches to statistics—the arithmetic approach and the geometric approach. The arithmetic approach is based on abstract numbers; the geometric approach involves spatial relationships. Spatial relationships entail a visual, or pictorial, representation. For those who are statistically unsophisticated, pictures lend themselves more readily to intuitive understanding than do numbers.

A picture shows me at a glance
what it takes dozens of pages
of a book to expound.
—Ivan Sergeyevich Turgenev

Spatial representations involve dimensions and any discrete observation (datum point) can be described by its location in a theoretically unlimited number of dimensions. In a three-dimensional world, visual representation is practically limited to three dimensions and two-dimensional representation, such as on a graph with an "x" dimension (axis) and a "y" dimension (axis) is generally the norm.

In the analysis of a data series (a collection of multiple data points—such as all of the individual scores for a specific HISS scale), a basic geometric description of the series involves two factors: (1) its location and (2) its dispersion (or variation) around that location. The location of a data series is a function of its central tendency or middle, usually its arithmetic "mean" (the sum of the values of all its data points divided by the number of data points—often spoken of as the "average"). Other common measures of central tendency are the "median" (that value in the series where half of the data points have a higher value and half have a lower value) and the "mode" (that value in the series which occurs most frequently). When data are spoken of as being "normally distributed," it signifies that their mean, their median and their mode are collocated and have the same value. Plotting normally distributed data (such as the height or weight of individuals in a normal population) on a graph results in a "normal" (or bell-shaped) curve, the appearance of which is similar to that of the curve illustrated in Figure 13.1., below. In this hypothetical example, "Scale Scores" are plotted on the "x" axis and the "Number of Subjects" who received each score is plotted on the "y" axis.

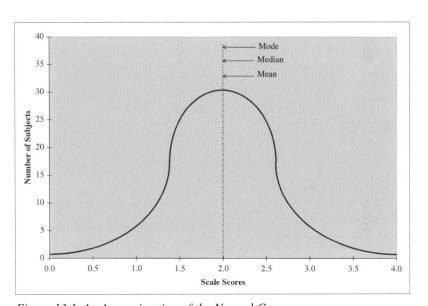

Figure 13.1. An Approximation of the Normal Curve

When the data points are *not* normally distributed, the shape of their graphed curve differs from that of the normal curve (usually involving a loss of symmetry), with the result that the mean, median and mode have different values and are no longer located together. Figure 13.2, next page, illustrates a case in which there are a disproportionately large number (relative to a normal curve) of low-value data points. In a case such as this, the curve (or data) is said to "have a left skew." The data for the majority of actual HISS scales have a strong left skew. When a large number of data points is involved, the statistical errors introduced by this "non-normal" distribution of data are of no great import and the assumption of normal distribution is acceptable.

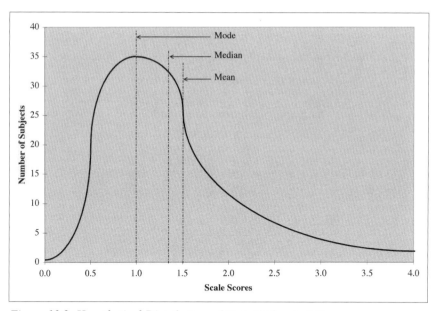

Figure 13.2. Hypothetical Distribution of Data With a Left Skew

The second basic factor used to describe a data series is the dispersion of its points around its mean. The concept of "dispersion" (statistical terms with similar meanings include "variation," "distribution," "deviation," "variability," and "variance") has to do with how far away from their mean the individual data points are located. An illustration will help here.

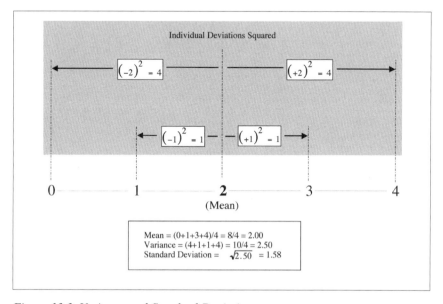

Figure 13.3. Variance and Standard Deviation

Assume that on a scale, four subjects had individual scores of 0, 1, 3 and 4. The arithmetic mean ("average") of their scores is (0+1+3+4)/4, or 2. The four scores deviate from their mean by -2, -1, +1 and +2, respectively. The sum of these deviations is 0. Since, by definition, the sum of the individual deviations for any set of data has the same value of 0, this sum statistic provides no useful information. However, if each deviation is squared (thereby eliminating the minus signs), then their squares are summed and the sum of the squares is divided by the number of data

> *The whole of science
> is nothing more than
> a refinement of
> everyday thinking.*
> *—Albert Einstein*

points—$[(-2)^2+(-1)^2+(+1)^2+(+2)^2]/4$—the result is a meaningful number (2.50) that is commonly called "variance." Although variance has theoretical meaning, it has little practical utility because, while the original data points and their mean are expressed in units, variance is expressed in units squared. That problem can be resolved by taking the square root of the variance ($\sqrt{2.50}$) to arrive at a useful number (1.58), which is commonly called "standard deviation." Since the standard deviation, like the individual data points and their mean, is expressed in units, it can be used, along with the mean, to visualize and describe the data series. All that business about squares and square roots can be very confusing, but it truly is required to arrive at a useful number. Statistical mumbo-jumbo

> *I have yet to see any problem,
> however complicated,
> which, when you look at it in
> the right way,
> did not become
> still more complicated.*
> *—Paul Anderson*

aside, the standard deviation is nothing more than a mathematical convention used to indicate the average distance of the individual data points from their mean.

With normally distributed data, it can be determined that 68.27% of the data points fall within +/- 1 standard deviation, 95.45% fall within +/- 2 standard deviations and 99.73% fall within +/- 3 standard deviations of their mean. Figure 13.4, below, illustrates this distribution. The concept of standard deviations is especially important relative to the HISS data, because HISS scale scores are considered to be anomalously high if they are two or more standard deviations above the mean (i.e., in approximately the top 2%)—and the Anomalously Sensitive Person (ASP) is defined as an individual whose scores on both the first-level Predispositions (PRE) scale and the first-level Indicators (IND) scale are anomalously high.

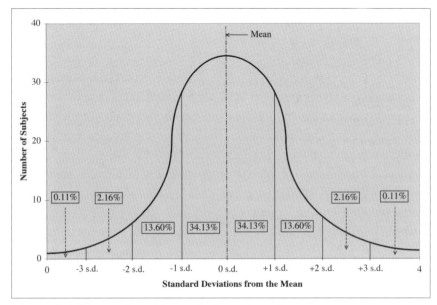

Figure 13.4. Distribution of Scores Under a Normal Curve

CORRELATIONS

Description of the individual data series provides the springboard from which to launch into an analysis of the ways in which different data series are related to each other. "Relationships," "relations," "co-relations," and "correlations" are all the same thing. They have to do with how the different series of data co-relate, with how they co-vary. Correlation is a simple concept and, because of its simplicity, those who equate statistical complexity and sophistication with the validity of the results frequently overlook its efficacy. While it is true that some statistical techniques are better than others at unearthing subtleties hidden within the data, most of the relationships among the HISS data are anything but subtle and the simplest technique—the analysis of correlations—appeared to be the most appropriate one.

The specific methodology used for analysis of correlations within the HISS data was the "Pearson Product-Moment Coefficient of Correlation of Paired Data." The Pearson Technique is designed to generate a single, meaningful, numerical value—called the "coefficient of correlation" (mathematically represented as "r")—that indicates the strength of the correlation between two data series. It is simply a quantification of the linear relationship that exists between two series of paired data—and has a two-decimal numerical value between +1.00 and -1.00. The closer that number ("r" value) is to 1 (either plus or minus), the stronger is the correlation (either positive or negative) it represents.

251

The formula for the Pearson Technique is even more daunting than is its formal name, but using it is simple, thanks to the wizardry of personal computers and the Microsoft® Excel spreadsheet program. The program can do the calculations with just a couple of mouse-clicks and it can generate what is called a "scatter diagram" of the relationship between the two data series, as well. The scatter diagram is a two-dimensional graphical representation of the distribution of one data series (plotted on the "x" axis) in relation to the other data series (plotted on the "y" axis). A best-fit "line of regression," the formula for that line and the value of "r^2" (to be discussed shortly), can also be added to this scatter diagram. The whole procedure is commonly spoken of as "regression analysis." It requires some further explanation, but first it would be helpful to establish context by looking at the example in Figure 13.5., below—a regression analysis

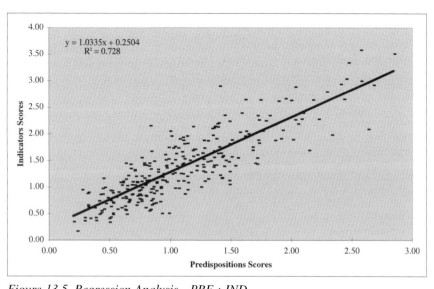

Figure 13.5. Regression Analysis—PRE : IND

of the relationship between the actual scores for the HISS first-level Predispositions (PRE) and Indicators (IND) scales.

The coefficient of correlation, "r" (in this case with a value of .85), as previously mentioned, is a measure of the linear relationship between the "x" and "y" variables. The nature of that relationship is further described by the formula for the best-fit line of regression— a line drawn on the scatter diagram in such a way that the dispersion of the data points around that line is minimized.[†] The best-fit line of regression is a graphical tool that can be used for predicting "y" axis values from "x" axis values (or vice-versa)—by locating the point on the line of regression that corresponds to the specific "x" axis value (PRE score) and then locating the "y" axis value (IND score) that corresponds to that point on the line of regression. The higher the "r" value, the greater will be the level of accuracy of the prediction.

Perfect correlation (r = 1.00) allows for perfect (100% reliable) prediction, but perfect correlation seldom occurs in the real world and almost never in the world of the social sciences. When the value of "r" is anything less than 1.00, it is not directly indicative of the predictive reliability of the relationship— an "r" of .85, as in the PRE : IND relationship, for example, does not mean that a specific PRE score can predict a specific IND score at an 85% level of accuracy. Squaring "r," however, results in a number (in this case .73) that does provide a more appropriate assessment of predictive reliability. Again, though, this does not mean that a specific PRE score can predict a specific IND score at a 73% level of accuracy. What it does mean is that 73% of the variability in one set of scores can be accounted for by the variability in the other set of scores. For linguistic simplicity, however, the "r^2" value will be spoken of as the "predictive reliability" inherent in a relationship. Graphically, "r^2" is the scatter (or lack of it) of the individual data points around the line of regression—the higher the "r^2" value, the less the scatter.

[†] The formula for the line of regression is, in its general form: $y = bx + a$. In this formula, "b" is the slope of the line and "a" is the point at which the line intersects the "y" axis.

The predictive reliability of a correlation is the basis for the concept of "correlational strength." For discussion purposes, the following qualitative terms for correlational strength will be used:

Correlation Coefficient (r)	Predictive Reliability (r^2)	Correlational Strength
.00 – .10	00% – 01%	None
.10 – .20	01% – 04%	Minimal
.20 – .40	04% – 16%	Weak
.40 – .60	16% – 36%	Moderate
.60 - .80	36% – 64%	Strong
.80 – 1.00	64% – 100%	Very Strong

Table 13.1. Predictive Reliability and Correlational Strength

In the context of this book, for a correlation between two HISS data series to be considered "strong" or better, it must have an "r" value of at least .60—that is, a predictive reliability ("r²") of 36% or higher. The previously discussed "r" value (correlation coefficient) of .85 between the HISS first-level PRE and IND scales yields an "r²" value (predictive reliability) of .73. That means that the predictive reliability of the relationship is 73% and the correlation can be considered to be "very strong."

PROBABILITIES

The final statistical concept to be dealt with here is that of probability—mathematically represented as "p." Probability goes hand-in-hand with the coefficient of correlation. If the coefficient of correlation between two data series and the number of data points in the series are both known,

The theory of probabilities
is at bottom
nothing but common sense
reduced to calculus.
—Pierre Simon de Laplace

the statistical probability of the chance occurrence of their relationship can be readily calculated. In academic papers, the correlation coefficient and its associated probability usually appear together like this: r = .19 (p < .001). This notation means that when the correlation coefficient between two series of paired data (in this case, HISS data with 295 data points in each series) has a value of .19, the probability of that correlation occurring by chance alone is less than 1 in 1000.

In the social sciences, a correlation with a probability of chance occurrence of less than 1 in 20 ($p < .05$) is generally considered to be a relatively uncommon occurrence and is said to be "statistically significant." A correlation with a probability of chance occurrence of less than 1 in 100 ($p < .01$) is considered to be a very uncommon occurrence and is said to be "statistically very significant."

This rule of thumb about degrees of uncommonness applies to a single specific correlation. In a study involving multiple correlations, the more of them there are, the greater is the likelihood that some of them will exhibit statistical significance strictly by chance. Among 20 correlations, chance occurrence is likely to result in 1 being statistically significant and among 100 correlations, chance occurrence is likely to result in 1 being statistically very significant. Among the 32 HISS scales in the first-, second- and third-level PRE and IND groupings, there are 527 possible correlations. On the basis of chance alone, 26 of them are likely to be statistically significant and 5 of them are likely to be statistically very significant. Because of the large number of correlations among the HISS data, relatively stringent criteria for statistical significance seemed to be called for. After calculating the probabilities associated with various "r" values for 295 paired data points (the higher the number of data points, the greater the statistical significance associated with a given "r" value), the following qualitative criteria for statistical significance in the HISS data appeared to be appropriate:

> *Life is finite. Time is infinite.*
> *The probability that I am alive today is zero.*
> *In spite of this, I am now alive.*
> *Now how is that?*
> —*Albert Einstein*

Correlation Coefficient (r)	Probability (p)	Statistical Significance
< .10	> .05	Not Significant
.10	< .05	Minimally Significant
.15	< .01	Moderately Significant
.19	< .001	Quite Significant
.23	< .0001	Very Significant

Table 13.2. Statistical Significance of HISS Correlation Coefficients

Note that "correlational strength" (or "predictive reliability") and "statistical significance" are two very different concepts. A relationship between two series of HISS paired data with a correlation coefficient of .23 is statistically very significant (with a probability of chance occurrence of less than 1 in 10,000), but its correlational strength is weak (with a predictive reliability of only 5%). In other words, while the relationship is a very uncommon occurrence, it is not sufficiently uncommon to have any utility in making

I am from Missouri.
You have got to show me.
—William Duncan Vandiver

255

statistical predictions. By now it has probably become clear that the use of ordinary language to discuss mathematical constructs can be very confusing. That is why abbreviated mathematical notations— such as "r = .xx (p < .yyy)"—are commonly used. Such notations, however, mean little to those who don't use them regularly. Therefore, whenever practicable, I shall try to present important findings from the HISS data in geometric (graphical) form as well as in the more common arithmetic form.

Among the second-level HISS scales encompassed by the Predispositions grouping—Biological (BIO), Trauma and Abuse (TAB) and Temperament Type Preferences (TTP)—and the Indicators grouping—Physiological (PHS), Cognitive (COG), Emotional (EMO), Altered States of Consciousness (ASC) and Transpersonal Experiences (TPE)—the lowest correlation coefficient value for any two sets of scores is .38. The probability of chance occurrence at that "r" value is less than 1 in a billion. The 28 correlations among those eight scales have an average "r" value of .63. The probability of chance occurrence at that "r" value is unknown because my computer stops calculating beyond a probability of less than 1 in a trillion (p < .000,000,000,001), where, with 295 data points in a series, the "r" value is .40. A probability smaller than that is considered to be effectively a probability of zero. Correlations for almost all the third-level and fourth-level scales in the PRE and IND groupings, as well as many of the individual questions, have "r" values considerably greater than the very significant .23—they are statistically very, very significant, or very, very, very significant, or…The repetition of "verys" with increasing orders of magnitude could quickly become overwhelmingly cumbersome—in many cases, there would be 20 or more of them. Suffice it to say that the correlations among the vast majority of the various HISS scales are such that their statistical significance is not open to question and little more will be said on this subject—except in cases where relationships are

256

Mathematics may be defined as the subject in which we never know what we are talking about, nor whether what we are saying is true.
—Bertrand Russell

exceptionally strong (r > .80) or relatively weak (r < .19) compared to the others. In any event, most discussions of the data will be couched in the language of "predictive reliability" ("r²" value)—a concept that is likely to make more sense to the layperson.

For most people, with numbers such as a million (1,000,000), a billion (1,000,000,000), or a trillion (1,000,000,000,000), the meaning of all those zeros tends to get lost—in the words of one typical, non-mathematically-inclined, ASP, "After all, what is a zero? It's nothing."† That's why graphical representations of the relationships can be especially helpful. Instead of having to deal with a bunch of seemingly meaningless numbers, often involving long strings of zeros, one gets to look at a picture in which the relationships, the patterns, the peaks and valleys of the data can be perceived visually. While probabilities are easier to grasp, intuitively, than are correlation coefficients, they are, unfortunately, very awkward to use graphically. Therefore, "r"

Mathematics takes us still further from what is human.
—Bertrand Russell

values, rather than "p" values, will be used in subsequent graphical presentations, but there is no need to concern oneself with the actual numbers. It is the relationships that are important and the relationships will be immediately apparent in the pictorial representations. Particularly noteworthy relationships will also be discussed in the text.

† Here is an example: In Chapter 11, it was stated that the storage capacity of the brain is equivalent to that of one hundred and forty trillion high-density computer floppy disks. If all those disks were stacked on top of one another, how high would the stack reach? To the top of the Empire State Building? To the top of Mount Everest? To the Moon? Well, actually it would be a bit farther than that. 140,000,000,000,000 computer floppy disks, each 1/8" thick, would make a stack 1,400,000,000,000 feet high. That's 265,000,000 miles — or approximately 3 times the mean distance from the Earth to the sun.

ADDITIONAL POINTS

Before moving on to a discussion of what the HISS data reveal, there are a few more points about statistical methodologies and interpretation that warrant attention:

- As mentioned earlier, the Pearson Technique is a relatively simple and unsophisticated statistical tool. Some people object to its use because of its potential for being influenced by a few outlying data points. If the relationships being explored were at the 1 in 100 probability level, that would be a legitimate concern; at the 1 in 10,000 (and up) level, it can generally be dismissed.

- When required, additional statistical analysis tools such as the "chi square distribution," "analysis of variance," and "factor analysis" were used, but understanding them is not a prerequisite for understanding the findings.
- Twelve questionnaires were eliminated from among the 307 originally received—either because they were incomplete, or because the responses were internally inconsistent (see Appendix E, "Double-Checking," for a discussion of the Skew scales). Other than that, nothing has been done to make the data look better.
- Statistical weighting is often used to make a Reference Group more representative of the general population. With the HISS, weighting of the data was ruled out because the sample was too small to reasonably allow for extrapolation to the population at large, no matter what fancy statistical techniques might be used. Moreover, weighting would involve judgment calls that could lead to controversy and create needless red herrings.
- "Winsorizing" of data involves deleting a certain percentage of both the highest and lowest scores from a Reference Group, based on the assumption that those scores are statistical anomalies. Of particular interest in the HISS are those anomalously high scores (i.e., in the top 2%) that make the Anomalously Sensitive Person (ASP) anomalous. The Winsorizing procedure would have eliminated all ASPs from the Reference Group, so it was not used.
- Correlations, no matter how strong they might be, do not address issues of cause and effect. The labeling of one

258

grouping of scales as "Predispositions" and another grouping of scales as "Indicators," and the two groupings of scales being very strongly correlated at the level of r = .85, does not necessarily mean that Predispositions (toward sensitivities) cause Indicators (of sensitivities). The labels are nothing more than a reflection of the original hypothesis. Perhaps Indicators cause Predispositions, or perhaps neither causes the other—perhaps they are just co-related. To drive this point home, the following example is offered: Shoe size and handwriting quality are strongly correlated. Is there a cause and effect relationship? If not, why not ... and why do they happen to be co-related? (See the footnote below for the answer.[†])

• While the findings from the HISS data may *provide strong evidence* in support of the original ASP hypothesis, they actually *prove nothing*. Proof is a very slippery concept. At the very least it requires that the experimenter have control over and be able to manipulate, the variables—a situation that obviously did not pertain to the administration of the HISS. Most readers have probably seen tabloid headlines screaming something like: "SCIENTIFIC PROOF OF ABDUCTION BY ALIENS!" Rest assured, it is not.

There are quite a few very intriguing findings associated with the HISS data. The next chapter addresses the more significant ones among them.

[†] Up to a point, shoe size increases with age. Similarly, up to a point, handwriting quality increases with age. Shoe size and handwriting quality are strongly correlated.

CHAPTER SUMMARY

⇒ Two hundred and ninety-five questionnaires, each with 221 responses, generated 65,195 data points. Making sense out of all those data points required the use of statistical analysis techniques.

⇒ Statistical analysis can be approached either arithmetically or geometrically. The arithmetic approach is based on abstract numbers; the geometric approach is based on spatial relationships. For those who are statistically unsophisticated, the geometric approach is easier to grasp intuitively.

259

⇒ A datum *point* can be described geometrically by its location in two dimensions—the "x" dimension (axis) and the "y" dimension (axis) on a graph.

⇒ A data *series* can be described geometrically by: (1) the location of the arithmetic mean of its data points and (2) the dispersion (or variation) of the data points around that mean.

⇒ Most statistical analysis techniques are grounded in the theoretical assumption of "normally distributed" data—i.e., plotting the data points on a graph produces a "normal" (or bell-shaped) curve and their mean, median and mode are collocated and have the same value. In practice, data are often not normally distributed, but the resulting statistical errors are generally not cause for concern. Most of the HISS data have a strong "left skew"—that is, relative to normally distributed data, there are a disproportionately large number of low-value data points.

⇒ An Anomalously Sensitive Person (ASP) is defined, statistically, as an individual whose scores on both the first-level Predispositions (PRE) scale and the first-level Indicators (IND) scale are two or more standard deviations above the mean (i.e., roughly in the top 2%).

⇒ Correlations have to do with how two series of paired data are co-related—with how they fit together and vary together. Analysis of correlations (by way of the Pearson Technique) was the primary statistical technique used to explore the HISS data. The "coefficient of correlation" (mathematically represented by "r"), with a two decimal numerical value between +1.00 and -1.00, represents the strength of the correlation between two data series. The closer that number is to 1 (either plus or minus), the stronger is the correlation (either positive or negative).

260

⟹   Regression analysis, a statistical tool based on correlations, can be used to predict the value of one variable from the value of another variable. The "predictive reliability" (the variability in one data series that can be accounted for by the variability in the other data series) of a correlation, expressed as a percentage, is the square of its "r" value.

⟹   The probability of a correlation between two series of paired data occurring strictly by chance can be determined from the correlation's "r" value and the number of data points in the series. In the social sciences, a correlation with a probability of chance occurrence of less than 1 in 20 ($p < .05$) is said to be "statistically significant"; a correlation with a probability of chance occurrence of less than 1 in 100 ($p < .01$) is said to be "statistically very significant."

⟹   The "statistical significance" and "correlational strength" (or "predictive reliability") of a correlation are very different concepts. A correlation can be statistically very significant ($p < .0001$) while the predictive reliability of that correlation is weak ($r^2 = 5\%$). The probability of the correlation between scores on any two second-level HISS scales occurring strictly by chance, however, is less than 1 in a billion.

⟹   Very little was done to make the HISS data look better. Other than the elimination of twelve questionnaires, either because they were incomplete or because their responses were internally inconsistent, the data were analyzed as they originally appeared.

⟹   Correlations, no matter how strong they might be, do not address issues of cause and effect.

⟹   While findings from the HISS data *provide strong evidence* in support of the original **ASP** hypothesis, they actually *prove nothing.*

Chapter 14

The Findings

There is something fascinating about science.
One gets such wholesale returns of conjecture
out of such trifling investment of facts.
—Mark Twain

Facts are stubborn things;
and whatever may be our wishes, our inclinations,
or the dictates of our passions, they cannot alter
the state of facts and evidence.
—John Adams

Age, occupation and education are three demographic variables inquired about in most questionnaires. The HISS is no exception. These factors, however, are considered to be neither Predispositions (PRE) toward sensitivities nor Indicators (IND) of sensitivities and hence are not emcompassed by any HISS scale. Nevertheless, they were included so as to determine what relationships, if any, they might have with the scaled variables.

Age wasn't significantly correlated with anything—but then

there were only fourteen subjects in the Reference Group who were less than 21 years old.

Occupation, by "Strong Vocational Inventory Blank (SVIB)" categories, showed clear-cut differences in scores on the PRE, IND and TPE (and presumably most, if not all, other) scales (the patterns for each being similar). On the IND scale, for example, mean scores for the occupational categories were, in descending order: Artistic (music, dramatics, art, writing, etc.)—1.62, Investigative (science, medical science, mathematics, etc.)—1.43, Social (social service, religion, athletics, domestic arts, etc.)—1.27, Enterprising (public speaking, politics, merchandising, sales, business management, etc.)—1.21, Conventional (office practices, etc.)—1.14 and Realistic (agriculture, nature, military, mechanical, etc.)—1.00. Figure 14.1, below, illustrates this ranking graphically.[†]

262

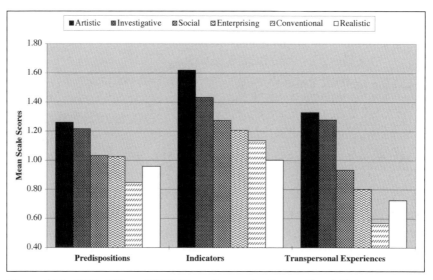

Figure 14.1. PRE, IND and TPE Mean Scores By Occupational Category

Educational level, on the surface, did not appear to show meaningful relationships with PRE, IND, or TPE scores. This may have been due, in part, to the "ceiling effect" (to be discussed shortly) resulting from the Reference Group being extremely well educated—

[†] PRE scores and TPE scores for the "Conventional" category are somewhat suppressed relative to the IND scores. Most likely, this is a statistical artifact resulting from the small number (19) of subjects in that category.

most subjects had at least some college education. There were, however, some indirect clues in the data to the effect that individuals with higher education levels might have an elevated frequency of Transpersonal Experiences (TPEs). For example, subjects in the three occupational categories with the highest TPE scores (mean of 1.02) had a mean educational level of 16.01 years, while those in the three occupational categories with the lowest TPE scores (mean of 0.71) had a mean education level of 15.21 years. Statistically, the difference is insignificant, but it is suggestive when considered together with other similarly subtle findings.

263

An exemplary Reference Group is randomly selected and is representative of the population at large, but such an ideal is seldom attainable. In the HISS project, as with most other research efforts in the social sciences, it was necessary to settle for a sample of convenience. As a result, the Reference Group had some compositional imbalances. The most obvious of these were that it was:

- too female—62% were female;
- too white—86% were of full European ethnicity;
- too educated—41% had some graduate-level education and the mean education level was 15.7 years; and
- too human-services oriented—66% had "Social" occupations.

The available data suggest that all four of these factors are, to a certain extent, associated with high HISS scores. Correction of the sampling imbalances (either by weighting of scores or by obtaining additional questionnaires from selected new subjects) would, then, increase the left skews of the various HISS scale scores, rather than making the distribution of the data more normal. That would result in a further lowering of mean scores, with scores that are high (in absolute terms) becoming even more anomalous.

One of the primary reasons for imposing normalization criteria on a Reference Group is to legitimize the use of statistical techniques for extrapolating results from that group to the entire population, but such an extrapolation is risky under the best of circumstances—and given that the HISS Reference Group is not truly representative of any population other than itself, it seemed best to avoid doing that. A reminder is therefore in order: The use of the term "Anomalously Sensitive Persons (ASPs)" is technically appropriate only when referring to those ten individuals in the Reference Group who scored two or more standard deviations above the mean on both the first-level Predispositions (PRE) scale and the first-level Indicators (IND) scale. Other people in the general population who have

There are three kinds of untruths; lies, damn lies, and statistics.
—Benjamin Disraeli
(attributed)

characteristics similar to those ten may, indeed, be ASPs, but such an assumption is not entirely valid from a statistical perspective.

OVERVIEW

Establishing a context for discussion of the findings arising out of the HISS data requires a bit more discussion of the difference between mean scores and mode scores. The statistical analysis of the data, as stated in Chapter 13, was performed on the basis of mean scores and standard deviations. Since the mean score is generally spoken of as the "average" score, one is inclined to think of it as representing the "average" person—which it does—but most people tend to think of the "average" person as the one who is "normal," "ordinary," or "most frequently represented" … and that would be the person whose scores fall at the mode of the data.

With data that is normally distributed, this differentiation would be irrelevant because the mean and the mode scores would have the same value. With the strong left skew in the HISS data, however, mode scores are considerably lower than mean scores. Consider the HISS first-level IND scale, for example. If the data were normally distributed in the range of possible scores from 0 to 4, the mode, median and mean would all be 2.00. However, the actual mode score for the Reference Group is 1.09, the actual median score is 1.27 and the actual mean score is 1.36—and the actual standard deviation from the mean is 0.62. A similar pattern holds for most other HISS scales—the data for the PRE, IND and TPE scales in Table 14.1., below, being illustrative. What this suggests is that the

	PRE	IND	TPE
Mode	0.76	1.09	0.11
Median	0.96	1.27	0.67
Mean	1.08	1.36	0.90
Std. Deviation	0.51	0.62	0.85

Table 14.1. Modes, Medians, Means and Standard Deviations—PRE, IND and TPE Scales

individual who scores at the mean of the IND scale is actually considerably more sensitive (25%) than the (modal) "norm"—and this effect is magnified enormously on the TPE scale.

The mode scores being substantively lower than the mean scores is indicative of the disproportionately large number (relative to a normal curve) of scores that fall toward the lower end of the score range (both possible and actual). This distribution of scores is illustrated in Figure 14.2, below—a plot of the Reference Group's scores on the PRE, IND and TPE scales. Observe that TPE scores have a stronger left skew than do PRE scores and that PRE scores have a stronger left skew than do IND scores. In terms of absolute values, high IND scores are relatively uncommon, high PRE scores are more uncommon and high TPE scores are the most uncommon of all. The amount of skew for a given scale reflects the degree of uncommonness (among the Reference Group) of the traits or experiences that scale represents.[†]

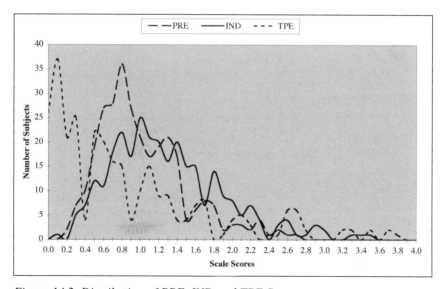

Figure 14.2. Distribution of PRE, IND and TPE Scores

[†] Interestingly, on an earlier version of the HISS, scores for beliefs in the objective reality of transpersonal *phenomena* had a right skew rather than a left skew. This finding appears to affirm anecdotal observations to the effect that beliefs are not a key factor influencing frequency of Transpersonal Experiences.

This clustering of scores in a very narrow low-end range results in something called the "floor effect"—meaning that there simply isn't enough room for strong correlations to come into play in that portion of the score range. A similar "ceiling effect" can also occur at the high end. Illustratively, for the Reference Group the overall correlation between the PRE and IND scale scores has an "r" value of .85 (72% predictive reliability). When the Reference Group is divided into thirds (by high, mid-range and low absolute scores for the IND scale), the "r" values of the correlations for the high and low thirds are substantially lower—for the high third it becomes .70 (49% predictive reliability) and for the low third it becomes .49 (24% predictive reliability).

Another consequence of the floor effect is that a relatively small number of scores fall one or more standard deviations below the mean.† With a normal curve, 16% of the scores on a scale (47 Reference Group subjects) would be one or more standard deviations below the mean. Because of the HISS data's left skew, however, only 4.7% (14 Reference Group subjects) of the TPE scale scores, for example, are that low. Similarly, with a normal curve, 16% of the scores on a scale would fall one or more standard deviations above the mean and 2% (6 Reference Group subjects) would fall two or more standard deviations above the mean (the criterion for an anomalously high score). Whereas the left skew of the data reduces the number of anomalously low scores, it increases the number of anomalously high scores. This results in 5.8% (17) of the Reference Group subjects having anomalously high scores on the first-level PRE scale and 5.8% (17) of the Reference Group subjects having anomalously high scores on the first-level IND scale. Ten (3.4%) of the Reference Group subjects have anomalously high scores on both of these scales—and thus meet the statistical criteria by which the basic **Anomalously Sensitive Person (ASP)** has been defined.

As previously stated, the correlations among scores for the various HISS scales are unusually strong relative to most statistical findings in the social sciences. The weakest correlation between scores on any two second-level scales (the BIO : TTP correlation) has an "r" value of .38, which indicates a probability of chance occurrence

---

† Note, in Table 14.1., page 264, that it is essentially impossible to score more than two standard deviations below the mean on the Predispositions and Indicators scales, or one standard deviation below the mean on the Transpersonal Experiences scale.

of less than one in a billion (p < .000,000,001). Table 14.2., below, delineates the "r" values for all 45 of the correlations among first- and second-level scales in the PRE and IND groupings.[†]

| | #100 | #110 | #120 | #130 | #200 | #210 | #220 | #230 | #240 | #250 |
	PRE	BIO	TAB	TTP	IND	PHS	COG	EMO	ASC	TPE
PRE	1.00	.81	.89	.76	.85	.80	.66	.71	.78	.77
BIO		1.00	.63	.38	.63	.65	.51	.53	.54	.55
TAB			1.00	.52	.74	.69	.52	.60	.71	.69
TTP				1.00	.73	.64	.60	.64	.68	.66
IND					1.00	.94	.77	.88	.92	.86
PHS						1.00	.68	.83	.84	.75
COG							1.00	.63	.67	.50
EMO								1.00	.75	.66
ASC									1.00	.78
TPE										1.00

Table 14.2. Correlation Coefficients Among First- and Second-Level PRE and IND Scales

267

A graphical representation might also be helpful in understanding the meaning of these data. In developing Figure 14.3., next page, the Reference Group subjects were broken out into high, middle and low thirds (by their absolute scores on the TPE scale) and the mean scores for each third on each of the first- and second-level PRE and IND scales were then plotted on the graph. For every scale represented, those subjects who had high TPE scores (solidly shaded columns) scored higher, on average, than did those who had mid-range TPE scores (crosshatched columns) and those who had mid-range TPE scores scored higher, on average, than did those who had low TPE scores (unshaded columns). The same pattern would hold if the breakout into thirds had been handled by scores on any of the other represented scales. All correlations among these scales are statistically very significant and most of them have strong or very strong predictive reliability for one another.

Clearly the scale scores do not exhibit *statistical* independence—their covariance (the degree to which the scores on one scale vary with variance in the scores on another) is extremely

[†] Note that the numbers in the cells of this and other, tables (in keeping with convention) are "r" values (i.e., coefficients of correlation), whereas "r²" values (predictive reliability) are spoken of in the text (because they are likely to be more meaningful to the layperson.) The format of this table will be used for all similar tables (in this chapter and in Appendix E, "Double-Checking") showing correlation coefficients. Scale numbers and scale name abbreviations appear in the top two rows; scale name abbreviations appear in the left column. See Appendix B, "Index of HISS Scales" for all scale numbers, names (which, remember, are only convenient labels, not definitive theoretical constructs) and name abbreviations. See Appendix C, "Composition of HISS Scales" for a listing of the responses that comprise each scale.

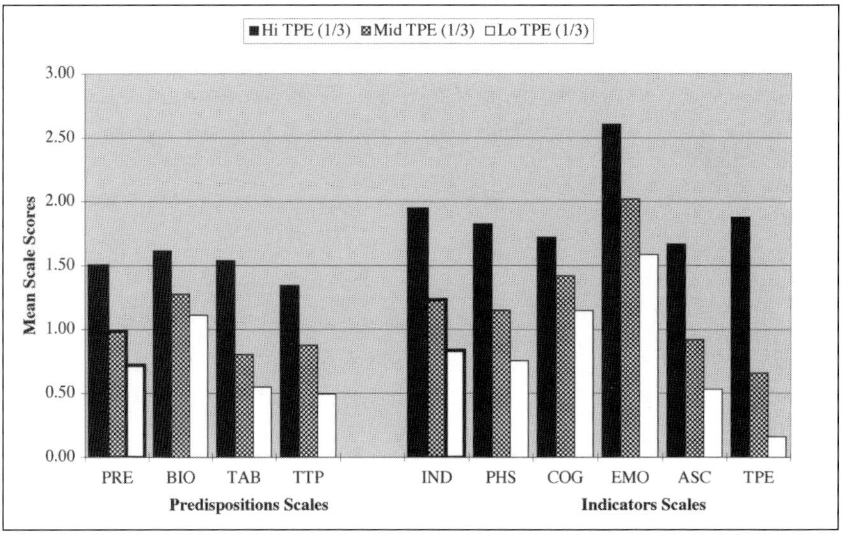

Figure 14.3. Mean Scale Scores By Hi/Mid/Lo Thirds (TPE)

high. That's appropriate; that's what strong correlations are all about. From a purely statistical perspective, it can be said that the HISS scales are measuring the same thing—they are measuring sensitivities (either Predispositions toward sensitivities or Indicators of sensitivities).

The correlational strengths are so high, however, as to raise some concerns about their *functional* independence—as to whether or not the sensitivities they are measuring are truly different types of sensitivities. An example of this issue, at the level of the individual question, might be helpful. Experiencing, for no apparent reason, the sensation of a strong unpleasant taste (HISS question #129) and experiencing, for no apparent reason, the sensation of a strong unpleasant odor (HISS question #139), are most likely not functionally independent variables. Both involve sensory processing, the gustatory and olfactory senses are closely linked and both sensations occur in the apparent absence of corresponding stimuli in consensus reality. Because the variables appear not to be functionally independent, the responses to the questions are scored in the same HISS scale (Hallucination [HAL]).

On the other hand, being born as one of a set of twins, triplets, etc. (HISS question #[6]) and frequency of experience of alien contact (HISS question #181) definitely appear to be functionally independent variables and they are scored in different scales (the former is scored in the Biological [BIO] scale and the latter is scored in the Transpersonal Experiences [TPE] scale). Nevertheless, the responses to these questions are correlated at an "r" value of .28 (a probability of chance occurrence of less than 1 in 100,000). One would be hard pressed to argue that multiple births and alien contact experiences are essentially the same thing (but then again, some UFO researchers...). There is no clear-cut resolution to this issue. Ultimately it ends up being a judgment call (even more so for scales than it is for responses to individual questions).

The most merciful thing in the world, I think, is the inability of the human mind to correlate all its contents.
—*H. P. Lovecraft*

269

While it seems clear that the organization of the HISS scales in the PRE and IND groupings meets any reasonable criterion for functional independence, exploring the issue inevitably leads one to the recognition that neurophysiological structuring (specifically whether or not the brain is Less Strongly Lateralized [LSL] than the norm) appears to be a significant factor influencing scores on all of the scales. Consider, for example:

- Biological predispositions involve factors such as sex and handedness, both of which have neurological implications;
- Trauma and Abuse have been shown to be associated with Temporo-Limbic Epilepsy and with dissociation, both of which are influenced by neurology;
- Temperament Type Preferences involve Introverted/Extraverted Orientation, iNtuitive/Sensate strategies for Perceiving and Feeling/Thinking strategies for Judging, all of which are affected by the way one is "wired up";
- Physiological indicators include sensitivities to external stimuli and sensitivity to psychogenic illness, both of which involve neurological mechanisms;
- Cognitive indicators include Learning, Attention and Mnemonic style differences, all of which clearly have neurological components;

- Emotional indicators include both Intrapersonal and Interpersonal sensitivities and are presumably strongly influenced by the limbic system;
- Altered States of Consciousness indicators include sensitivities to Dissociation, Hallucination, Sleep/wake overlap, Association and Suggestibility, all of which are heightened by increased inter-hemispheric communication; and
- Transpersonal Experiences indicators are associated with Temporo-Limbic Epilepsy and with hypnogogia, both of which are characterized by anomalous brainwave patterns.

270

Given that every one of the 45 relationships among the first- and second-level PRE and IND scales is statistically very significant, it is informative to explore their *relative* significance—so as to determine which of the second-level scales have notably stronger, or notably weaker, relationships with the others than the norm. Figure 14.4, below, proves helpful in this respect by illustrating graphically the "peaks and valleys" in the correlational strengths.

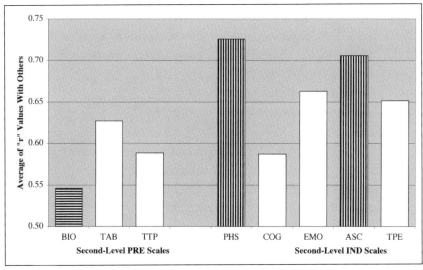

Figure 14.4. Average Correlational Strength of Each Second-Level PRE and IND Scale with the Others

The "y" axis value for each represented scale is the mean of its correlation coefficients ("r") with all other second-level PRE and IND scales. Those scales with a "y" axis value of one or more standard deviations above the mean of the "y" axis values of all represented scales are represented by vertically striped columns and can be considered to have notably stronger correlations than the norm. Those scales with a "y" axis value one or more standard deviations below the mean are represented by horizontally striped columns and can be considered to have notably weaker relationships than the norm. Those scales with no noteworthy (less than one standard deviation) difference from the norm are represented by unshaded columns. Physiological (PHS) indicators and Altered States of Consciousness (ASC) indicators form the two true peaks; Biological (BIO) predispositions form the one true valley.

271

The relatively low correlational strengths of the BIO predispositions scale are to be expected. The nature of the questions included in that scale is qualitatively different from that of the questions included in the other scales. The questions in the BIO scale have to do with objective, physical data; the questions in the other scales have to do with subjective experiences, perceptions and preferences.

The relatively high correlational strengths of the PHS and ASC indicators scales will be discussed in some depth shortly, but for now suffice it to say that they probably reflect the especially significant import of the neurophysiological structuring factor in those realms. Admittedly, there is only circumstantial evidence to go on, but …

> *Some circumstantial evidence is very strong,*
> *as when you find a trout in the milk.*
> *—Henry David Thoreau*

A variety of statistical tools were used to check the validity and reliability of the HISS. Discussion of them is likely to be of interest only to researchers and has, therefore, been relegated to Appendix E, "Double-Checking."

The rest of this chapter will be devoted to discussing the more noteworthy HISS findings. It will be divided into sections that correspond to the second-level scales in the Predispositions (PRE) and Indicators (IND) groupings and the third-level scales in the Explanatory (EXP) grouping.

Biological (BIO) Scale Scores

The second-level Biological (BIO) predispositions scale (see Chapter 4 for additional information) encompasses two third-level scales: Anomalous Cerebral Laterality (ACL) and Star (STR). Questions in the ACL scale have to do with such things as sex, birth order and handedness and were suggested primarily by Geschwind and Galaburda's Anomalous Cerebral Laterality (ACL) research. Questions in the STR scale have to do with such things as body temperature and blood pressure and were suggested by Steiger's "Star People" research. The correlation coefficients between the various BIO scales and other selected scales are shown in Table 14.3., below.

	#111 ACL	#112 STR	#110 BIO	#100 PRE	#250 TPE	#200 IND
ACL	1.00	.35	.69	.59	.46	.47
STR		1.00	.92	.73	.46	.57
BIO			1.00	.81	.55	.63

Table 14.3. Correlation Coefficients of Biological Scales

The predictive reliability of scores on the BIO scale for scores on the first-level IND scale is a strong 40%. Of all the second-level scales, however, the BIO scale scores have the weakest average correlational strength with the others—presumably because, as previously explained, its questions are about objective, physical data rather than about subjective experiences, perceptions and preferences. Factor analysis shows that, unlike most other scales, the individual items in the BIO scale appear to represent separate and distinct variables.

> *It is a test of true theories not only to account for but to predict phenomena.*
> *— William Whewell*

Among the ACL-related questions in the BIO scale, some had utility in the HISS findings and some didn't. Those that didn't were:

- Season of Birth—showed no significant correlation with anything else in the HISS;

- Latitude of Birth, Ethnicity and Pigmentation—Reference Group data was not sufficiently distributed to determine if significant relationships existed; and
- Birth Order and Parity—An error in the development of the HISS questionnaire occurred with respect to this item. The ACL theory appears to suggest that people who were either first-born, or were born four or more years after their next older sibling, would show elevated IND scores —but the reverse was found to be true. A review of the theory indicated that maternal age at birth is hypothesized to be a more influential factor than birth order and parity—the higher the maternal age, the higher the expected scores. First-borns (who are heavily represented in the Reference Group), however, are usually born to young mothers and the HISS had not even asked about maternal age. This error has been corrected in subsequent versions of the HISS.

273

The capacity to leap across mountains of information
to land lightly on the wrong side
represents the highest of human endowments.
—Lewis Thomas

Some of the useful items in the BIO scale, derived from the ACL theory, were two-point variables—that is, only two response options were available. For statistical reasons, a tool known as analysis of the "Chi Squared Distribution" (rather than the Pearson Technique) was employed to determine their significance. As shown in Table 14.4., next page, the last line of which indicates the probability of chance occurrence for the difference in the mean Indicators scale scores, it was found that in the Reference Group mean scores are:

- higher for women than they are for men;
- higher for Non-Right-Handers than they are for right-handers;
- higher for those who were born as one of a multiple birth (twins/triplets/etc.) than they are for those who had a solo birth; and
- higher for those whose sexual orientation is other-than-conventionally heterosexual than they are for those whose sexual orientation is conventionally heterosexual.

	Sex		Handedness		Birth Type		Sexual Orient.	
	Female	Male	NRH	RH	Multi.	Solo	Other	Conv.
PRE	1.18	0.79	1.26	0.85	1.47	0.93	1.43	0.99
IND	1.34	1.08	1.38	1.13	1.62	1.16	1.55	1.21
TPE	1.04	0.68	1.08	0.76	1.48	0.77	1.41	0.86
Prob.	< .05		< .05		< .005		< .006	

Table 14.4. PRE, IND and TPE Scores by Two-Point Biological Variables

TRAUMA AND ABUSE (TAB) SCALE SCORES

The second-level Trauma and Abuse (TAB) predispositions scale (see Chapter 5 for additional information) encompasses two third-level scales: Trauma (TRM) and Abuse (ABU). Questions in the TRM scale have to do with such things as accidents, injuries, illnesses and psychological shocks (e.g., being raped, seeing a loved-one killed, being in a fire). Questions in the ABU scale have to do with instances of childhood abuse—Sexual Abuse, Mental Abuse and Abusive Punishments. The correlation coefficients between the various TAB scales and other selected scales are shown in Table 14.5, below.

	#121	#122	#120	#100	#250	#200
	TRM	ABU	TAB	PRE	TPE	IND
TRM	1.00	.49	.90	.80	.66	.68
ABU		1.00	.82	.74	.52	.58
TAB			1.00	.89	.69	.74

Table 14.5. Correlation Coefficients of Trauma and Abuse Scales

The predictive reliability of scores on the TAB scale for scores on the first-level IND scale is a strong 46%.

Scores on the TAB scale also show strong predictive reliability for scores on the second-level ASC scale (50%) and the second-level TPE scale (48%). These findings accord well with (but do not demonstrate cause and effect) hypotheses in the extant literature of links between childhood abuse (especially Sexual Abuse) and both dissociation and alien contact experiences. The HISS data suggest, however, that the specific emphasis placed on childhood Sexual Abuse may require some rethinking. On the one hand, it is true that within the Reference Group, three (all women) of the ten ASPs reported experiencing significant childhood Sexual Abuse, that women are four times more likely than men (8 versus 2) to be ASPs and that, overall, women are three times more likely than men (5.46% versus

1.79%) to have experienced significant Sexual Abuse. On the other hand, while scores on both the second-level ASC scale and the second-level TPE scale are strongly correlated with scores on the third-level TRM scale, they are only moderately correlated with scores on the third-level ABU scale. Moreover, factor analysis shows that the statistical behavior of scores for childhood Sexual Abuse is more like that of scores for items in the Trauma scale than it is like that of scores for other items in the Abuse scale (i.e., Mental Abuse and Abusive Punishment).

275

Interestingly, as strong as the correlations are between scores on the second level TAB scale and scores on both the second-level ASC scale (50% predictive reliability) and the second-level TPE scale (48% predictive reliability), they are even stronger (56% predictive reliability) with scores on the third-level Somatic (SOM) scale (which is encompassed by the second-level Physiological [PHS]) scale. This finding suggests that Trauma and Abuse have negative implications for physical health, presumably either because they stimulate stress hormones that compromise the immune system, or because they contribute to psychogenic illness factors, or both.

TEMPERAMENT TYPE PREFERENCES (TTP) SCALE SCORES

The second-level Temperament Type Preferences (TTP) predispositions scale (see Chapter 6 for additional information) encompasses four third-level scales: Orientation (ORN), Perceiving (PER), Judging (JUD) and Preference (PRF). Questions in the ORN scale have to do with Orientation toward either Introversion or Extraversion. Questions in the PER scale have to do with Perceiving strategies—either iNtuitive or Sensate. Questions in the JUD scale have to do with Judging strategies—either Feeling or Thinking. Questions in the PER scale have to do with organization and planning and reflect an exhibited Preference for either the Judging strategy or the Perceiving strategy. The correlation coefficients between the various TTP scales and other selected scales are shown in Table 14.6., below.

	#131 ORN	#132 PER	#133 JUD	#134 PRF	#130 TTP	#100 PRE	#250 TPE	#200 IND
ORN	1.00	.36	.11	.08	.61	.56	.41	.46
PER		1.00	.55	-.32	.92	.65	.59	.66
JUD			1.00	-.15	.60	.51	.44	.59
PRF				1.00	-.21	-.09	-.16	-.13
TTP					1.00	.76	.66	.73

Table 14.6 Correlation Coefficients of Temperament Type Preferences Scales

The predictive reliability of scores on the TTP scale for scores on the first-level IND scale is a strong 53%. The negative correlation coefficients between scores on the PRF scale and scores on most other scales is a function of the complexity involved in scoring the TTP scales—PRF scores do not stand alone, but modify and are modified by, ORN scores. Factor analysis shows that the statistical behavior of scores on both the PRF scale and the ORN scale is quite different from that of scores on most other scales.

276

The third-level PER scale scores have their strongest correlation, among the second-level scales (exclusive of the TTP scale by which it is encompassed), with the ASC scale scores (37% predictive reliability). Since high scores on the PER scale are indicative of a Perceiving strategy based on iNtuition, this finding appears to suggest that Altered States of Consciousness are an important factor in iNtuitive Perceiving.

The third-level JUD scales scores have their strongest correlation, among the second-level scales (exclusive of the TTP scale by which it is encompassed), with the EMO scale scores (37% predictive reliability). Since high scores on the JUD scale are indicative of a Judging strategy based on Feeling, this finding appears to affirm the validity of both scales.

In Chapter 6, it was hypothesized that:

(1) All those who use an iNtuitive strategy for Perceiving will be more ASP-like than all those who use a Sensate strategy for Perceiving.

(2) Among those who use an iNtuitive strategy for Perceiving, all those with an Orientation toward Introversion will be more ASP-like than all those with an Orientation toward Extraversion.

(3) Among those Introverts who use an iNtuitive strategy for Perceiving, all those who use a Feeling strategy for Judging will be more ASP-like than all those who use a Thinking strategy for Judging.

(4) Among those Introverts who use an iNtuitive strategy for Perceiving and a Feeling strategy for Judging, all those with an *exhibited* Preference for their Judging function (an actual Preference for their Perceiving function) will be more ASP-like than all those with an *exhibited* Preference for their Perceiving function (an actual Preference for their Judging function).

Accordingly, the Introverted, iNtuitive, Feeling type with an exhibited Preference for the Judging function (that is, the INFJ), would be expected to have the highest mean IND (and other) scale score of all the types and the Extraverted, Sensate, Thinking type, with an actual preference for the Judging function (that is, the ESTJ), would be expected to have the lowest mean IND (and other) scale score of all the types. Scores for the other fourteen types would be surmised to fall in between these extremes in an order consistent with the hypothesis. That's what the HISS data show…well, almost. Figure 14.5., below, displays the 16 temperament types on the "x" axis in the order, from left to right, of their hypothesized mean Indicators scale scores. The "y" axis value shows their actual mean Indicators scale scores. A similar pattern is exhibited for scores on the TPE scale and most other scales.

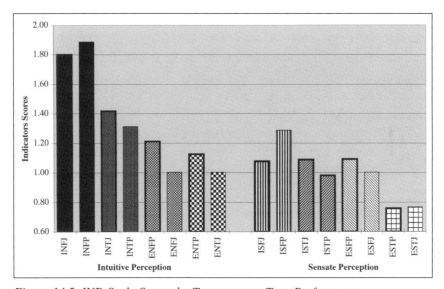

Figure 14.5. IND Scale Scores by Temperament Type Preferences

PHYSIOLOGICAL (PHS) SCALE SCORES

The second-level Physiological (PHS) indicators scale (see Chapter 7 for additional information) encompasses two third-level scales: Somatic (SOM) and Sensory (SEN). Questions in the SOM scale have to do with such things as immune disorders and physiological responses to substances, Electro-Magnetic Radiation and psychological stress. Questions in the SEN scale have to do with reactions to intrusive sensory stimuli (loud noises, bright lights, etc.) and responses to more subtle aesthetic stimuli. The correlation coefficients between the various PHS scales and other selected scales are shown in Table 14.7., below.

	#211	#212	#210	#250	#200	#100
	SOM	SEN	PHS	TPE	IND	PRE
SOM	1.00	.76	.92	.73	.89	.84
SEN		1.00	.96	.69	.87	.69
PHS			1.00	.75	.96	.80

Table 14.7. Correlation Coefficients of Physiological Scales

The predictive reliability of scores on the PHS scale for scores on the first-level IND scale is a very strong 92%. Of all the second-level scales, the PHS scale scores have the strongest average correlational strength with the others. Moreover, scores on the third-level SOM scale have a stronger average correlational strength with scores on all of the second-level scales (exclusive of PHS by which it is encompassed) than do scores on any of the other second-level scales except PHS. Finally, scores on the fourth-level Electro-Magnetic Radiation (EMR) scale (which is encompassed by the third-level SOM scale) have a stronger average correlational strength with scores on all the second-level scales (exclusive of PHS) than do scores on the majority of the second-level scales.

The correlational strengths of scores on the fourth-level EMR scale are quite extraordinary! What is more, factor analysis shows that the statistical behavior of its scores fits as well with the statistical behavior of the ASC scale scores as it does with that of the PHS scale scores. These findings suggest a vital role for EMR in explaining anomalous sensitivities. In order to facilitate analysis and discussion, the EMR scale has been replicated in the Explanatory (EXP) grouping of scales with the title "Electro-Magnetic Sensitivity (EMS)"—and it will be discussed later in that context.

The third-level SEN scale encompasses two fourth-level scales: Sensory-Aesthetic (AES) and Sensory-Overload (OVR). Questions in the AES scale have to do with responses to Aesthetic stimuli. Questions in the OVR scale have to do with experiencing Overload from intrusive stimuli such as loud noises and bright lights. The patterns of correlational strengths for these two scales are quite similar, except that scores on the AES scale have substantially stronger correlations, than do scores on the OVR scale, with scores on the third-level Perceiving (PER) scale (encompassed by the second-level

Temperament Type Preferences [TTP] scale) and the third-level Association (ASN) scale (encompassed by the second-level Altered States of Consciousness [ASC] scale). This finding may suggest an important role for Altered States of Consciousness in Aesthetic sensitivities. Additionally, factor analysis shows that the AES scale encompasses two separate factors (not previously identified as such) that may be spoken of as "Artistic sensitivities" and "Synesthetic sensitivities."†

279

Cognitive (COG) Scale Scores

The second-level Cognitive (COG) indicators scale (see Chapter 8 for additional information) encompasses three third-level scales: Attention (ATT), Learning (LRN) and Mnemonic (MNE). Questions in the ATT scale have to do with concentration and distractibility. Questions in the LRN scale have to do with strengths and weaknesses in mathematics, reading and spelling. Questions in the MNE scale have to do with strengths and weaknesses in remembering. The correlation coefficients between the various COG scales and other selected scales are shown in Table 14.8., below.

	#221	#222	#223	#220	#250	#200	#100
	ATT	LRN	MNE	COG	TPE	IND	PRE
ATT	1.00	.58	.46	.82	.37	.59	.53
LRN		1.00	.52	.87	.31	.59	.49
MNE			1.00	.77	.55	.78	.62
COG				1.00	.49	.78	.66

Table 14.8. Correlation Coefficients of Cognitive Scales

The predictive reliability of scores on the COG scale for scores on the first-level IND scale, while lower than that of all second-level scales except Biological (BIO), is nevertheless still a strong 59%.

The correlational strength of scores on the third-level MNE scale with scores on most other HISS scales is higher than is that of scores on either the third-level ATT scale or the third-level LRN scale. The strength of the correlation between scores on the third-level MNE scale and scores on the fourth-level Psychogenic (PSY) scale

---

† Six of the ten ASPs in the Reference Group had very high levels of Synesthetic sensitivities. As discussed previously, synesthesia is the spontaneous association of a sensation being activated by an external stimulus with another sensation of a different kind. Synesthetic sensitivities are more strongly correlated with Altered States of Consciousness sensitivities than are either Artistic or Overload sensitivities.

(encompassed by the third-level Somatic [SOM] scale, which is, in turn, encompassed by the second-level Physiological [PHS] scale) is unusually strong (52% predictive reliability), given the low hierarchical level of those scales—and suggests that memory may somehow play an important role in stress-related illness.

Of the fourth-level scales encompassed by the third-level MNE scale—Amnesia (AMN) and Hypermnesia (HYP)—the AMN scale scores have a higher correlational strength with scores on most other HISS scales than do HYP scale scores. Not surprisingly, the biggest difference is with scores on the third-level Attention (ATT) scale where the predictive reliability of AMN scores is 36% and the predictive reliability of the HYP scores is only 3%. Paradoxically, AMN scores are correlated with HYP scores (12% predictive reliability). While the strength of this correlation is considered weak by HISS standards, it nevertheless has a probability of chance occurrence of less than one in a billion. This finding, coupled with the noteworthy strength of the correlation between scores on the MNE scale and scores on the second-level ASC scale (53% predictive reliability), presumably speaks to the issue of state-dependent memory—and has implications for the theory of the Fantasy Prone Personality and the theory of False Memory Syndrome (both discussed in Chapter 2).

EMOTIONAL (EMO) SCALE SCORES

The second-level Emotional (EMO) indicators scale (see Chapter 9 for additional information) encompasses two third-level scales: Intrapersonal (TRA) and Interpersonal (TER). Questions in the TRA scale have to do with attunement to one's own emotions. Questions in the TER scale have to do with attunement to the emotions of others. The correlation coefficients between the various EMO scales and other selected scales are shown in Table 14.9., below:

	#231 TRA	#232 TER	#230 EMO	#250 TPE	#200 IND	#100 PRE
TRA	1.00	.64	.90	.51	.78	.63
TER		1.00	.92	.68	.82	.66
EMO			1.00	.66	.88	.71

Table 14.9. Correlation Coefficients of Emotional Scales

The predictive reliability of scores on the EMO scale for scores on the first-level IND scale is a very strong 77%.

The strength of the correlations between scores on the EMO scale and scores on the third-level Judging (JUD) scale, the fourth-level Psychogenic (PSY) scale, the fourth-level Aesthetic (AES) scale, the fourth-level Overload (OVR) scale and the third-level Association (ASN) scale are noteworthy (given the low hierarchical levels of those scales), all having a predictive reliability of 37% or better. These findings presumably speak to the role of Emotions in the creative process and the potential for sensory Overload being a concomitant of the creative individual's temperament.

The pattern of correlational strengths for scores on the third-level TRA scale and scores on the third-level TER scale, with other HISS scales is quite similar, but there is one notable exception. TER scale scores have a predictive reliability for TPE scale scores of 46%, whereas TRA scale scores have a predictive reliability for TPE scale scores of only 26%. This finding suggests that Interpersonal sensitivity (empathy) might appropriately be thought of as a transpersonal ability.

ALTERED STATES OF CONSCIOUSNESS (ASC) SCALE SCORES

The second-level Altered States of Consciousness (ASC) indicators scale (see Chapter 10 for more information) encompasses five third-level scales: Dissociation (DSN), Hallucination (HAL), Sleep/Wake Overlap (SWO), Association (ASN) and Suggestibility (SUG). Questions in the DSN scale have to do with psychological fragmentation, depersonalization and derealization. Questions in the HAL scale have to do with sensory perceptions that have no apparent corresponding stimuli in consensus reality. Questions in the SWO scale have to do with patterns of sleeping and dreaming. Questions in the ASN scale have to do with imagination, daydreaming and fantasies. Questions in the SUG scale have to do with matters completely irrelevant to sensitivities—but a *pattern* of consistently high responses to those questions implies that the subject is highly suggestible. The correlation coefficients between the various ASC scales and other selected scales are shown in Table 14.10., below.

| | #241 | #242 | #243 | #244 | #245 | #240 | #250 | #200 | #100 |
	DSN	HAL	SWO	ASN	SUG	ASC	TPE	IND	PRE
DSN	1.00	.77	.63	.80	.67	.89	.74	.82	.70
HAL		1.00	.63	.73	.64	.88	.68	.80	.68
SWO			1.00	.68	.53	.81	.57	.74	.62
ASN				1.00	.66	.91	.72	.86	.75
SUG					1.00	.81	.65	.75	.62
ASC						1.00	.78	.92	.78

Table 14.10. Correlation Coefficients of Altered States of Consciousness Scales

281

The predictive reliability of scores on the ASC scale for scores on the first-level IND scale is a very strong 85%. Of all the second-level scales, scores on the ASC scale have the highest correlational strength with scores on the second-level Transpersonal Experiences (TPE) scale (61% predictive reliability).

Scores on the ASC scale also show noteworthy correlational strength (37% predictive reliability) with scores on the third-level Perceiving (PER) scale. As stated before, this finding is perhaps suggestive of Altered States of Consciousness playing an important role in iNtuitive strategies for Perceiving.

The strength of the correlation between scores on the ASC scale and scores on the third-level Somatic (SOM) scale is striking (67% predictive reliability). This strength is primarily attributable to the impressive strength of the correlations between scores on the ASC scale and scores on two of the fourth-level scales encompassed by the SOM scale—the Psychogenic (PSY) scale (61% predictive reliability) and the Electro-Magnetic Radiation (EMR) scale (62% predictive reliability). The finding with respect to the PSY scale suggests a role for Altered States of Consciousness in psychogenic illness (and perhaps in psychogenic healing as well). The finding with respect to the EMR scale reflects, as previously mentioned, factor analysis having shown that the statistical behavior of the EMR scale scores fits equally as well with the statistical behavior of the ASC scale scores as it does with the statistical behavior of the PHS scale scores.

Of the third-level scales encompassed by the ASC scale, the ASN scale scores show a higher correlational strength with scores on most other HISS scales than do scores on the DSN, HAL, SWO and SUG scales. This finding suggests that it is the associative aspects of Altered States of Consciousness that are especially important in the manifestations of sensitivities.

TRANSPERSONAL EXPERIENCES (TPE) SCALE SCORES

The second-level Transpersonal Experiences (TPE) indicators scale (see Chapter 11 for more information) encompasses two third-level scales: T/P Experiences-Verifiable (X-V) and T/P Experiences-Unverifiable (X-U). Questions in the X-V scale have to do with experiences of transpersonal (or Extra Sensory) Perception (ESP) and experiences of transpersonal influence or PsychoKinesis (PK)—that is, with psi experiences. Questions in the X-U scale have to do

282

with experiences of transpersonal manifestation of mind (e.g., apparition, alien contact, spirit possession)—that is, with psi-related experiences. The correlation coefficients between the various TPE scales and other selected scales are shown in Table 14.11., below.

	#251	#252	#250	#200	#100
	X-V	X-U	TPE	IND	PRE
X-V	1.00	.86	.96	.82	.72
X-U		1.00	.97	.84	.76
TPE			1.00	.86	.77

Table 14.11. Correlation Coefficients of Transpersonal Experiences Scales

283

The predictive reliability of scores on the TPE scale for scores on the first-level IND scale is a very strong 74%. As was mentioned previously, the correlational strength of scores on the TPE scale is higher with scores on the second-level ASC scale (61% predictive reliability) than it is with scores on any other second-level scale—presumably an indication of the special importance of the role of Altered States of Consciousness in Transpersonal Experiences.

Earlier in this chapter, it was pointed out as being noteworthy that scores on the TPE scale are more strongly correlated with scores on the third-level Trauma (TRM) scale than they are with scores on the third-level Abuse (ABU) scale (both encompassed by the second-level Trauma and Abuse [TAB] scale). It was also pointed out as being noteworthy that scores on the TPE scale are more strongly correlated with scores on the third-level Interpersonal (TER) scale than they are with scores on the third-level Intrapersonal (TRA) scale (both encompassed by the second-level Emotional [EMO] scale). Finally, it should be noted that scores on the TPE scale are more strongly correlated with scores on the fourth-level Electro-Magnetic Radiation (EMR) scale (59% predictive reliability) than they are with scores on its encompassing third-level Somatic (SOM) (53% predictive reliability) and second-level Physiological (PHS) (56% predictive reliability) scales as well as with scores on all the second-level scales except the Altered States of Consciousness (ASC) scale (61% predictive reliability). This very important finding with respect to EMR will be further discussed later in this chapter.

The pattern of correlational strengths shown by scores on the third-level T/P Experiences-Verifiable (X-V) scale (that is, experience of transpersonal perception and transpersonal influence) with scores on all other HISS scales is almost identical to the pattern of correlational strengths shown by scores on the third-level T/P

Experiences-Unverifiable (X-U) scale (that is, experiences of transpersonal manifestation of mind) with those same scales. This finding suggests that there is very little difference between the dynamics underlying verifiable Transpersonal Experiences (collectively) and the dynamics underlying unverifiable Transpersonal Experiences (collectively)—and perhaps between the individual experiences themselves.

284

In-depth analysis of the data shows that, relative to the other second-level scales, TPE scale scores are clearly a dependent variable. This means that changes in scores on the other scales are likely to be accompanied by changes in scores on the TPE scale, but that changes in scores on the TPE scale are not so likely to be accompanied by changes in scores on the other scales. This same analysis shows that, relative to the other second-level scales, Biological (BIO) scale scores are clearly an independent variable. This means that changes in scores on the BIO scale are likely to be accompanied by changes in scores on the other scales, but that changes in scores on the other scales are not so likely to be accompanied by changes in scores on the BIO scale. Given the data available, this analysis is as close as it is possible to get to a determination of cause and effect. In other words, it would not be *entirely* unwarranted to suggest that Biological predispositions *cause* the other factors and that Transpersonal Experiences sensitivities *are caused by* the other factors. The complete results are illustrated graphically in figure 14.6., below.

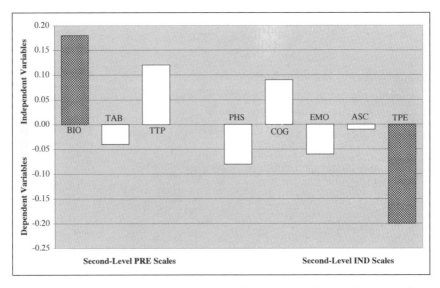

Figure 14.6. Independent/Dependent Variable Analysis—Second-Level Scales

In the graph above, the numbers on the "y" axis are raw scores for the independent/dependent variable relationship. Those scales for which the column is above the 0.00 line are considered to be independent variables and those scales for which the column is below the 0.00 line are considered to be dependent variables. The cross-hatching in the columns for the BIO and TPE scales signifies that their independent/dependent variable relationship scores are more than one (but less than two) standard deviation above (for the former) or below (for the latter) the mean of the scores for all the scales shown.

285

The same type of analysis of scores for each of the individual **Transpersonal Experiences** relative to the others results in the graphical illustration shown in Figure 14.7., below.

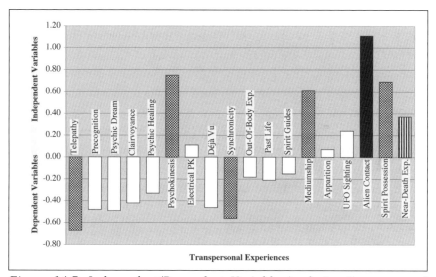

Figure 14.7. Independent/Dependent Variable Analysis—Transpersonal Experiences

Again, those individual experiences for which the column is above the 0.00 line are considered to be independent variables and those experiences for which the column is below the 0.00 line are considered to be dependent variables. The experiences that are considered to be independent variables are those for which changes in their scores are likely to be accompanied by (but not so likely to accompany) changes in the scores for other experiences and the experiences that are considered to be dependent variables are those for which changes in the scores for other experiences are likely to be accompanied by (but not so likely to accompany) changes in their scores.

The column for the alien contact experience is solidly shaded to signify that its independent/dependent variable relationship raw score is more than two standard deviations above the mean of the raw scores for all the individual experiences. The columns for the PsychoKinesis, mediumship and spirit possession experiences are crosshatched to signify that their independent/dependent variable relationship raw scores are more than one (but less than two) standard deviation above the mean. The column for the Near-Death Experience is vertically striped to signify that its independent/dependent variable relationship raw score would presumably be more than one standard deviation above the mean but for a formatting error in the questionnaire (since corrected) that resulted in positive responses to the question about that experience being substantially understated.

The columns for the telepathy and synchronicity experiences are crosshatched to signify that their independent/dependent variable relationship raw scores are more than one (but less than two) standard deviation below the mean of the raw scores for all the individual experiences. In part, their low scores may reflect their commonness— that is, the high frequency with which subjects reported having those experiences. The mean HISS score for frequency of the telepathic experience is 1.48 and for the synchronicity experience is 2.06, as compared to the mean score for all of the **Transpersonal Experiences**, collectively, of 0.90. The mean score for the frequency of the déjà vu experience, however, is the highest of all at 2.42 and its independent/dependent variable relationship raw score is less than one standard deviation below the mean.

EXPLANATORY (EXP) SCALES SCORES

The Other (OTH) grouping of scales encompasses the Internal Checks (CHK) grouping of scales (see Appendix E, "Double-Checking, for further discussion) and the Explanatory (EXP) grouping of scales. The three independent scales in the EXP grouping (see Chapter 11 for more information), each of which is scored alone, are: Electro-Magnetic Sensitivity (EMS), Temporo-Limbic Epilepsy (TLE) and Kundalini Arousal (KUN). Questions included in these scales can be determined by reference to Appendix C, "Composition of HISS Scales." The correlation coefficients between the various EXP scales and other selected scales are shown in Table 14.12., below.

	#311	#312	#313	#210	#240	#250	#200	#100
	EMS	TLE	KUN	PHS	ASC	TPE	IND	PRE
EMS	1.00	.77	.76	.88	.79	.77	.87	.73
TLE		1.00	.95	.84	.94	.76	.91	.77
KUN			1.00	.81	.92	.78	.89	.76

Table 14.12. Correlation Coefficients of Explanatory Scales

The predictive reliability of scores on each of the three third-level scales in the EXP grouping of scales, for scores on the first-level IND scale, is very strong—for EMS it is 76%, for TLE it is 83% and for KUN it is 79%.

The strengths of these correlations and other correlations between scores on the three Explanatory scales and scores on various scales encompassed by the IND grouping of scales are somewhat artificially enhanced because of a duplication of questions. All six questions scored in the EMS scale, for example, are also scored in the Physiological (PHS) scale. Of the twenty questions scored in the TLE scale, ten are also scored in the Altered States of Consciousness (ASC) scale, five are also scored in the Physiological (PHS) scale and two are also scored in the Cognitive (COG) scale. Of the thirteen questions scored in the KUN scale, six are also scored in the Altered States of Consciousness (ASC) scale, three are also scored in the Physiological (PHS) scale and one is also scored in the Emotional (EMO) scale. The degree of artificial enhancement of correlational strengths is, however, less than one might expect. If the duplication of the six EMS questions in the PHS scale is eliminated, for example, the "r" value of the correlation between the scores of those two scales is only reduced to .84 (from .88)—a meaningless change from the perspective of statistical significance. In the HISS scoring, the Explanatory scales are not treated as Indicators of sensitivities. They are, rather, handled separately and are considered to be theoretical constructs by which the Indicators of sensitivities—Physiological, Cognitive, Emotional, Altered States of Consciousness and Transpersonal Experiences—can be explained.

The correlations among scores on the three Explanatory scales—EMS, TLE and KUN—are sufficiently strong that their similarities as theoretical constructs are affirmed. The strength of the correlation between scores on the TLE scale and scores on the KUN scale (90% predictive reliability) suggests that they are essentially identical. That correlational strength is, in part, attributable to the two scales having seven questions in common—a situation that was unavoidable because the symptoms of each, as described in the relevant literature, are almost indistinguishable. There are, however, six questions in the KUN scale that are not duplicated in the TLE scale and scores for those six questions, collectively, nevertheless have a very strong (76%) predictive reliability for scores on the TLE scale.

288

It is noteworthy that the predictive reliabilities of scores on the EMS, TLE and KUN scales for scores on the second-level Transpersonal Experiences (TPE) scale (59%, 58% and 61% respectively) are effectively as strong as that of the second-level Altered States of Consciousness (ASC) scale (61% predictive reliability) and are stronger than that of any second-level scale other than the ASC scale.

Also noteworthy is that the strength of the correlations between scores on each of the Explanatory scales and scores for all except one of the individual Transpersonal Experiences are almost identical. While the correlational strengths with the UFO sighting, alien contact, spirit possession and Near-Death Experiences are somewhat reduced, that can readily be explained by the "floor effect."

The one significant (and logical) exception to this finding is that the correlational strength between scores on the Electro-Magnetic Sensitivity (EMS) scale and scores for the Electrical PsychoKinesis experience is relatively elevated. It appears, however, that Electro-Magnetic Sensitivity plays much the same role in each of the other Transpersonal Experiences and there is nothing in the HISS data to support claims made by some that the dynamics of certain specific Transpersonal Experiences (notably the Near-Death Experience and the alien contact experience) are such as to *cause* experiencers to develop Electro-Magnetic Sensitivity.

What is most obvious may be most worthy of analysis.
—L. L. White

In the final analysis, the HISS data appear to support the arguments that have been presented in this book about the factors involved in the occurrence of Transpersonal Experiences including:

- Certain individuals have brains (specifically Less Strongly Lateralized brains) that are more sensitive to stimuli (especially stressful stimuli) than the norm.
- Repeated exposure to such stimuli, of which Electro-Magnetic Radiation is a representative example, results in the development of neuronal hypersynchrony in the temporal lobes and the limbic system of the brain.
- Neuronal hypersynchrony (which, in extreme instances, is spoken of by some as "Temporo-Limbic Epilepsy" and by others as "Kundalini Arousal") manifests as Altered States of Consciousness (specifically, under certain circumstances, as Transpersonal Consciousness).
- Altered States of Consciousness establish pathways by which the sub-cortical structures of the brain (notably the limbic system) can experience direct (unmediated by the cortex) interaction with the environment.
- Subcortical experiences are characterized by their transcendence of the ordinary differentiated boundaries of ego, space and time—and therefore qualify as Transpersonal Experiences.
- Such experiences, when they occur above the threshold of awareness are sufficiently uncommon (anomalous) that they are considered not to be a part of consensus reality.
- That, however, does not necessarily mean that they are fictive.

289

RECAPITULATION

By way of bringing this discussion to closure, the ASP hypothesis, which was originally presented in the Introduction to this book, is reiterated below. It is followed by a brief recapitulation of the operative mechanisms that appear to underlie anomalous sensitivities.

Certain individuals—who will be spoken of as Anomalously Sensitive Persons (ASPs)—in addition to being anomalously sensitive to stimuli in the Transpersonal Experiences realm, are also anomalously sensitive to stimuli in the Physiological, Cognitive, Emotional and Altered States of Consciousness realms. These individuals are predisposed toward being anomalously sensitive by various Biological ("nature"), Trauma and Abuse ("nurture") and Temperament Type Preferences ("personality") factors.

290

In humans, genetic influences and biochemical influences can lead to physiological anomalies, immunological anomalies and neurophysiological anomalies (especially in the temporal lobes and limbic system of the brain). The manifestations of physiological anomalies include, among other things, hypopigmentation and biochemical anomalies. The manifestations of immunological anomalies include, among other things, allergies and autoimmune disorders.The manifestations of neurophysiological anomalies include, among other things, Temperament Type Preferences, Non-Right-Handedness, a brain that is Less Strongly Lateralized than the norm and the full spectrum of human sensitivities (Physiological, Cognitive, Emotional, Altered States of Consciousness and Transpersonal Experiences).

The effects of neurophysiological anomalies can be amplified (through neuronal hypersynchrony) by stressors (both psychological and physiological) as well as by hypnosis, meditation and training.

Neurophysiological anomalies play a key role in sensitivity to Altered States of Consciousness (specifically Transpersonal Consciousness). ASCs, in turn, are involved in anomalously high levels of all the other sensitivities,

> *The whole of science consists of data that, at one time or another, were unexplainable.*
> —*Brendan O'Regan*

most especially in Transpersonal Experiences sensitivities. It is only in an ASC that an individual is able to experience stimuli arising out of the implicate order (imaginal realm).

For those (especially ASPs) who prefer a visual explanation, this recapitulation is presented in diagrammatic form in Figure 14.8., next page.

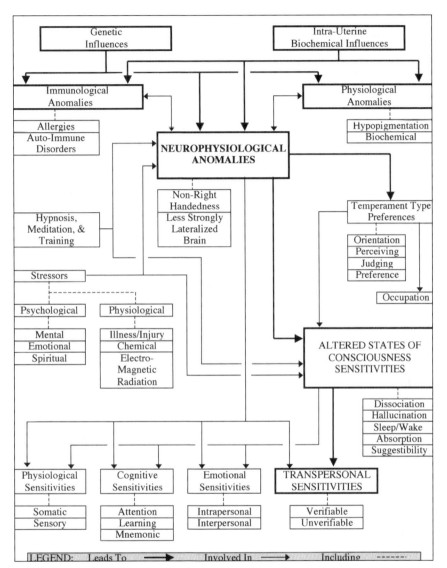

Figure 14.8. The Origins and Manifestations of Anomalous Sensitivities

CHAPTER SUMMARY

⇒   There are clear-cut differences in scores on the HISS Indicators (IND) scale across "Strong Vocational Inventory Blank (SVIB)" occupational categories. In descending order of IND scores, the ranking of categories is: Artistic, Investigative, Social, Enterprising, Conventional and Realistic.

⇒   Compositional imbalances in the Reference Group included: too female, too white, too educated and too human-services oriented.

⇒   The mean of scores on the IND scale is 25% higher than the mode.

⇒   The correlations among the scores for the first- and second-level scales in the Predispositions (PRE) and Indicators (IND) groupings are very strong. The weakest correlation among scores on the second-level scales has a probability of chance occurrence of less than one in a billion.

⇒   Neurophysiological structuring (specifically whether or not the brain is Less Strongly Lateralized [LSL] than the norm) appears to be a significant factor influencing scores on all of the HISS scales.

⇒   A comparison of the average correlations among all second-level HISS scales reveals that those for the Biological (BIO) scale are notably lower and those for both the Altered States of Consciousness (ASC) and Physiological (PHS) scales are notably higher, than the norm.

⇒   The predictive reliability of scores on the second-level Biological (BIO) predispositions scale for scores on the first-level IND scale is strong. Two point variables included in the BIO scale show that among the Reference Group, mean scores are higher: for women than for men; for Non-Right-Handers than for right-handers; for those who were born as one of a set of twins/triplets/etc. than for those who had a solo birth; and for those whose sexual orientation is other-than-conventionally heterosexual than for those whose orientation is conventionally heterosexual.

⇒   The predictive reliability of scores on the second-level Trauma and Abuse (TAB) predispositions scale for scores on the first-level IND scale is strong. Scores on the TAB scale also show strong predictive reliability for scores on the second-level ASC scale and

292

the second-level TPE scale (the third-level Trauma [TRM] scale scores having stronger correlations than the third-level Abuse [ABU] scale scores). TAB scores showed an unusually strong correlation with scores on the third-level Somatic (SOM) scale (which is encompassed by the second-level Physiological [PHS] scale).

⇒   The predictive reliability of scores on the second-level Temperament Type Preferences (TTP) predispositions scale for scores on the first-level IND scale is strong. High IND scores are related to: (1) an iNtuitive strategy for Perceiving, (2) an Orientation toward Introversion, (3) a Feeling strategy for Judging and (4) an *exhibited* preference for the Judging function over the Perceiving function.

293

⇒   The predictive reliability of scores on the second-level Physiological (PHS) indicators scale for scores on the first-level IND scale is very strong. The correlational strengths of scores on the fourth-level Electro-Magnetic Radiation scale (encompassed by the third-level Somatic [SOM] scale) are quite extraordinary and suggest a vital role for EMR in explaining anomalous sensitivities.

⇒   The predictive reliability of scores on the second-level Cognitive (COG) indicators scale for scores on the first-level IND scale is strong. The correlational strength of scores on the third-level Mnemonic (MNE) scale with scores on most other scales is higher than is that of scores on either the third-level Attention (ATT) scale or the third-level Learning (LRN) scale.

⇒   The predictive reliability of scores on the second-level Emotional (EMO) indicators scale for scores on the first-level IND scale is very strong. Scores on the third-level Interpersonal (TER) scale have a higher predictive reliability for scores on the second-level Transpersonal Experiences (TPE) scale than do scores on the third-level Intrapersonal (TRA) scale. This suggests that interpersonal sensitivity (empathy) might appropriately be thought of as a transpersonal ability.

⇒   The predictive reliability of scores on the second-level Altered States of Consciousness (ASC) indicators scale for scores on the first-level IND scale is very strong. Of all the second-level scales, scores on the ASC scale have the highest correlational strength with scores on the second-level Transpersonal Experiences (TPE) scale. Of the third-level scales encompassed by the ASC scale, the scores on the Association (ASN) scale show the highest correlational strength with scores on most other scales—thus suggesting that it is the associative aspects of Altered States of Consciousness that are especially important in the manifestations of anomalous sensitivities.

⟹ The predictive reliability of scores on the second-level Transpersonal Experiences (TPE) indicators scale for scores on the first-level IND scale is very strong. The correlational strength of scores on the TPE scale is higher with scores on the ASC scale than it is with scores on any other second-level scale. Relative to scores on the other second-level scales, scores on the TPE scale are a dependent variable.

⟹ Relative to scores for the other individual TPEs, scores for the alien contact, PsychoKinesis, mediumship, spirit possession and Near-Death Experiences are independent variables and scores for the telepathy and synchronicity experiences are dependent variables.

⟹ The predictive reliability of scores on each of the three third-level scales in the Explanatory (EXP) grouping of scales—Electro-Magnetic Sensitivity (EMS), Temporo-Limbic Epilepsy (TLE) and Kundalini Arousal (KUN)—for scores on the first-level IND scale, is very strong.

⟹ The correlations among scores on the three scales in the EXP grouping—EMS, TLE and KUN—are sufficiently strong that their similarities as theoretical constructs are affirmed. The extraordinary strength of the correlation between scores on the TLE scale and scores on the KUN scale suggests that the two scales are measuring the same thing.

⟹ The HISS data appear to support the following arguments about the factors involved in the occurrence of TPEs: (1) Less Strongly Lateralized (LSL) brains are more sensitive to stimuli than the norm, (2) repeated exposure to stimuli leads to the development of neuronal hypersynchrony, (3) neuronal hypersynchrony manifests as ASCs, (4) ASCs establish pathways by which sub-cortical structures can experience direct interaction with the environment, (5) sub-cortical experiences can transcend the ordinary differentiated boundaries of ego, space and time—they are Transpersonal Experiences, (6) TPEs are considered not to be a part of consensus reality and (7) TPEs are not necessarily fictive.

⟹ The various operative mechanisms underlying anomalous sensitivities include these: (1) genetic influences and biochemical influences can lead to physiological, immunological and neurophysiological anomalies, (2) the manifestations of neurophysiological anomalies include the full spectrum of human sensitivities (Physiological, Cognitive, Emotional, Altered States of Consciousness and Transpersonal Experiences), (3) ASCs are involved in anomalously high levels of all the other sensitivities, especially TPE sensitivities and (4) only in an ASC can an individual experience stimuli arising out of the implicate order (imaginal realm).

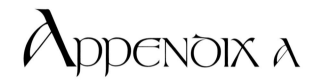

Appendix A

The Hiss Questionnaire

HOLISTIC INVENTORY OF STIMULUS SENSITIVITIES
Rev. VI.A. — 2/99

The ASP Project
Orient, New York

Some line items in the "Holistic Inventory of Stimulus Sensitivities" were adapted from various sources, including:

"Dissociative Experiences Survey (DES)"— Eve Carlson & Frank Putnam. 1986
"Experiences of Absorption Survey" — Auke Telegren & Gilbert Atkinson. 1974
"Hartmann Boundary Questionnaire" — Ernest Hartmann. 1991
"Inventory of Childhood Memories & Imaginings (ICMI)"— Steven Lynn & Judith Rhue. 1986.
"Kiersey Temperament Sorter" — David Kiersey & Marilyn Bates. 1984.
"Myers-Briggs Type Indicator - Abbreviated (MBTI)" — Consulting Psychologists Press. 1983
"Myers-Briggs Type Indicator - Form J (MBTI)" — Consulting Psychologists Press. 1984.
"Omega Home Environment Questionnaire" — Kenneth Ring. 1992.
"Physio-Kundalini Syndrome Index" — Bruce Greyson. 1993.
"Unusual Personal Experiences ('The Roper Poll')" — Bigelow Holding Corporation. 1992.

298

HOLISTIC INVENTORY OF STIMULUS SENSITIVITIES

Rev. VI.A. —2/99

299

Current Date: _____ Address: _____

Name: _____

Tel. No.: _____

GENERAL:

Instructions: This inventory is designed to help develop an awareness of your sensitivities to a variety of stimuli in several different areas including the physiological, the immunological, the neurological, the psychological, and the "transpersonal". Your results may be useful to you in understanding the ways you react to things, in managing stress, and in making effective choices about your lifestyle. There are no "right" or "wrong" responses.

There are two major sections, each with three parts, and each part has its own set of instructions. Begin with Section I, Part A, and move through the sections and parts, <u>in the order in which they appear</u>, until you have completed Section II, Part C. Completion time should be about forty minutes, preferably all in one sitting. A long break, such as overnight, could adversely affect the validity of your results. If you need to take a brief break, try to do so at the end of a part.

Please mark your responses to each statement clearly. Editorial comments, while perhaps helpful to you in relieving tension, cannot be scored. Feel free to make them if you wish, but be sure to <u>circle the appropriate letter or number response</u> as well. A red ballpoint pen is the ideal writing instrument to use, but is not required.

SECTION I: PERSONAL & FAMILIAL DATA

Instructions: In this section, which has three parts (A, B, and C), you are asked to respond (generally by circling a letter or number response option in the right-side columns) to statements about yourself and/or your relatives. The method of responding in each of the three parts varies, so please read the instructions for each part carefully.

Please respond to <u>all</u> of the statements even if "it depends" and/or you are not absolutely sure of the precisely accurate response. When asked to select among specified response options, pick <u>one and only one</u> of the options. If your <u>most accurate</u> response would fall between two options, pick that <u>one</u> option of the two which is the <u>more accurate.</u>

Part A: Demographic and Biological

Instructions: In this part, respond to each statement either by writing on the blank line or by circling that <u>single</u> response option letter in <u>the right-side columns</u> which corresponds to that specified option which <u>most accurately</u> applies to you. Note that not all statements offer the same number of response options.

STATEMENT: RESPONSE:

1. The date of my birth was:

_____

(fill in line above)

2. The place of my birth (i.e., city & state) was:

_____

(fill in line above)

3. My occupation is/was (<u>if retired or unemployed</u>)/

will be (<u>if student</u>):

_____

[Note: If full-time homemaker, so state.]   (fill in line above)

4. The highest level formal education I have completed is:

[A = didn't finish high school, B = high school graduate,

C = some college, D = college graduate, E = graduate school] .... A   B   C   D   E

5. My sex is: [A = male, E = female] .... A   E

6. I was born as one of a set of twins/triplets/etc.

[A = no, E = yes] .... A   E

[<u>Only</u> if "yes," specify by circling number: 1 = Fraternal, 3 = Identical.] ...   *1*   *3*

7. I was born: [A = less than 4 years after my next older sibling,

C = 4 or more years after my next older sibling,

E = a first-born or only child] .... A   C   E

8. My <u>biological</u> mother's age when I was born was:

[A = < 25, B = 25–29, C = 30–34, D = 35–39, E = >40] .... A   B   C   D   E

9. My <u>biological</u> mother's primary ethnic origins are/were:

[A = African, B = Asian, C = European, D = Latino, E = Amerindian] .... A   B   C   D   E

10. My <u>biological</u> father's primary ethnic origins are/were:

[A = African, B = Asian, C = European, D = Latino, E = Amerindian] .... A   B   C   D   E

11. My natural complexion is/was:

[A = very dark, B = dark, C = medium, D = fair, E = very fair] .... A   B   C   D   E

12. My natural eye color is/was:

[A = black, B = brown, C = hazel, D = green, E = blue/gray] .... A   B   C   D   E

13. My natural hair color is/was:

[A = black, B = dark brown, C = light brown, D = blond, E = red] ....A   B   C   D   E

14. My blood type is:

[A = A, B = B, C = AB, D = O, E = Unknown] .... A   B   C   D   E

15. My blood rhesus factor is: [A = Rh+, C = Rh-, E = Unknown] .... A   C   E

16. My natural handedness is/was:

[A = fully right, C = fully left, E=mixed]. ....A   C   E

17. My sexual orientation is:

[A = conventionally heterosexual, E = other] .... A   E

Part B: Historical

Instructions: In this part, respond to each statement by circling that <u>single</u> response option number which <u>most accurately</u> reflects the statement's applicability to you. The specified meaning for each response option number is as follows:

> *0 = Definitely <u>does not</u> apply to me.*
> *1 = Generally <u>does not</u> apply to me.*
> *2 = Minimally applies to me.*
> *3 = Generally applies to me.*
> *4 = Definitely applies to me.*

STATEMENT: RESPONSE:

18. I have/had chronic severe headaches (e.g.: migraines,

   clusters, etc.). 0   1   2   3   4

19. I have/had chronic sinus problems (i.e., infections,

   post-nasal drip, etc.). 0   1   2   3   4

20. I have/had a chronic food intolerance/food allergy. 0   1   2   3   4

21. I have/had a chronic atopic disorder/allergy (e.g.: asthma,

   hay fever, hives, eczema). 0   1   2   3   4

22. I have/had chronically <u>low</u> blood pressure. 0   1   2   3   4

23. I have/had a chronically <u>low</u> "normal" body temperature. 0   1   2   3   4

24. I have/had a chronic <u>low</u> thyroid condition (<u>hypo</u>thyroidism). 0   1   2   3   4

25. I have/had a chronic <u>high</u> thyroid condition (<u>hyper</u>thyroidism). 0   1   2   3   4

26. I have/had a chronic <u>low</u> blood sugar condition (<u>hypo</u>glycemia). ... 0   1   2   3   4

27. I have/had a chronic <u>high</u> blood sugar condition (<u>diabetes</u>). 0   1   2   3   4

28. I have/had a chronic gastrointestinal disorder (e.g.: regional ileitis,

   ulcerative colitis, celiac disease). 0   1   2   3   4

29. I have/had a chronic autoimmune disorder (e.g.: myasthenia

   gravis, rheumatoid arthritis, lupus erythematosus). 0   1   2   3   4

30. I have/had a chronic unusual health problem (e.g.: Lyme disease,

   Epstein-Barr virus, chronic fatigue syndrome, fibromyalgia). 0   1   2   3

31. I have/had a chronic sleep disorder (e.g.: insomnia, hypersomnia,

   myoclonus, sleepwalking, nightmares, narcolepsy, apnea, etc.). 0   1   2   3   4

32. I have/had a chronic developmental learning disorder

   (e.g.: dyslexia, Tourette's syndrome, attention deficit disorder, etc.). 0   1   2   3   4

33. I have/had a chronic developmental speech disorder

   (e.g.: delayed speech, stuttering, hesitation, lisp, etc.). 0   1   2   3   4

Part C: Familial

Instructions: In this part, you are asked to provide information about your <u>first-degree</u> <u>biological relatives</u> — parents, siblings, and offspring … <u>only</u> those to whom you are <u>genetically</u> related. Half-siblings qualify, but adopted- or step-siblings (or children, or parents) do not. If an individual is deceased, respond for when s/he was living. If you are uncertain about something, respond to the best of your ability.

Each statement should be read as if it were preceded by the words "I believe, <u>as compared</u> <u>to the population at large</u>, a higher than 'normal' percentage of these relatives …"

Respond to each statement by circling that <u>single</u> response option number which <u>most accurately</u> reflects the statement's applicability to you. "Accuracy" in responding has more to do with your subjective perception than it does with objective reality. The specified meaning for each response option number is as follows:

302

> *0 = Definitely <u>does not</u> apply to me.*
> *1 = Generally <u>does not</u> apply to me.*
> *2 = Minimally applies to me.*
> *3 = Generally applies to me.*
> *4 = Definitely applies to me.*

STATEMENT: RESPONSE:

["A higher than 'normal' percentage of these relatives …"]

34. …have/had very fair or fair complexions. 0   1   2   3   4

35. …have/had blue, gray, or green eyes. 0   1   2   3   4

36. …have/had naturally red or blond hair. 0   1   2   3   4

37. …are/were left-handed or ambi-dexterous. 0   1   2   3   4

38. … have/had a chronic learning disorder and/or

   a speech disorder. 0   1   2   3   4

CONTINUE ON TO SECTION II.

SECTION II: EXPERIENCES & PREFERENCES

Instructions: In this section, which has three parts (A, B, and C), you are asked to respond (by circling a number in the right-side columns) to statements having to do with your experiences and preferences . The meanings specified for the response option numbers in "Part A" differ from the meanings specified for the response option numbers in "Part B" and "Part C", so be sure to read the instructions for each part carefully.

Please respond to <u>all</u> of the statements even if "it depends" and/or you are not absolutely sure of the precisely accurate response. When asked to select among specified response options, pick <u>one and only one</u> of the options. If your <u>most accurate</u> response would fall between two options, pick that <u>one</u> option of the two which is the <u>more accurate.</u> "Accuracy" in responding has more to do with your subjective perception than it does with objective reality. Your responses should reflect only those times when you were <u>not under the influence</u> of drugs or alcohol.

303

Read each statement carefully, but don't spend too much time deciding on your response. Remember, your initial response is likely to be the more accurate one, so please don't review and "correct" your responses later.

Part A: Applicability

Instructions: In this part, respond to each statement by circling that <u>single</u> response option number that <u>most accurately</u> reflects the statement's applicability to you. The specified meaning for each response option number is as follows:

> *0 = Definitely <u>does not</u> apply to me.*
> *1 = Generally <u>does not</u> apply to me.*
> *2 = Minimally applies to me.*
> *3 = Generally applies to me.*
> *4 = Definitely applies to me.*

STATEMENT: RESPONSE:

1. I believe I am more sensitive to loud noises than the average person. ..0   1   2   3   4

2. Growing up, I was not one of the "popular" kids. 0   1   2   3   4

3. I tend to think in concrete, practical terms. 0   1   2   3   4

4. I tend to have trouble following verbal instructions. 0   1   2   3   4

5. I don't care to know what other people really think of me. 0   1   2   3   4

6. I spend a lot of time putting my personal thoughts and feelings on

    paper (e.g.: journals, poems, pictures, songs) 0   1   2   3   4

7. In the morning, I wake up easily and am quickly fully alert. 0   1   2   3   4

8. I have a lot of difficulty doing rote memorization. 0   1   2   3   4

9. At least once, I have become temporarily blind, deaf, paralyzed,

    or numb without any logical medical explanation 0   1   2   3   4

10. Sometimes I feel happy and sad all at once. 0   1   2   3   4

0 = definitely <u>does not</u> apply; 1 = generally <u>does not</u> apply; 2 = minimally applies;
3 = generally applies; 4 = definitely applies

STATEMENT: RESPONSE:

11. I believe I am more sensitive to temperature and/or humidity
extremes than the average person. 0   1   2   3   4
12. I am more drawn to "the touching" than I am to
"the convincing." 0   1   2   3   4
13. It is very difficult for me to imagine myself as an animal or
what being an animal might be like. 0   1   2   3   4
14. I have a tendency to start things and then not finish them. 0   1   2   3   4
15. I like to keep my options open as long as possible, not making
decisions until I absolutely must. 0   1   2   3   4
16. My dreams are often so vivid as to later be indistinguishable
from waking reality. 0   1   2   3   4
17. I can easily maintain my focus and concentration without
being distracted. 0   1   2   3   4
18. Daydreaming has been an effective tool in solving many of
my problems. 0   1   2   3   4
19. When I am "stressed out," I develop physical symptoms
(e.g.: ulcers, headaches, hives, asthma, heart palpitations). 0   1   2   3   4
20. I am especially fond of the color magenta. 0   1   2   3   4
21. I believe I am more sensitive to bright lights and/or flashing lights
than the average person. 0   1   2   3   4
22. If I were a teacher, I would rather teach theory courses than
fact courses. 0   1   2   3   4
23. When emotionally drained, I can best recharge by spending
time with a group of friends 0   1   2   3   4
24. When several people are talking, I tend to have difficulty
focusing on just one person's words. 0   1   2   3   4
25. I am a list maker. 0   1   2   3   4
26. I believe I would be a good psychotherapist. 0   1   2   3   4
27. Generally speaking, I am quite well coordinated. 0   1   2   3   4
28. I have/had trouble counting change and/or balancing a checkbook. ...0   1   2   3   4
29. I have/had unusual reactions to coffee or tea. 0   1   2   3   4
30. At least once, from a medical perspective, I almost died. 0   1   2   3   4
31. I believe I am more sensitive to colors than the average person. 0   1   2   3   4
32. I can be more impressed by people's emotions than by their
principles. 0   1   2   3   4
33. I have not always been honest with myself. 0   1   2   3   4
34. I have trouble organizing my thoughts and/or setting priorities 0   1   2   3   4
35. My strengths lie more in dealing with the unexpected than they
do in following detailed plans. 0   1   2   3   4
36. Others sometimes comment that I seem to be off in another world. .0   1   2   3   4

304

0 = definitely <u>does not</u> apply; 1 = generally <u>does not</u> apply; 2 = minimally applies;
3 = generally applies; 4 = definitely applies

<u>STATEMENT:</u>   <u>RESPONSE:</u>

37. My approach toward others tends to be more objective
    than it is personal. 0   1   2   3   4
38. I am emotionally quite sensitive. 0   1   2   3   4
39. I have/had unusual reactions to alcohol. 0   1   2   3   4
40. The phrase *"mel-tahn-doe"* (phonetic spelling) stimulates unusual
    feelings in me. 0   1   2   3   4
41. I believe I am more sensitive to thunderstorms than the
    average person. 0   1   2   3   4

42. Within my group, I'm among the last to know what
    everybody is doing. 0   1   2   3   4
43. I am better served by having a strong sense of reality than I am by
    having a vivid imagination. 0   1   2   3   4
44. In reading, I tend to mix up letters like p and q or
    numbers like 2 and 5. 0   1   2   3   4
45. When I am aware that other people are talking privately,
    I make it a point never to eavesdrop. 0   1   2   3   4
46. I can sense another person's thoughts or feelings with
    nothing being said. 0   1   2   3   4
47. I believe I had an easier childhood than most people. 0   1   2   3   4
48. Over the course of a normal week, I recall several of my dreams. ...0   1   2   3   4
49. I have/had unusual reactions to marijuana. 0   1   2   3   4
50. I have experienced one or more electrical shocks sufficiently
    severe to have physiological consequences (i.e., knockdown,
    unconsciousness, etc.) 0   1   2   3   4
51. I believe I am more sensitive to crowds than the average person. ... 0   1   2   3   4
52. I am more interested in possibilities than I am in facts and data. 0   1   2   3   4
53. I have a very clear and distinct sense of time. 0   1   2   3   4
54. I have a tendency to get confused between left and right. 0   1   2   3   4
55. I do not like surprises and/or changes in routine. 0   1   2   3   4
56. As a child, I lived in a make-believe world much/most of
    the time. 0   1   2   3   4
57. I generally have an easy time memorizing things by rote. 0   1   2   3   4
58. I would rather be known for my sensitivity than for my
    reasonableness. 0   1   2   3   4
59. My senses tend to get jumbled up together (i.e., sounds seem to
    have a color, textures to have a tone, or tastes to have a shape). 0   1   2   3   4
60. I especially like the smell of damp fur. 0   1   2   3   4
61. I believe I am more sensitive to rhythmic sounds than the
    average person. 0   1   2   3   4
62. There are very few people with whom I can get along really well. ..0   1   2   3   4
63. I don't always know the reasons why I do the things I do. 0   1   2   3   4
64. In reading, I tend to make mistakes like reading "unclear"
    as "nuclear." 0   1   2   3   4
65. I never take things that don't belong to me. 0   1   2   3   4

0 = definitely <u>does not</u> apply; 1 = generally <u>does not</u> apply; 2 = minimally applies;
3 = generally applies; 4 = definitely applies

STATEMENT:			RESPONSE:		

66. I am very attuned to other people's feelings. 0   1   2   3   4

67. I find daydreaming to be a waste of time. 0   1   2   3   4

68. I tend to be highly distractible and/or easily sidetracked. 0   1   2   3   4

69. Sometimes I experience colors as having "sounds" or
"tonal qualities." 0   1   2   3   4

70. I have experienced one or more traumas with significant
psychological consequences
(e.g.: being raped, seeing somebody killed, being in a fire). 0   1   2   3   4

71. I believe I am more sensitive to fluorescent lights than the
average person. 0   1   2   3   4

72. I believe there are times when "common sense" is anything but 0   1   2   3   4

73. In making decisions, I tend to be guided more by reason, logic, and
objective standards than by subjective feelings and personal values.. 0   1   2   3   4

74. I tend to get confused about the order of the letters in the alphabet. 0   1   2   3   4

75. Making lists would cramp my style. 0   1   2   3   4

76. I vividly "remember" things I know couldn't "really" have
happened. 0   1   2   3   4

77. I am pretty adept at handling routine mathematical things like
balancing a checkbook or dealing with cash. 0   1   2   3   4

78. I drop things and/or bump into things a lot. 0   1   2   3   4

79. Sometimes, a piece of music will stimulate a "light show"
in my mind. 0   1   2   3   4

80. I am especially drawn to things that have a hexagonal
(six-sided) shape. 0   1   2   3   4

81. I believe I am more sensitive to textures and/or tactile
sensations than the average person. 0   1   2   3   4

82. I am generally more interested in what people have to say about
concepts and ideas than in what they have to say about people,
places, and things. 0   1   2   3   4

83. I am more a practical sort of person than I am an
imaginative sort. 0   1   2   3   4

84. I read very slowly and/or often lose my place when reading. 0   1   2   3   4

85. I prefer to make decisions as quickly as practicable rather than
keeping my options open as long as possible. 0   1   2   3   4

86. I have/had a well-developed talent/ability in one or more of the
arts (i.e., musical, graphic, literary, dramatic). 0   1   2   3   4

87. I have a "thick skin" — my feelings are not easily hurt 0   1   2   3   4

88. I am more likely to be personal than objective in my approach
to others. 0   1   2   3   4

89. I am bothered by chronic body pain (especially in the
joints, neck, back). 0   1   2   3   4

90. I believe I've had "more than my share of" serious accidents,
injuries, and/or illnesses. 0   1   2   3   4

306

0 = definitely <u>does not</u> apply; 1 = generally <u>does not</u> apply; 2 = minimally applies;
3 = generally applies; 4 = definitely applies

STATEMENT: RESPONSE:

91. I believe I am more sensitive to psychological stress than the
    average person. 0   1   2   3   4
92. I tend to identify with other people so strongly that I take on their
    emotions, problems, or illnesses as my own. 0   1   2   3   4
93. At times, I have taken unfair advantage of other people. 0   1   2   3   4
94. My spelling is terrible. 0   1   2   3   4
95. Surprises/unexpected events are, for me, a welcome change
    from routine. 0   1   2   3   4
96. When I'm speaking, my mind sometimes goes blank and/or I
    lose my train of thought. 0   1   2   3   4
97. I seldom recall my dreams. 0   1   2   3   4
98. I had a difficult, complicated, and/or stressful childhood. 0   1   2   3   4
99. I can easily recapture an event in memory and relive it as if
    I were there. 0   1   2   3   4
100. I believe I've had "more than my share of" hospitalizations
    and/or major surgeries. 0   1   2   3   4
101. I believe I am more sensitive to moving water than the
    average person. 0   1   2   3   4
102. I have deep friendships with very few people rather than broad
    friendships with many different people. 0   1   2   3   4
103. I can remember (almost) nothing, from before I was three
    years old. 0   1   2   3   4
104. I have trouble following directions and/or often get lost. 0   1   2   3   4
105. I find I deal better with detailed plans than I do with the
    unexpected. 0   1   2   3   4
106. I have done "inspirational writing" (i.e., poems, prayers,
    songs, etc.) and felt it wasn't I who was doing the writing. 0   1   2   3   4
107. In relating to others, I believe that reasonableness takes one
    further than does sensitivity. 0   1   2   3   4
108. In the morning, it takes a few minutes before I am sure I'm
    really awake. 0   1   2   3   4
109. I can vividly re-experience physical sensations in my imagination
    (i.e., a gentle breeze, soft fur, cool grass, the warmth
    of the sun, etc.). 0   1   2   3   4
110. Sometimes, for no apparent reason, I have "attacks" of
    panic or anxiety. 0   1   2   3   4
111. I believe I'm more sensitive to smells and/or tastes than the
    average person. 0   1   2   3   4
112. In doing something challenging which others have done before,
    I like to invent my own way rather than following the
    "tried and true" method. 0   1   2   3   4

307

Part B: Frequency

Instructions: In this part, some statements address your perceptions of how you were treated by your parents or primary caretakers. If you were raised by somebody other than one or both of your biological parents, please respond in terms of the person(s) who had primary responsibility for your upbringing. Where a statement refers to the behavior of both caretakers and they differed in their behavior, respond in terms of that caretaker whose behavior was the more severe or worse.

Respond to each statement by circling that <u>single</u> response option number that <u>most accurately</u> reflects the frequency with which you have had the experience referred to in the statement. Each statement should be read as if it were preceded by the words, "At times,…", and each response option should be read as if it were preceded by the words "I have (had) this experience…". The specified meaning for each response option number is as follows:

<u>*["I have (had) this experience …"]*</u>

0 = Never
1 = Rarely
2 = Occasionally
3 = Often
4 = Regularly

STATEMENT: RESPONSE:
["At times …"]   ["I have (had) this experience …"]

113. … growing up, I was physically mistreated. 0   1   2   3   4
114. … I have blank spells and do things without conscious
     awareness. 0   1   2   3   4
115. … I have experienced episodes of twitching, jerking, shaking, or
     vibrating in my body and/or extremities. 0   1   2   3   4
116. … growing up, I experienced traumatic or upsetting sexual
     experiences that I couldn't talk about with adults. 0   1   2   3   4
117. … I have experienced episodes of staring off into space,
     thinking of nothing, and being unaware of the passage of time. 0   1   2   3   4
118. … I have trouble distinguishing my inner reality from
     outer reality. 0   1   2   3   4
119. … I have experienced "flashbacks" (i.e., where memories come
     flooding back all at once—sometimes in ways that are
     overwhelming). 0   1   2   3   4
120. … electrical or electronic equipment will malfunction in
     my presence. 0   1   2   3   4
121. … for no apparent reason, I experience sudden intense feelings
     of ecstasy, bliss, peace, love, devotion, joy, or cosmic harmony. 0   1   2   3   4
122. … I have experienced the feeling that I was actually flying
     through the air, although I didn't know why or how. 0   1   2   3   4
123. … growing up, when I was punished, I understood the
     reason(s) why. 0   1   2   3   4
124. … for no apparent reason, my body seems to change size
     and/or shape. 0   1   2   3   4

0 = never; 1 = rarely; 2 = occasionally; 3 = often; 4 = regularly

STATEMENT: RESPONSE:
["At times …"]   ["I have (had) this experience …"]

125. … I have heard internal sounds — such as ringing, buzzing, whistling, or chirping — with no logical explanation for them. 0   1   2   3   4

126. … growing up, my relationship with a parent(s) involved a sexual experience(s). 0   1   2   3   4

127. … in the early morning hours (@2:00 AM to 4:00 AM), I have unusual experiences that are especially meaningful to me. 0   1   2   3   4

309

128. … I have gone from one room to another, then forgotten why I went 0   1   2   3   4

129. …for no apparent reason, I have experienced a strong, unpleasant taste in my mouth...0   1   2   3   4

130. … for no logical reason, my fingernails grow unusually fast. 0   1   2   3   4

131. … my breathing will spontaneously become rapid, or shallow, or deep, or even stop altogether for an extended period of time. 0   1   2   3   4

132. … I have found puzzling scars on my body and neither I nor anyone else could remember how or where I got them. 0   1   2   3   4

133. … growing up, I was severely punished when I didn't follow the rules. 0   1   2   3   4

134. … I have had the feeling that I was no longer real, or not the same person, or that I had suddenly become changed, distorted, or transformed. 0   1   2   3   4

135. … for no apparent reason, feelings of extreme heat or cold move through my body. 0   1   2   3   4

136. … I engaged in sexual activity with an adult before I was 14 years old. 0   1   2   3   4

137. … I have experienced some person, place, or situation as being strangely familiar — despite my never having been exposed to it before. 0   1   2   3   4

138. … I have sensed, with no "ordinary" way of knowing, that someone I cared about was in danger or hurt, and I later found out it was true. 0   1   2   3   4

139. … for no logical reason, I have experienced the sensation of smelling a strong unpleasant odor (e.g.: sewage, ammonia, "rotten eggs"). 0   1   2   3   4

140. … electric lights mysteriously turn on, off, or blow out in my presence. 0   1   2   3   4

141. … inner voices distract me from what other people are saying. 0   1   2   3   4

142. … I have experienced a period of an hour or more, in which I was apparently lost, but I could not remember why, or where I had been. 0   1   2   3   4

143. … growing up, when punished, I felt "the punishment fit the crime." 0   1   2   3   4

144. … I have found myself in some place or situation and have been unable to figure out how I got there. 0   1   2   3   4

145. … for no apparent reason, I have experienced the sensation of tickling, itching, or crawling under my skin. 0   1   2   3   4

0 = never; 1 = rarely; 2 = occasionally; 3 = often; 4 = regularly

STATEMENT: RESPONSE:

["At times …"]   ["I have (had) this experience …"]

146. … growing up, I was told to ignore or overlook things I
knew were true. 0   1   2   3   4
147. … for no apparent reason, I have had the strong feeling of being
watched by an unseen "presence." 0   1   2   3   4
148. … I experience things as if they were "more real than real." 0   1   2   3   4
149. … for no logical reason, I have felt rising or sinking sensations
in my stomach — as if I were on a roller coaster or an elevator. 0   1   2   3   4
150. … growing up, my parents accused me of lying when I knew
I was not. 0   1   2   3   4
151. … I experience energy discharges or currents flowing through
my body. 0   1   2   3   4
152. … I have had the experience of waking up paralyzed with a sense
of a strange person or presence or something else in the room. 0   1   2   3   4
153. … growing up, my parents hit or beat me when
I did not expect it. 0   1   2   3   4
154. … for no logical reason, a person, place, or thing will seem to
me to have suddenly become changed, distorted, or transformed. 0   1   2   3   4
155. … I have heard a voice calling my name or repeating a phrase
and have been uncertain whether it was real or imagined. 0   1   2   3   4
156. … growing up, I felt disliked, unwanted, or emotionally
neglected by one or both of my parents. 0   1   2   3   4
157. … I have experienced a familiar person, place, or situation as
being unfamiliar, different, or changed — almost as if I 'd never
been exposed to it before. 0   1   2   3   4
158. … I don't know if I have actually done something, or have just
thought about doing it (e.g.: mailing a letter). 0   1   2   3   4
159. … I have experienced unexplained episodes of dizziness/loss
of balance. 0   1   2   3   4
160. … I experience noticeable physical sensations around electrical
transmission lines and/or electrical/electronic equipment. 0   1   2   3   4
161. … my body will spontaneously assume and hold strange
positions. 0   1   2   3   4
162. … I have seen lights or balls of light without knowing what
was causing them or where they came from. 0   1   2   3   4
163. … growing up, when I was punished, I felt I deserved it. 0   1   2   3   4
164. … people whom I feel certain I don't know will insist that we
have met before and/or call me by a name other than my own. 0   1   2   3   4
165. … I have experienced the sensation of my consciousness
leaving my physical body and being able to see my body from
another location. 0   1   2   3   4

310

Part C: Transpersonal Experiences

Instructions: In this part, you are asked to provide information about your personal experiences of the "transpersonal" ("anomalous", "metaphysical", or "paranormal") kind. Respond to each statement by circling that single response option number that most accurately reflects the frequency with which you have had the experience. Spontaneous experiences should be weighted more heavily than those that were deliberately cultivated — use your best judgment in responding. Each statement should be read as if it were preceded by the words "With respect to …", and each response should be read as if it were preceded by the words "I have (had) this experience …". The specified meaning for each response option number is as follows:

["I have (had) this experience …"]
0 = Never
1 = Rarely
2 = Occasionally
3 = Often
4 = Regularly

STATEMENT: RESPONSE:
["With respect to …"]   ["I have (had) this experience …"]

166. *Déjà-vu:* (the strong feeling that one has experienced some person, place, or situationbefore, even though the experience is, "in reality," occurring for the first time.). 0   1   2   3   4

167. Synchronicity: (the occurrence of a pattern of significant events, apparently causally unrelated, the connections among which seem to be too meaningful to be mere coincidence.). 0   1   2   3   4

168. Telepathy: (transmission and/or reception of thoughts with another person without normal communication or clues.). 0   1   2   3   4

169. Precognition: (accurate knowledge of an event that will take place in the future and could not be predicted by logical means.). 0   1   2   3   4

170. Psychic dream: (a dream which matches in detail an event the dreamer did not know about or have reason to expect at the time of the dream.). 0   1   2   3   4

171. Clairvoyance/Clairaudience/Clairsentience: (accurate awareness of events at a distance which are not available to usual sensory impressions.). 0   1   2   3   4

172. Psychic healing: (healing of an injury or illness through non-physical means such as prayer, meditation, laying on of hands, therapeutic touch, etc.). 0   1   2   3   4

173. Psychokinesis: (the causing of changes in the location or state of a physical object—metal bending, fire starting, things falling to the floor, etc. — through no "natural"physical means.). 0   1   2   3   4

174. Electrical psychokinesis: (the influencing of electrical and/or electronic equipment — causing lights to go on and off, causing malfunctions in watches, calculators, computers, etc. — through no "natural" physical means.). 0   1   2   3   4

175. Out-of-body experience: (the sense that one's consciousness or mind has moved outside the physical body to a different location and the body can actually be seen from that location — other than during a near-death experience which is covered below.). 0   1   2   3   4

0 = never; 1 = rarely; 2 = occasionally; 3 = often; 4 = regularly

STATEMENT:				RESPONSE:	
["With respect to …"]			["I have (had) this experience …"]		

176. Past-life recall: (the recollection of details and/or emotions of what apparently was another lifetime occurring before the experiencer was born into her/his current body.) 0   1   2   3   4

177. Contact with spirit guides: (mental contact with "spirits" or "higher beings" in which the individual receives information or guidance while remaining aware of what is happening.). 0   1   2   3   4

178. Mediumistic episode: (communication of information or guidance by a "spirit" using the voice — "trance channeling," or hand — "automatic writing," of the experiencer who is in a trance and has little awareness afterwards of what was communicated.). 0   1   2   3   4

179. Apparition: (a vision, while awake, of another person, living or dead, who is not physically, or "objectively," present.) 0   1   2   3   4

180. UFO sighting: (the observation of a UFO—["flying saucer"] — and/or its occupants without actual contact taking place.). 0   1   2   3   4

181. Alien contact: (actual contact with "extraterrestrial beings" — often involving being taken aboard a UFO — frequently against the experiencer's will.). 0   1   2   3   4

182. Spirit possession: (the feeling that another consciousness— demon, spirit, soul of someone living or dead — is attempting to take over control of the experiencer's body and will.). 0   1   2   3   4

Instructions: For the following item only, circle "0" if you have never had the experi-ence, circle "3" if you have had the experience once, and circle "4" if you have had the experience two or more times.

183. Near-death experience: (coming very close to death— and experiencing such classical NDE phenomena as leaving the body, journeying through a tunnel, entering a world of light, perceiving a presence, etc.—but ultimately surviving). 0   3   4

Instructions: In the space provided below, please make whatever comments you feel are appropriate about your experience of completing this inventory:

_____

_____

_____

_____

_____

THE END — THANK YOU!

312

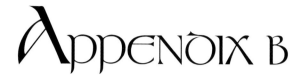

Appendix B

Index Of Hiss Scales

244	ASN	ASSOCIATION
245	SUG	SUGGESTION
<u>250</u>	<u>TPE</u>	<u>TRANSPERSONAL EXPERIENCES</u>
251	X-V	T/P EXPERIENCES - VERIFIABLE
252	X-U	T/P EXPERIENCES - UNVERIFIABLE

FOURTH-LEVEL PRE & IND SCALES (11)

Scale #	*Abbr.*	*Nomenclature*
122a	Sex	Abuse - Sexual
122b	Men	Abuse - Mental
122c	Pun	Abuse - Punishment
211a	Imm	Somatic - Immune
211b	Psy	Somatic - Psychogenic
211c	Sub	Somatic - Substance
211d	Emr	Somatic - Electro-Magnetic Radiation
212a	Aes	Sensory - Aesthetic
212b	Ovr	Sensory - Overload
223a	Amn	Mnemonic - Amnesia
223b	Hyp	Mnemonic - Hypermnesia

314

OTHER SCALES (7 Scored)

Scale #	*Abbr.*	*Nomenclature*
300	***OTH***	***OTHER***
310	*EXP*	*EXPLANATORY*
311	EMS	ELECTRO-MAGNETIC SENSITIVITY
312	TLE	TEMPORO-LIMBIC EPILEPSY
313	KUN	KUNDALINI AROUSAL
320	*CHK*	*INTERNAL CHECKS*
321	*TST*	*TEST ITEMS*
322	*SKU*	*SKEW*
322a	Out	Skew — Outliers
322b	Rev	Skew — Reversals
322c	Sdr	Skew — Socially Desirable Responses

Appendix C

Composition Of Hiss Scales

Note: [ ] = responses from Section I; { } = average of included responses; 315 *all other responses are from Section II.*

#	ABBR.	NOMENCLATURE & RESPONSES

100 PRE PREDISPOSITIONS
110 BIO BIOLOGICAL
111 ACL ANOMALOUS CEREBRAL LATERALITY
    [1] [2] [5] [6] {[11] + [12] + [13]} [16]
    [17] [32] [33]
112 STR STAR
    [19] [22] [23] 89

120 TAB TRAUMA AND ABUSE
121 TRM TRAUMA
    30 50 70 90 100
122 ABU ABUSE
122a Sex Abuse — Sexual
    116 126 136
122b Men Abuse — Mental
    47 98 146 150 156
122c Pun Abuse — Punishment
    113 123 133 143 153 163

130 TTP TEMPERAMENT TYPE PREFERENCES
131 ORN ORIENTATION
    2 23 42 62 82 102
132 PER PERCEIVING
    3 18 22 43 52 67 72 83
112
133 JUD JUDGING
    12 32 37 58 73 88 92 107
134 PRF PREFERENCE
    15 25 35 55 75 85 95 105

#	ABBR.	NOMENCLATURE & RESPONSES

200   **IND**   **INDICATORS**

210   PHS   PHYSIOLOGICAL

211   SOM   SOMATIC

211a   Imm   Somatic — Immune
     [18]   [28]   [29]   [30]

211b   Psy   Somatic — Psychogenic
     9   19   115   135   145   149   159

316   211c   Sub   Somatic — Substance
     [20]   [21]   29   39   49

211d   Emr   Somatic — Electro-Magnetic Radiation
     41   71   101   120   140   160

212   SEN   SENSORY

212a   Aes   Sensory — Aesthetic
     31   59   61   69   79   86

212b   Ovr   Sensory — Overload
     1   11   21   81   111

220   COG   COGNITIVE

221   ATT   ATTENTION
     4   14   17   24   27   34   53   68   78

222   LRN   LEARNING
     8   28   44   54   57   64   74   77   84
     94   104

223   MNE   MNEMONIC

223a   Amn   Amnesia
     96   128   157   158

223b   Hyp   Hypermnesia
     99   103   109   119

230   EMO   EMOTIONAL

231   TRA   INTRAPERSONAL
     10   38   87   91   110   121

232   TER   INTERPERSONAL
     26   46   51   66   138

#	ABBR.	NOMENCLATURE & RESPONSES							

<u>240</u>   ASC   <u>ALTERED STATES OF CONSCIOUSNESS</u>

241   DSN   DISSOCIATION

114	124	134	141	142	144	154	164	165

242   HAL   HALLUCINATION

125	129	139	155	162

243   SWO   SLEEP/WAKE OVERLAP

[31]	7	16	48	97	108	122	127

244   ASN   ASSOCIATION

13	36	56	76	106	117	118	148

245   SUG   SUGGESTIBILITY

20	40	60	80	130

<u>250</u>   TPE   <u>TRANSPERSONAL EXPERIENCES</u>

251   X-V   T/P EXPERIENCES — VERIFIABLE

166	167	168	169	170	171	172	173	174

252   X-U   T/P EXPERIENCES — UNVERIFIABLE

175	176	177	178	179	180	181	182	183

300   ***OTH***   ***OTHER***

<u>*310*</u>   *EXP*   *EXPLANATORY*

311   EMS   ELECTRO-MAGNETIC SENSITIVITY

41	71	101	120	140	160

312   TLE   TEMPORO-LIMBIC EPILEPSY

6	115	117	119	125	127	129	134	135
137	139	145	147	149	154	155	157	159
162	165							

313   KUN   KUNDALINI AROUSAL

115	121	122	125	131	135	141	145	151
155	161	162	165					

#	**ABBR.**	**NOMENCLATURE & RESPONSES**								
320	*CHK*	*CHECKS, INTERNAL*								
321	*TST*	*TEST ITEMS*								
		[1]	[1A]	[3]	[4]	[6A]	[7]	[8]	[9]	[10]
		[14]	[15]	[24]	[25]	[26]	[27]			
322	SKU	SKEW								
322a	Out	Skew — Outliers								
322b	Rev	Skew — Reversals								
		3	7	13	17	23	27	37	43	47
		53	57	67	73	77	83	87	97	103
		107	123	143	163					
322c	Sdr	Skew — Socially Desirable Responses								
		5	33	45	63	65	93			

318

Appendix D

The Hiss EMS Scale

The six questions below comprise the HISS Electro-Magnetic Sensitivity explanatory scale. Answer the questions in each group according to the instructions, do the math and your score will provide a reasonably accurate indication of whether or not you're an ASP.

Answer the following three questions on an "applicability" basis.
0 = Definitely <u>does not</u> apply to me, 1 = Generally <u>does not</u> apply to me,
2 = Minimally applies to me,
3 = Generally applies to me, 4 = Definitely applies to me.

- I believe I am more sensitive to thunderstorms than
  is the average person. 0   1   2   3   4
- I believe I am more sensitive to fluorescent lights than
  is the average person. 0   1   2   3   4
- I believe I am more sensitive to moving water than
  is the average person. 0   1   2   3   4

Answer the following three questions on a "frequency" basis.
0 = Never, 1 = Rarely, 2 = Occasionally, 3 = Often, 4 = Regularly.

- At times, electrical or electronic equipment will
  malfunction in my presence. 0   1   2   3   4
- At times, electric lights mysteriously turn on, off,
  or blow out in my presence. 0   1   2   3   4
- At times, I experience noticeable physical sensations
  around electrical transmission lines and/or
  electrical/electronic equipment. 0   1   2   3   4

TOTAL (of scores for the 6 questions above):   _____

EMS SCALE SCORE ("TOTAL" divided by 6):   _____

The Reference Group's mean score on this scale is 1.16; its standard deviation is 1.03. If your score is more than 2.19 (+1 s.d.), you scored high; if your score is more than 3.22 (+2 s.d.), you scored very high. The predictive reliability of EMS scores for PRE scores is 53% and for IND scores is 76%. If your score on the EMS scale is very high (3.22 or higher), you *might* meet the criteria for being a basic ASP.

320

Appendix E

Double-Checking

The findings from the HISS data were internally consistent and logically congruent, but the more checking that could be done to ensure the validity and reliability of the questionnaire itself, the better. The Skew (SKU) scales (encompassed by the second-level Internal Checks, [CHK] grouping of scales, which is, in turn, encompassed by the first-level Other [OTH] grouping of scales)—was built into the HISS from the outset and was designed to identify individual questionnaires that appeared to be potentially invalid because of inconsistencies in the pattern of responses. Additionally, after the Reference Group data had been analyzed, test/retest reliability was explored to determine the constancy of individual responses over time. Finally, the results for the HISS were compared to results for other questionnaires that presumably measured some similar variables.

Skew Scales

Some people claim that the results of a self-reporting questionnaire (such as the HISS) cannot be believed because there is no objective confirmation of the subjects' responses. The accuracy of the responses for any one individual's questionnaire is, of course, always open to question, but with a large enough number of subjects, it is unlikely that a meaningful percentage of questionnaires will contain major inaccuracies. Moreover, from a practical perspective, it must be remembered that two widely used and highly respected questionnaires, the "Myers-Briggs Type Indicator (MBTI)" and the "Minnesota Multiphasic Personality Inventory (MMPI)," are both of the self-reporting genre. The former was discussed in some depth in Chapters 6 and 14. The latter is regularly employed as a screening instrument for such things as security clearances, access to nuclear materials and airline pilot qualifications. As far as I am concerned, if the self-reporting format is good enough for the MBTI and the MMPI, it's good enough for the HISS.

Nevertheless, it is true that responses given to the questions

322

in the HISS were entirely subjective and it seemed appropriate to have an objective basis on which to eliminate individual questionnaires that showed strong evidence of potentially being invalid. Subjects might give invalid responses either unconsciously (as a result of mind-set, suggestibility, or the like) or consciously (because they wanted to appear either more or less sensitive than they really are). The Skew scales were designed to address these issues. Three fourth-level scales—Skew - Outliers (Out), Skew - Reversals (Rev) and Skew - Socially Desirable Responses (Sdr)—are encompassed by the third-level Skew (SKU) scale. Each is discussed below.

The fourth-level Skew - Outliers (Out) scale was designed to identify those questionnaires in which there is an unusually large difference (in either direction) between the subject's scores on the first-level Indicators (IND) scale and the first-level Predispositions (PRE) scale. A high score on the Skew - Outliers scale might indicate a respondent who wants to appear more sensitive than s/he really is; a low score might indicate a respondent who wants to appear less sensitive than s/he really is. Scores on this scale are correlated with IND scores at an "r" value of .61. As expected, relative to the norm, those in the Reference Group who are highly predisposed toward sensitivities appear to overstate and those who are not highly predisposed toward sensitivities appear to understate, their actual sensitivities.

The fourth-level Skew - Reversals (Rev) scale was designed to identify questionnaires in which the respondent appeared to have a mind-set that resulted in a generalized response bias toward either high scores or low scores. Ten percent (22) of the HISS questions are reverse-worded and reverse-scored. Scores for this scale are based on a comparison of the subject's mean score for the reversed questions with her/his score for the Indicators scale. The correlation between scores on this scale and scores on the IND scale has an "r" value of .56 and, as expected, indicates that a mind-set response bias does exist within the Reference Group.

My expectation was that any such bias would be in the high-scoring direction. The HISS was, after all, developed as part of a project to study people with anomalously high levels of sensitivities and my own mind-set might well have introduced an upside bias with leading questions—perhaps resulting in mean scale scores in the 2.0 – 3.0 range. Such was not the case, however. The mean score for all second-level PRE and IND scales combined is only 1.22—and just one of those scales, Emotional indicators, has a mean score greater than 2.0 (specifically 2.07).

Also contrary to expectations was the finding that the correlation between Skew - Reversals (Rev) scores and IND scores is caused more by a downside mind-set on the part of low scorers than it is by an upside mind-set on the part of high scorers. Whereas the reversal responses for low scorers were substantially understated, the reversal responses for high scorers were somewhat overstated—indicating emphatic disagreement with the reverse-worded questions as they were presented.

The fourth-level Skew - Socially Desirable Responses (Sdr) scale was designed to identify those questionnaires in which there was a bias toward the reporting of conventional socially desirable (or, conversely, undesirable) behaviors. It consists of questions addressing such behaviors directly. Scores on this scale are somewhat negatively correlated with scores on the IND scale, the "r" value of the correlation being -.19. While there was no significant difference, with respect to claims of socially desirable behavior, between those who had high IND scores and those who had low IND scores, high scorers more readily admitted to socially undesirable behaviors.

The scoring for all of the Skew scales is quite complex, but simplistically it can be said that individual scores for the third-level Skew (SKU) scale are the sum of the absolute values of the standard deviations of the individual scores for its three underlying fourth-level scales—in other words, three separate and distinct factors are involved. When a subject's score on the third-level Skew (SKU) scale was two or more standard deviations above the mean score of that scale, the questionnaire was presumed to be invalid. In keeping with that criterion, eight of the questionnaires originally submitted were rejected as being internally inconsistent and were not included in the Reference Group data.

TEST/RETEST RELIABILITY

The HISS was administered a second time (about six months after it was first completed) to a group of 41 Reference Group subjects. The purpose of doing this was to determine what degree of constancy existed in an individual's responses over time. For an $n = 41$, an $r = .55$ results in a $p < .0001$. The correlations between the first-time and second-time scores on all first-, second- and third-level PRE and IND scales as well as the third-level Explanatory scales were statistically very significant. The relevant "r" values are shown in Table E.1., below.

HISS TEST/RETEST CORRELATION COEFFICIENTS								
Predispositions Group			**Indicators Group**			**Explanatory Group**		
#	Abbr.	Coeff.	#	Abbr.	Coeff.	#	Abbr.	Coeff.
100	PRE	.80	200	IND	.83	311	EMS	.67
110	BIO	.82	210	PHS	.77	312	TLE	.72
111	ACL	.78	211	SOM	.81	313	KUN	.76
112	STR	.65	212	SEN	.65			
120	TAB	.72	220	COG	.92			
121	TRM	.67	221	ATT	.89			
122	ABU	.81	222	LRN	.87			
130	TTP	.82	223	MNE	.75			
131	ORN	.77	230	EMO	.72			
132	PER	.78	231	TRA	.72			
133	JUD	.69	232	TER	.72			
134	PRF	.75	240	ASC	.77			
			241	DSN	.78			
			242	HAL	.72			
			243	SWO	.75			
			244	ASN	.76			
			245	SUG	.65			
			250	TPE	.84			
			251	X-V	.84			
			252	X-U	.82			

Table E.1. HISS Test/Retest Correlation Coefficients

COMPARISON WITH OTHER QUESTIONNAIRES

Three other questionnaires—the "Dissociative Experiences Survey (DES)," the "Limbic System Checklist (LSCL-33)" and the "Kiersey Temperament Sorter (KTS)"—that measure variables similar to some of those measured by the HISS were administered to 36 HISS Reference Group subjects. The correlation coefficients between the subjects' scores on those instruments and their scores on the comparable HISS scales were then determined—and are shown in Table E.2., Table E.3. and Table E.4., below. For an n = 36, an r = .35 results in a p < .05, an r = .40 results in a p < .01, an r = .50 results in a p < .001 and an r = .55 results in a p < .0001. The most relevant correlation coefficients are shown in bold-faced type.

325

COMP. QUEST.	HISS SCALES			
	#240 ASC	#200 IND	#100 PRE	#250 TPE
D.E.S.	**.66**	.65	.57	.51

Table E.2. HISS Correlation Coefficients with Dissociative Experiences Survey Scores

COMP. QUEST.	HISS SCALES			
	#312 TLE	#100 PRE	#200 IND	#250 TPE
L.S.C.L.-33	**.67**	.48	.63	.45

Table E.3. HISS Correlation Coefficients with Limbic System Checklist Scores

COMP. QUEST.	Equivalent Sub-Scales	HISS SCALES						
		#131 ORN.	#132 PER.	#133 JUD.	#130 TTP	#100 PRE	#200 IND	#250 TPE
KTS		.46	.51	.39	**.65**	.30	.35	.12
	ORN	**.37**	-.20	-.26	-.03	-.23	-.11	-.24
	PER	.35	**.66**	.40	.69	.41	.44	.27
	JUD	.12	.34	**.66**	.44	.22	.19	.10

Table E.4. HISS Correlation Coefficients with Kiersey Temperament Sorter Scores

The "Dissociative Experiences Survey (DES)" measures variables that are similar to those measured by the HISS Altered States of Consciousness (ASC) indicators scale. The correlation of scores between the two was statistically very significant.

The "Limbic System Checklist (LSCL-33)" measures variables that are similar to those measured by the HISS Temporo-Limbic Epilepsy (TLE) explanatory scale. The correlation of scores between the two was statistically very significant.

326

The "Kiersey Temperament Sorter (KTS)" measures variables that are similar to those measured by the HISS Temperament Type Preferences (TTP) predispositions scale. There were some surprises here. The correlation between the overall KTS scores and the HISS TTP scale scores was statistically very significant ... but the correlations between the overall KTS scores and the HISS PRE, IND and TPE scales scores were not statistically significant. Moreover, while scores on the KTS equivalent (of the HISS TTP Orientation [ORN] scale) were positively correlated with scores on the HISS TTP Orientation scale at a level that was statistically minimally significant, scores on the KTS equivalent showed slight negative correlations with scores on the HISS PRE, IND and TPE scales. Apparently, the HISS TTP Orientation scale and its KTS equivalent are measuring somewhat different variables. The nature of that difference, however, remains unclear.

Appendix F

Resources For The ASP

327

Anomalously high levels of sensitivities, by societal convention, are likely to be perceived as symptoms of disorders. Organizations that will help one to "understand" such "disorders," and that will suggest "treatments" for their "symptoms" are relatively easy to locate. Organizations that consider such symptoms to be evidence of potential abilities (when properly managed) are few and far between. Presented below are brief profiles of a few organizations that might prove to be helpful to those who choose to take a self-empowering approach to anomalous sensitivities.

EEG Spectrum
16500 Ventura Blvd., Suite 418
Encino, CA 91436
Tel: (818) 789-3456
E-mail: info@eegspectrum.com
Web Site: http://www.eegspectrum.com

This organization was formed in 1988 to promote all aspects of EEG biofeedback—clinical service delivery, training of professionals, controlled research in universities, clinical research and publications. Its stated vision is "to promote the advancement of full human potential through brain-based self-regulation techniques and to help evolve human consciousness through the exploration and development of advanced technologies for self-regulation, self-awareness and self-knowledge." EEG Spectrum has more than 150 affiliate offices in the United States and more than 60 affiliates in 20 other countries.

Foundation for Shamanic Studies
P.O. Box 1939
Mill Valley, CA 94924
Tel: (415) 380-8282
E-mail: info@shamanicstudies.com
Web Site: http://www.shamanism.org

328

This non-profit, educational and research organization was incorporated in 1985 and is dedicated to the preservation, study and teaching of shamanic knowledge. Through its Foundation Field Associates, when invited, the Foundation assists native peoples in saving, maintaining and reviving their own shamanic traditions. Through its Shamanism and Health Program, the Foundation conducts research on the effects of shamanic healing practices. Through its Mapping of Nonordinary Reality Project, the Foundation gathers data for use in constructing a cross-cultural map of the hidden universe discovered and rediscovered by shamans through the ages. The Foundation offers an educational program of workshop and training courses, from basic to advanced, providing rigorous training in core shamanism—the universal, or near-universal, methods of shamanism not bound to any specific cultural group or perspective.

Problems > Solutions > Innovations
37 Camino Ranchitos
Alamogordo, NM 88310
Tel: (505) 437-8285
E-mail: psi@crviewer.com
Web Site: http://www.crviewer.com

P>S>I was established in 1992 by Lyn Buchanan, an early army Controlled Remote Viewer, after his retirement from the military. The company specializes in providing CRV services and CRV training to both individuals and organizations. As a public service, P>S>I also provides, free of charge, CRV consultations to law enforcement agencies through its "Assigned Witness Program."

Spiritual Emergence Network
SEN at CIIS
1453 Mission Street
San Francisco, CA 94103
Tel: (415) 648-2610
E-mail: sen@ciis.edu
Web Site: http://www.senatciis.org

This non-profit organization was founded in 1978 by psychiatrist Stanislav Grof and his wife Christina. It is currently affiliated with the California Institute of Integral Studies. SEN @ CIIS is an information and referral service offering support and resources for individuals experiencing difficulties with their spiritual growth. Trained graduate students in the CIIS School of Professional Psychology respond to each caller, providing assistance and educational information regarding spiritual emergence. They can also make referrals, in the caller's area, to licensed mental health professionals who have demonstrated a capacity to work with clients experiencing psychospiritual difficulties.

International Association for Regression Research and Therapies
(Formerly Association for Past-Life Research and Therapies)
P.O. Box 20151
Riverside, CA 92516-0151
Tel: (909) 784-1570
E-mail: pastlife@empirenet.com
Web Site: http://www.aprt.org

This non-profit, international organization was founded in 1980 by a group of psychotherapists, as a networking resource. It is dedicated to increasing the acceptance and use of responsible regression therapy through education, association and research. Most of its almost 1000 members in 20 countries are psychotherapists, but membership is also open to interested laypersons. Two conferences (open to the public) are presented each year, as well as seminars, workshops and training programs. The refereed "Journal of Regression Therapy" is published annually. Lists, for referral to regression therapists by locale, are available upon inquiry.

Kundalini Research Network
c/o Lawrence Edwards, Ph.D.
66 Main Street
Bedford Hills, NY 10507
Tel: (914) 241-8510
E-Mail: ledwards@bestweb.net
Web Site: http://www.kundalininet.org

This organization was founded in 1990 to: (1) establish a network of scientists, professionals and individuals interested in kundalini research, (2) contact, establish and expand linkages with other groups sharing an interest in kundalini research, (3) share and exchange information by means of a newsletter and by annual meetings or conferences, (4) encourage and collaborate in kundalini research and resulting publications and (5) disseminate information on kundalini to health care professionals and to people experiencing this process.

Institute of Noetic Sciences
101 San Antonio Road
Petaluma, CA 94952
Tel: (707) 775-3500
E-mail: membership@noetic.org
Web Site: http://www.noetic.org

This non-profit research, education and membership organization, founded in 1973, has a membership exceeding 50,000. It conducts and sponsors research and education relating to the workings and powers of the mind, including perceptions, beliefs, attention, intention and intuition. One of its primary stated goals is "to expand our understanding of human possibility by investigating aspects of reality—mind, consciousness and spirit—that include, but potentially go beyond, physical phenomena." It supports community building through community groups, online discussion groups, the "Pathfinding" project and other networking opportunities. Education of the public occurs through publications, conferences and the IONS web site. Six main areas of focus are: spirituality, "Pathfinding" (social transformation), healing, science, creativity and human potential and consciousness.

International Society for the Study of
Subtle Energies and Energy Medicine
11005 Ralston Road - Suite 100D
Arvada, CO 80004
Tel: (303) 425-4625
E-mail: issseem@compuserve.org
Web Site: http://www.issseem.org

This non-profit organization was founded in 1989 to improve human health and welfare through the advancement of education, practice, training and research in the field of subtle energies and energy medicine by: (1) increasing knowledge, (2) improving applications, (3) promoting exploration and (4) disseminating information. Current membership is more than 1300. It publishes an annual peer-reviewed journal, "Subtle Energies and Energy Medicine," and a quarterly magazine, "Bridges." It also sponsors an annual conference.

Highly Sensitive Person
The Comfort Zone
P.O. Box 460564
San Francisco, CA 94146-0564
Web Site: http://www.hsperson.com

This is not an organization, per se. It is, rather, a web site and a quarterly newsletter, "The Comfort Zone," that arose out of Elaine Aron's very successful book entitled *The Highly Sensitive Person.* The concept of the "Highly Sensitive Person," very similar to that of the "Anomalously Sensitive Person," is focused primarily on sensory sensitivities and emotional sensitivities. Local support groups and e-mail chat rooms that develop on an ad-hoc basis can be found by subscribing to the newsletter.

Electrical Sensitivity Network
P.O. Box 4146
Prescott, AZ 86302

This organization was formed in 1994 as a United States support and advocacy group for people who are especially sensitive to Electro-Magnetic Radiation. Its goals are: (1) to assist those who are electrically sensitive in locating medical, legal, housing and EMR reduction resources, (2) facilitate idea sharing on a regional basis, (3) inform the public about the health hazards of EMR and (4) encourage the development of EMR reduction technology. It publishes a newsletter, "Electrical Sensitivity News," and makes available regional networking lists.

Exceptional Human Experience Network
414 Rockledge Road
New Bern, NC 28562
E-mail: rhea@ehe.org
Web Site: http://www.ehe.org

This organization was founded as an educational, research and information resource organization studying all types of anomalous experiences. The organization's philosophy is: (1) anomalous experiences are potential starting points for positive, personal, life-enriching and even life-changing growth, (2) by valuing these experiences and sharing them with others, experiencers gain meaningful insights, (3) when insight occurs, experiencers find a way to grow that enables them to integrate and internalize their experiences and (4) what was an anomaly becomes an Exceptional Human Experience, or EHE.

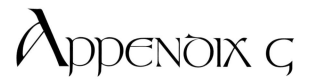

Appendix G

Other Questionnaires

333

*Note: Items appearing in **bold print** were administered separately to some subjects.*

1. "Cognitive Failures Questionnaire (CFQ)."
   Broadbent, D.E., P.F. Cooper, et. al. 1982.
2. **"Confidential Client Intake Information Form (CCIIF)."**
   Ritchey, D.. 1993.
3. "Dissociative Disorders Interview Schedule (DDIS)."
   Ross, C. & S. Heber. 1988.
4. **"Dissociative Experiences Scale (DES)."**
   Carlson, E. & F. Putnam. 1986.
5. "Electrical Sensitivity Questionnaire."
   Pursglove, P. D. Date unknown.
6. **"Experiences of Absorption Survey (EAS)."**
   Telegren, A. & G. Atkinson. 1974.
7. "Gregorc Style Delineator."
   Gregorc, A. 1985.
8. **"Hartmann Boundary Questionnaire (HBQ)."**
   Hartmann, E. 1991.
9. "Hermann Brain Dominance Instrument (HBDI)."
   Hermann, N. 1990.
10. **"Holistic Inventory of Stimulus Sensitivities (HISS) — Rev. 6/96."**
    Ritchey, D. 1996.
11. **"Holistic Inventory of Stimulus Sensitivities (HISS) — Rev. 12/96."**
    Ritchey, D. 1996.
12. **"Holistic Inventory of Stimulus Sensitivities (HISS) — Rev. 9/97."**
    Ritchey, D. 1997.

13. **"Inventory of Anomalous Cerebral Laterality Characteristics (IACLC)."**
Ritchey. D. 1993.

14. **"Inventory of Childhood Memories and Imaginings (ICMI)."** Lynn, S. & J. Rhue. 1986.

15. **"Kiersey Temperament Sorter (KTS)."**
Kiersey, D. & M. Bates. 1984.

16. **"Learning Style Screening Instrument (LSSI)."**
Ritchey, D. 1993.

17. **"Limbic System Checklist (LSCL-33)."**
Teicher, M., C. Glod, et. al. 1993.

18. "Minnesota Multiphasic Personality Inventory (MMPI)."
Hathaway & McKinley. 1940.

19. "Myers-Briggs Type Indicator (MBTI) - Abbr."
Consulting Psychologists Press. 1983.

20. "Myers-Briggs Type Indicator (MBTI) - Form J."
Consulting Psychologists Press. 1984.

21. **"Omega Home Environment Questionnaire."**
Ring, K. 1992.

22. "Omega Psychic Experiences Inventory."
Ring, K. 1984.

23. **"Omega Psychological Inventory (of Dissociation)."**
Wogan, M. 1992.

24. "Physio-Kundalini Syndrome Index."
Greyson, B. 1993.

25. "Psychic Experiences Questionnaire."
Richards, D. 1991.

26. "Psychological Sensitivity Inventory (PSI)."
Ring, K. Date unknown.

27. "Questionnaire for Episodic Psychic Experiences."
Ardila, A., C. Nino, et. al. 1993.

28. "The Roper Poll."
Hopkins, B., et. al. 1992.

29. "Star People Questionnaire."
Steiger, B. & S.H. Steiger. 1992.

30. "Sixteen Personality Factors Questionnaire (16PF)."
Cattell, R.B. 1971.

31. "Strong Vocational Inventory Blank (SVIB)."
Consulting Psychologists Press. 1985.

32. "The Twenty-Five Questions."
Budden, A. 1998.

GLOSSARY

"When I use a word,"
Humpty Dumpty said, in a rather scornful tone,
"it means just what I choose it to mean
—nothing more nor less."
—Lewis Carroll
(Through the Looking Glass)

This glossary is more about the meanings (connotations intended to be conveyed) of terms than it is about the definitions (precise unambiguous explanations) of terms. While the meanings provided for terms used in the text are, in most cases, standard and conventional (or at least relatively so), there are some notable exceptions. Terms (and their abbreviations) that have been assigned non-standard meanings appear in {{this non-standard typeface}}, rather than in {{this standard typeface}}. Other terms, the *precise* (even if standard) meanings of which are especially important, are handled in the same way. See the Preface for further discussion of this convention.

Altered State of Consciousness (ASC): Any State of Consciousness that differs substantively (whether or not that difference can be noticed by the experiencer or an observer) from the three theoretically discrete "ordinary" States of Consciousness— that is, waking consciousness, dreaming consciousness and sleeping consciousness. The number of possible ASCs is presumably infinite. See text, Chapter 10. See also, "consciousness," "State of Consciousness" and "Transpersonal Consciousness."

amnesia: A loss of, or gap in memory. See also, "cryptomnesia" and "hypermnesia."

anomalous: Inconsistent with, or deviating from what is usual, normal, or expected. While "anomalous" can suggest a qualitative difference, in this text it is primarily used to suggest a quantitative difference—in statistical terms, two or more standard deviations removed from the mean—and, under no circumstances is it intended to imply "weird" or "strange." See also, "mean" and "standard deviation."

Anomalous Cerebral Laterality (ACL): (1) From a structural perspective—an enlargement of portions of the right cerebral hemisphere and/or diminution of portions of the left cerebral hemisphere, such that standard hemispheric asymmetry ceases to exist and (2) from a functional perspective—a greater than normal participation of the right cerebral hemisphere in functions normally under the purview of the left cerebral hemisphere (notably language and motor control for handedness). Believed to be the result of an anomalously high level, in utero, of the hormone testosterone. See text, Chapter 4. See also, "anomalous," "brain," "cerebrum," "cortex," "corpus callosum," "Less Strongly Lateralized," "temporal lobe" and "testosterone."

Anomalously Sensitive Person (ASP): A person who has anomalously high levels of sensitivity in the Physiological, Cognitive, Emotional, Altered States of Consciousness and/or Transpersonal Experiences realms; statistically, one who scores two or more standard deviations above the mean on both of the first-level HISS scales, Predispositions (toward sensitivities) and Indicators (of sensitivities). See also, "anomalous," "Holistic Inventory of Stimulus Sensitivities," "mean" and "standard deviation."

Asperger's Syndrome: A mild form of autism characterized by: (1) impairment in social interaction, (2) speech and/or language difficulties, (3) problems with non-verbal communication, (4) restricted, repetitive and stereotyped patterns of behaviors, interests and activities and (5) motor clumsiness. See text, Chapter 8.

association: A mental process involving the joining together of behaviors, affects, sensations, or knowledge that are normally dissociated in ordinary waking consciousness; unification and incorporation. The inhibition of normal subject/object ("self/not-self") differentiation; the perceptual/experiential incorporation of that which is generally agreed to be (part of) "not-self" into that

336

which is generally agreed to be (part of) "self." See text, Chapter 10. See also, "Altered State of Consciousness," "consciousness," "dissociation," "hallucination," "hypnosis," "regression," "State of Consciousness" and "Transpersonal Consciousness."

biological clock: A colloquial term referring to an inherent timing mechanism responsible for controlling various physiological and behavioral cycles. Its measurement of time facilitates the nervous system's integration of the needs of the body with the demands of the environment. Light (especially), temperature, electric fields and magnetic fields, are its primary cueing stimuli. In human beings, the biological clock is believed to be controlled by the suprachiasmatic nucleus located within the hypothalamus. See text, Chapter 4. See also, "Electro-Magnetic Sensitivity," "limbic system" and "pineal gland."

brain: The principal structure of the central nervous system, it has four lobes, is located in the cranium and is composed primarily of neurons and their supportive and nutritive structures. The brain is generally believed to be involved in environmental interaction activities, regulation of bodily functions activities and mind activities. See text, Chapters 4 and 10. See also, "cerebrum," "corpus callosum," "cortex," "limbic system," "pineal gland" and "temporal lobe."

brainwave coherence: Brainwaves from different parts of the brain having the same frequency and amplitude and being mutually entrained so that they operate together in a smooth, continuous pattern. The more focused one's attention is, the more coherent one's brainwaves are likely to be. The greater the communication between different parts of the brain, the greater is the opportunity for brainwave coherence to occur. See text, Chapters 10 and 11. See also, "Anomalous Cerebral Laterality," "brain," "electroencephalogram" and "Less Strongly Lateralized."

cerebrum: The expanded anterior portion of the brain, it overlies the rest of the brain. The cerebrum has two hemispheres that are connected by the corpus callosum and other structures of nerve fibers. It has two layers, an outer layer of gray matter (the cortex), surrounding a thicker layer of white matter. See text, Chapter 4. See also, "brain," "corpus callosum," "cortex" and "temporal lobe."

338

consciousness: A process arising out of one or more types of mind activities involving awareness and/or thought or neither. See Text, Chapter 10. See also, "Altered State of Consciousness," "State of Consciousness" and "Transpersonal Consciousness."

coefficient of correlation: A number, mathematically represented by "r," that is a quantification of the linear relationship that exists between two sets of paired data or two random variables. It is equal to their covariance divided by the product of their standard deviations and has a two-decimal value ranging between -1.00 and +1.00. The nearer the number is to 1.00 (plus or minus), the stronger is the correlation (either positive or negative). See text, Chapter 13. See also, "correlated," "mean," "predictive reliability," "regression" and "standard deviation."

consensus reality: That reality, or those aspects of reality, that are, by general agreement (consensus), said to be "really real." See text, Chapter 10. See also, "explicate order," "really real," "hallucination" and "implicate order."

Controlled Remote Viewing (CRV): Clairvoyance (with its various sub-categories) performed under controlled conditions using stringent, structured protocols. See text, Chapter 12.

corpus callosum: The primary bundle of nerve fibers connecting the two cerebral hemispheres and functioning as a conduit for the transfer of information between them. See also, "brain," "cerebrum," "cortex" and "temporal lobe."

correlated: Having a mutual or reciprocal relationship. Fitting together and varying together. See text, Chapter 13. See also, "coefficient of correlation," "mean," "regression" and "standard deviation."

cortex: The outer layer of the cerebrum, generally believed to be the organ from which arises logical, rational, linear thought and thus said to be the part of the brain that makes humans uniquely different from all other animals. Also called "neo-cortex," "neo-mammalian brain," "new brain," or "gray matter." See text, Chapters 4 and 10. See also, "brain," "cerebrum," "corpus callosum" and "temporal lobe."

cryptomnesia: Detailed and accurate recall of information that was previously learned, often unconsciously, and then forgotten. Literally means "hidden memory." See also, "amnesia" and "hypermnesia."

debunker: An individual who is committed to convincing others that one or more beliefs, theories, or phenomena are false or fraudulent. See text, Chapter 2. See also, "skeptic."

developmental learning disorder: A term applied loosely to a group of conditions with onset before puberty and characterized by difficulties in acquisition of speech or certain cognitive functions, or in anomalies of emotional development. Included are Reading Disorder, Mathematics Disorder and Disorder of Written Expression. Can also be considered to include stuttering, delayed speech, Attention-Deficit/Hyperactivity Disorder, Tourette's Disorder, Asperger's Syndrome and others. Previously believed to be outgrown, these disorders are now known often to continue into adulthood. See text, Chapter 4. See also, "Anomalous Cerebral Laterality" and "Asperger's Syndrome."

dissociation: A mental process involving the disjoining of behaviors, affects, sensations and knowledge that are normally associated in ordinary waking consciousness; separation and fragmentation. The exaggeration of normal subject/object ("self/not-self") differentiation; the perceptual/experiential disincorporation of that which is generally agreed to be (part of) "self" from that which is also generally agreed to be (part of) "self." See text, Chapters 5 and 10. See also, "Altered States of Consciousness," "association," "consciousness," "hallucination," "hypnosis," "regression," "State of Consciousness" and "Transpersonal Consciousness."

ElectroEncephaloGram (EEG): An instrument, using electrodes attached to the scalp, that measures the minute electrical currents (brainwaves) generated by brain cells, especially in the cerebral cortex. See also, "brain," "brainwave coherence," "cerebrum" and "cortex."

Electro-Magnetic Sensitivity (EMS): Sensitivity to Electro-Magnetic Radiation, often resulting in anomalies in psychological, neurological and immunological functioning. A potential kindling mechanism for Temporo-Limbic Epilepsy, it is thought to originate in the limbic system of the brain by way of the pineal gland and the hypothalamus. See text, Chapters 4 and 11. See also, "biological clock," "kundalini," "limbic system," "pineal gland," "temporal lobe" and "Temporo-Limbic Epilepsy."

experimenter effect: The effect that an experimenter's or observer's prior expectations can have on the outcome of an experiment. Positive expectations can lead to positive results; negative expectations can lead to negative results. See also, "Perky effect" and "placebo effect."

explicate order: The concrete, tangible, objective, independent reality of everyday life. Also called the "unfolded order." See text, Chapter 11. See also, "implicate order," "consensus reality" and "really real."

Extra-Sensory Perception (ESP): The perception of objects, thoughts, or events without the mediation of the known human senses, the use of information directly obtained from other people, or the direct use of conventional information accessing tools; perception from a perspective that is bounded by neither space nor time. In this text, ESP is also spoken of as "experiences of transpersonal perception." See text, Chapter 11. See also, "psi," "psi-related," "PsychoKinesis" and "Transpersonal Experiences."

False Memory Syndrome (FMS): A concept based on the hypothesis that memories of forgotten (repressed or dissociated) events that are recovered during psychotherapy (especially when hypnosis is used) are not memories at all, but rather fantasies that have been created as a result of the set and setting. One of the principal arguments of debunkers, used primarily to dismiss allegations of childhood sexual abuse. See text, Chapter 2. See also, "Altered State of Consciousness," "association," "debunker," "dissociation," "experimenter effect," "Fantasy-Prone Personality," "hallucination," "hypnosis" and "Perky effect."

Fantasy-Prone Personality (FPP): A concept based on the hypothesis that, since highly hypnotizable persons have a more profound fantasy life than the norm and because highly hypnotizable persons report having more Transpersonal Experiences than the norm, Transpersonal Experiences are nothing more than fantasies. Used by debunkers to pathologize and discredit those who report such experiences. See text, Chapter 2. See also, "Altered State of Consciousness, "association," "consensus reality," "debunker," "dissociation," "experimenter effect," "False Memory Syndrome," "hallucination," "hypnosis," "Perky effect," "really real," "Transpersonal Consciousness" and "Transpersonal Experiences."

Findings—Anomalous Group Sensitivities (FANGS): A graphical form used to report group mean HISS scores, in terms of standard errors from the Reference Group mean, on the first- and second-level Predispositions and Indicators scales. See text, Chapter 12. See also, "Holistic Inventory of Stimulus Sensitivities," "mean," "standard deviation" and "Tally of Applicable Individual Life Sensitivities."

hallucination: A perception that occurs in the apparent absence of a corresponding stimulus in consensus reality. See text, Chapter 10. See also, "consensus reality," "hypnogogia," "Perky effect" and "really real."

Holistic Inventory of Stimulus Sensitivities (HISS): A paper-and-pencil test instrument, consisting of 221 questions, used to measure an individual's Predispositions toward sensitivities and Indicators of sensitivities. Scores are broken out into 50 different scales. See text, Chapters 3 and 14 and Appendices A, B, C and E. See also, "Anomalously Sensitive Person," "Findings—Anomalous Group Sensitivities," and "Tally of Applicable Individual Life Sensitivities."

hormone: One of several chemical substances produced by cells of the endocrine system and secreted into the bloodstream to regulate the growth and/or function of a special organ or tissue in another part of the body. See text, Chapter 4. See also, "melatonin," "neurotransmitter," "neurohormone," "pineal gland" and "serotonin."

hypermnesia: Unusually vivid or complete memory of historical events or stimuli. See also, "amnesia" and "cryptomnesia."

hypnogogia: The period of drowsiness preceding sleep (or preceding full awakening—technically called "hypnopompia"). It involves dreaming consciousness overlapping onto prevailing waking consciousness. It is characterized by theta-predominant brainwaves, muscle atonia, myoclonic jerks, a loosening of ego boundaries, synesthesias, extremely vivid imagery and perceptual intermixing of dream stimuli with environmental stimuli. See text, Chapter 10. See also, "Altered State of Consciousness," "consciousness," "consensus reality," "hallucination," "hypnosis," "myoclonic jerks," "primary process cognition," "Perky effect," "really real," "secondary process cognition," "State of Consciousness," "synesthesia," "tertiary process cognition" and "whole brain cognition."

hypnosis: A strategy or technique, employing a suggestion given by oneself or another, used to facilitate entering into a "non-ordinary" (i.e., other than waking, dreaming and sleeping) State of Consciousness. The States of Consciousness accessed by way of hypnotic techniques are generally characterized by focused attention, suspension of critical judgment, heightened suggestibility, vivid mental imagery, a heightened sense of reality and the transformation of thoughts and ideas into actions, sensations and perceptions without the intervention of cortical (intellectual) inhibition. See text, Chapter 10. See also, "Altered State of Consciousness," "association," "consciousness," "cortex," "dissociation," "hallucination," "hypnogogia," "Perky effect," "regression," "State of Consciousness" and "Transpersonal Consciousness."

hypopigmentation: Having a lower than normal level of melanin pigment. Hypopigmented individuals generally have blond or red hair, blue or gray eyes and very fair or fair complexions. See text, Chapter 4. See also, "melanin."

imaginal realm: A third realm that lies between the empirical realm of the senses and the abstract realm of the intellect. It is posited to be ontologically real and suggested to be a realm in which imagination functions as an organ of perception. Said to be accessible only when one is in an Altered State of Consciousness. See text, Chapter 11. See also, "Altered State of Consciousness," "consciousness," "consensus reality," "explicate order," "implicate order," "really real," "State of Consciousness," "Transpersonal Consciousness" and "Transpersonal Experiences."

implicate order: A deeper order of existence underlying the "really real" explicate order (consensus reality). A vast, primary level of reality out of which arise all the objects and appearances of the physical world as we know it—in much the same way that a piece of holographic film gives rise to a hologram. What we see in the world of consensus reality is only the surface of the implicate order as it unfolds into the explicate order. Time and space are the forms of the unfolding process. Also called the "enfolded order." See text, Chapter 11. See also, "Altered State of Consciousness," "consciousness," "consensus reality," "explicate order," "imaginal realm," "really real," "State of Consciousness," "Transpersonal Consciousness" and "Transpersonal Experiences."

343

kundalini: In the Hindu tradition, said to be a subtle form of bioenergy lying dormant, coiled up like a sleeping serpent, at the base of the spine. When aroused, kundalini energy moves upward along the spine activating energy centers (called "chakras"). Kundalini arousal purportedly has the potential to transform the central nervous system in such a way as to result in spiritual enlightenment, but the experience can be profoundly destabilizing, both physiologically and psychologically. See text, Chapter 11. See also, "Electro-Magnetic Sensitivity" and "Temporo-Limbic Epilepsy."

Less Strongly Lateralized (LSL): In a standard brain, the left cerebral hemisphere is larger than the right. A Less Strongly Lateralized (one-sided) brain generally has greater hemispheric symmetry, a larger corpus callosum and greater inter-hemispheric communication, than the asymmetric norm. Anomalous Cerebral Laterality is a special case of a LSL brain—one that is said to result from anomalous hormonal influences in utero. See text, Chapter 4. See also, "Anomalous Cerebral Laterality," "brain," "brainwave coherence," "cerebrum," "cortex," "corpus callosum" and "temporal lobe."

limbic system: A complex set of linked structures in the mid-brain and fore-brain (specifically the thalamus, hypothalamus, amygdala and hippocampus), that is closely connected to the temporal lobes. The limbic system is believed to be responsible for emotions and to function as a conduit for transmittal of information from the brain's central core to the cortex. Also called the "animal brain" or the "paleomammalian brain." See text, Chapters 4 and 9. See also, "biological clock," "cerebrum," "cortex" and "temporal lobe."

manifestation: That which appears; that which is made evident to the mind and/or the senses.

mean: The sum of a set of values divided by the number of values summed. Commonly called "average," "mean" is a more specific term and is used to ensure its differentiation from "mode" and "median," other terms with similar, but somewhat different meanings. See text, Chapter 13. See also, "standard deviation."

melanin: A brown to black pigment that influences skin, hair and eye color. People with more melanin than the norm (hyperpigmented) generally have black hair, brown eyes and dark complexions. See text, Chapter 4. See also, "hypopigmentation."

melatonin: A hormone, chemically related to both the pigment melanin and the neurotransmitter serotonin, it is produced primarily in the pineal gland (in the absence of light) from the neurotransmitter serotonin. It appears to be the chemical agent for several functions of the pineal gland having to do with timing and cycles. A powerful anti-oxidant, it enhances the immune system and is involved in the regulation of other hormonal levels. See text, Chapter 4. See also, "hormone," "neurohormone," "neurotransmitter," "pineal gland" and "serotonin."

meta-: A prefix meaning a later, more comprehensive, transcending, or more highly organized version of something. Used with the name of a discipline to designate a new but related discipline designed to deal critically with the original one.

mind: The element, or complex of elements, in an individual, that feels, perceives, thinks, wills and reasons; the organized conscious, subconscious and unconscious adaptive mental activity of an organism. Believed by some to be nothing more than a product of the brain's electro-chemical activity; believed by others to have viability independent of the brain. Similar to, but more closely associated with the brain than is either spirit or soul. In the text, "mind" generally refers to the "mind/spirit/soul" complex. See text, Chapter 1. See also, "brain," "consciousness," "soul" and "spirit."

mnemonic: Of, or relating to, memory.

myoclonic jerks: Sudden, involuntary muscle contractions.

neurohormone: One of several chemicals blurring the distinction between neurotransmitters produced by neuron cells and hormones produced by endocrine cells. The central nervous system and the endocrine system are intimately interconnected. For example, the nervous system can stimulate the adrenal glands of the endocrine system to produce the hormone adrenaline, but some nerve cells can also secrete neurohormones that act much like adrenaline. One can think of the nervous system as a rapid-acting electrical system and the endocrine system as a slower-acting chemical system, the two systems being complementary to, rather than independent of, each other. See text, Chapter 4. See also, "hormone," "melatonin," "neurotransmitter," "pineal gland" and "serotonin."

neurotransmitter: One of several chemicals that serve as a vehicle of communication between nerve cells by mediating the transmission of nerve impulses across the synapses between adjacent neurons. See text, Chapter 4. See also, "melatonin," "hormone," "neurotransmitter," "pineal gland" and "serotonin."

Non-Right-Handed (NRH): Any degree of ambidexterity up to and including full left-handedness. See text, Chapters 4 and 7. See also, "Anomalous Cerebral Laterality" and "Less Strongly Lateralized."

Perky effect: The occurrence of vivid mental imagery, in any sensory modality, that, in the absence of cortical reality judgment, assumes the perceptual status of reality as opposed to fantasy and seems to be "more real than real." Because the human brain actively constructs perceptions and because perceptions and internally generated imagery utilize the same mental mechanisms, the differentiation of imagery as an internal event, from perception as an internal representation of an external event can become confounded. See text, Chapter 10. See also, "Altered State of Consciousness," "consensus reality," "hallucination," "hypnogogia," "hypnosis," "primary process cognition," "really real," "secondary process cognition," "tertiary process cognition," and "whole-brain cognition."

pineal gland: A tiny gland located in the middle of the brain, it is involved (in the presence of light through the eyes) in the conversion of the amino acid tryptophan into the neurotransmitter serotonin and (in the absence of light through the eyes) of the neurotransmitter serotonin into the hormone melatonin. Biologically, it is composed of nerve cells; functionally, it is considered to be a master gland of the endocrine system. In the brain, it has reciprocal links with the thalamus, hypothalamus, hippocampus and amygdala; in the endocrine system it has reciprocal links with the pituitary gland, thymus gland, thyroid gland, parathyroid glands and adrenal glands. It is involved in the regulation of cycles, immune system functioning and other hormones and is said to be extremely sensitive to Electro-Magnetic Radiation. See text, Chapter 4. See also, "biological clock," "Electro-Magnetic Sensitivity," "hormone," "melatonin," "neurohormone," "neurotransmitter" and "serotonin."

placebo effect: The effect a patient's expectations (or the expectations of medical personnel, as communicated to the patient) can have on the efficacy of a medication or other medical intervention. Positive expectations (the placebo effect) can lead to positive results, negative expectations (the nocebo effect) can lead to negative results. See also, "experimenter effect" and "Perky effect."

predictive reliability: A term used to refer to the square of the coefficient of correlation between two series of paired data, expressed as a percentage. It indicates the percentage of variability in one data series that can be accounted for by the variability in the other data series. See text, Chapter 13. See also, "coefficient of correlation" and "correlated."

primary process cognition: A cognitive process, generally associated with the right hemisphere and subcortical structures of the brain, it involves a richness of ideas and originality and is characterized by movement away from set patterns and goals. It includes as many stimuli as possible in its field of consideration; it is simultaneous, holistic, unconscious, non-logical, non-rational and impulse controlled; it perceives similarities and recognizes patterns; and it uses a strategy of incorporation and unification. See text, Chapter 8. See also, "cerebrum," "cortex," "limbic system," "secondary process cognition," "tertiary process cognition" and "whole brain cognition."

PsychoKinesis (PK): The movement or change in state of physical objects by the mind, without the use of physical means. When used broadly, the term's meaning also includes electrical PsychoKinesis and psychic healing. In the text, PsychoKinesis is also spoken of as "experiences of transpersonal influence." See text, Chapters 1 and 11. See also, "Extra-Sensory Perception," "psi," "psi-related" and "Transpersonal Experiences."

psi: The 23rd. letter of the Greek alphabet (ψ). Used to refer to theoretically verifiable Transpersonal Experiences—experiences of transpersonal perception (Extra-Sensory Perception [ESP]) and experiences of transpersonal influence (PsychoKinesis [PK])— collectively. See text, Chapters 1 and 11. See also, "Extra-Sensory Perception," "psi-related," "PsychoKinesis" and "Transpersonal Experiences."

psi-related: Connected to, or related to, psi. Used to refer to theoretically unverifiable Transpersonal Experiences—experiences of transpersonal manifestation of mind. See text, Chapters 1 and 11. See also, "psi" and "Transpersonal Experiences."

"really real": Having concrete, tangible, objective, independent existence. See also, "consensus reality" and "explicate order."

regression: (1) In a hypnotherapy context, "regression" refers to reversion to an earlier mental or behavioral level. Narrowly, it refers to age regression in which a subject relives or recalls an earlier experience, generally with all five senses functioning. Broadly, it refers to the accessing of prevailing cortical brainwave patterns that are slower than those of ordinary waking consciousness—the slower the brainwaves, the younger the corresponding age. See text, Chapter 10. See also, "Altered State of Consciousness," "consciousness," "hypnosis," "primary process cognition," "State of Consciousness" and "whole brain cognition." (2) In a statistical context, "regression" refers to finding the equation that represents the linear relationship between two correlated variables. This equation, the general form of which is $y = bx + a$, can be used to predict the value of one variable that corresponds to a known value of the other variable. See text, Chapter 13. See also, "coefficient of correlation" and "correlated."

Schumann Resonance Frequency: The "fundamental frequency of the Earth"—approximately 7.8 cycles per second—at which energy is able to travel vast distances without significant attenuation. See text, Chapter 11. See also, "Transpersonal Consciousness."

secondary process cognition: A cognitive process, generally associated with the left hemisphere and other cortical structures of the brain, it is analytical reasoning of the type measured by I.Q. tests and tends to use rationality to move toward a single goal. It excludes from its field of consideration as many extraneous stimuli as possible; it is sequential, reductionistic, logical, rational and deliberation controlled; it perceives differences and recognizes discrete entities; it uses a strategy of separation and differentiation. See text, Chapter 8. See also, "cerebrum," "cortex," "limbic system," "primary process cognition," "tertiary process cognition" and "whole brain cognition."

serotonin: A neurotransmitter produced primarily in the pineal gland (in the presence of light through the eyes) from the amino acid tryptophan. In the absence of light through the eyes, it is converted to the hormone melatonin. Serotonin conveys messages between neurons and plays a major role in dampening the brain's response to incoming stimuli (the "serotonin screening mechanism") so as to prevent overload. It is one of the primary neurotransmitters involved in moods and emotions. See text, Chapter 4. See also, "hormone," "melatonin," "neurohormone," "neurotransmitter" and "pineal gland."

shaman: A term from the language of the Tungus people in Siberia, used by anthropologists to encompass other terms such as "witch doctor," "medicine man," "wizard," "sorcerer," "medium" and "seer." Narrowly defined, it means: "One who, at will, enters into Transpersonal Consciousness and experiences her/his mind or spirit journeying to other, normally hidden, realities and interacting with other entities to acquire knowledge and power and to help other people." More broadly, it means: "one who, at will, enters into Altered States of Consciousness in service of her/his community." See text, Chapter 12. See also, "Altered State of Consciousness," "consciousness," "mind," "State of Consciousness," "Transpersonal Consciousness" and "Transpersonal Experiences."

skeptic: An individual who holds that true knowledge, or knowledge in a particular area, is uncertain. Often incorrectly used as a synonym for "debunker." See also, "debunker."

soul: The immaterial essence, animating principle, or actuating cause of an individual life. Similar to "mind" and to "spirit," but less closely associated with the brain than either and said to be able to survive (brain) death. See also, "brain," "consciousness," "mind" and "spirit."

spirit: An animating or vital principle held to give life to physical organisms; the immaterial, intelligent, or sentient part of a person Similar to, but less closely associated with the brain than is "mind"; similar to, but more closely associated with the brain than is "soul." See also, "brain," "consciousness," "mind" and "soul."

standard deviation (s.d.): Technically: "A measure of the dispersion of a frequency distribution that is the square root of the arithmetic mean of the squares of the deviation of each of the class frequencies from the arithmetic mean of the frequency distribution." More comprehensibly, a standard deviation score indicates the degree to which a specific value in a series falls above or below the arithmetic mean of all the values in that series. A value of +/- 1 s.d. is in the top/bottom 16%; a value of +/- 2 s.d. is in the top/bottom 2%, a value of +/- 3 s.d. is in the top/bottom 0.14%. See text, Chapter 13. See also, "mean."

state-dependent memory: The proposition that the accessing of the memory of an experience is dependent (at least to some degree) on recreation of the specific State of Consciousness in which the experience originally occurred. See text, Chapters 2, 8 and 10. See also, "amnesia," "cryptomnesia," "hypermnesia," "regression," "State of Consciousness" and "Transpersonal Consciousness."

State of Consciousness (SOC): A specific set of mind activities with a specific pattern of awareness and/or thought. A specific SOC may be characterized by a specific (but not necessarily measurable) set of brainwave patterns. The four theoretically discrete SOCs are waking consciousness, dreaming consciousness, sleeping consciousness and Transpersonal Consciousness—but SOCs are seldom (if ever) pure, discrete, or clearly boundaried. Any SOC that differs substantively from the three "ordinary" SOCs (i.e., waking, dreaming and sleeping consciousness) can be thought of as "Altered State of Consciousness" (of which there are presumably an infinite number). See text, Chapter 10. See also, "Altered State of Consciousness," "consciousness" and "Transpersonal Consciousness."

synesthesia: The spontaneous association of a sensation being activated by an external stimulus with another sensation of a different kind. For example, hearing a sound in association with the visual perception of a color, or smelling an odor in association with the tactile perception of a texture. See text, Chapter 7. See also, "hallucination," "hypnogogia" and "Perky effect."

Tally of Applicable Individual Life Sensitivities (TAILS): A graphical form used to report individual HISS scores, in terms of standard deviations from the Reference Group mean, on the first- and second-level Predispositions and Indicators scales. See text, Chapters 3. See also, "Findings—Anomalous Group Sensitivities," "Holistic Inventory of Stimulus Sensitivities," "mean" and "standard deviation."

temporal lobe: One of the four primary lobes, or divisions, of the cerebral hemispheres (the others being the frontal lobe, parietal lobe and occipital lobe), it is located behind the temple of the cranium. It has tight reciprocal links (especially in the right hemisphere) with the limbic system that presumably give rise to its involvement in emotions. It is also involved in hearing and memory and the senses of time and individual identity. See text, Chapter 4. See also, "brain," "cerebrum," "corpus callosum," "cortex" and "limbic system."

Temporal-Lobe Epilepsy (TLE): See "Temporo-Limbic Epilepsy."

Temporo-Limbic Epilepsy (TLE): A neurological condition involving sudden discharges of excess electrical activity in the temporal lobes and limbic system of the brain. Symptoms are hallucinatory, emotional, physical, motor, sensory and experiential in nature, but do not involve the convulsions associated with classical grand mal seizures. Also called "Temporal Lobe Epilepsy," "complex partial seizures," "psychic seizures" and "psychomotor epilepsy." See text, Chapter 11. See also, "biological clock," "Electro-Magnetic Sensitivity," "kundalini," "limbic system," "pineal gland" and "temporal lobe."

tertiary process cognition: A cognitive process involving the coupling of or cycling between primary process cognition and secondary process cognition, it is central to the creative process. In tertiary process cognition, the full range of human intelligences can manifest in useful and productive form. See text, Chapter 8. See also, "cerebrum," "cortex," "limbic system," "primary process cognition," "secondary process cognition" and "whole brain cognition."

testosterone: A hormone produced primarily by the mammalian testes, it is responsible for the growth and development of male sex organs and male secondary sexual characteristics. In utero, small amounts of testosterone are present in female fetuses, having been produced by the mother, but the level is much higher in males once the testes are formed. Testosterone is thought to be the biochemical factor responsible for Anomalous Cerebral Laterality in that it may affect prenatal growth of the cerebral hemispheres and may be responsible for differences between male and female brains. See text, Chapter 4. See also, "Anomalous Cerebral Laterality" and "hormone."

352

Transpersonal Consciousness (TPC): A theoretically discrete State of Consciousness involving awareness, but not thought—pure awareness. TPC is complementary to the three "ordinary" (and theoretically discrete) States of Consciousness—waking consciousness (awareness and thought), dreaming consciousness (thought, no awareness) and sleeping consciousness (no thought, no awareness). See text, Chapter 10. See also, "Altered State of Consciousness," "consciousness" and "State of Consciousness."

Transpersonal Experiences (TPEs): "Experiences that occur beyond the ordinary differentiated boundaries of ego, space and time; experiences that suggest the interconnectedness (and/or absolute unity) of all that ever was, is, or will be; experiences that imply the existence of mind (as distinct from brain), of spirit, of soul." TPEs can be logically grouped into three categories: (1) experiences of transpersonal perception (déjà vu, synchronicity, telepathy, precognition, psychic dream and clairvoyance), (2) experiences of transpersonal influence (psychic healing, electrical PsychoKinesis and PsychoKinesis) and (3) experiences of transpersonal manifestation of mind (contact with spirit guides, Out-Of-Body Experience, past-life recall, apparition, mediumistic episode, UFO sighting, Near-Death Experience, spirit possession and alien contact). See text, Chapters 1 and 11. See also, "Extra-Sensory Perception," "mind," "PsychoKinesis," "psi," "psi-related," "soul" and "spirit."

whole brain cognition: A variant of tertiary process cognition, whole brain cognition is a cognitive process involving the *simultaneous* functioning of both primary process cognition and secondary process cognition. It utilizes both the cortical structures and the subcortical structures of the brain. It is characterized by slow (theta-predominant) cortical brainwave patterns, a high level of brainwave coherence and enhanced communication between the different parts of the brain—thus permitting a greater-than-normal two-way communication between subcortical brain structures and the environment. See text, Chapter 10. See also, "Altered State of Consciousness," "brainwave coherence," "cerebrum," "cortex," "limbic system," "primary process cognition," "secondary process cognition" and "tertiary process cognition."

wyrd: An Anglo-Saxon term having to do with a way of life governed by the beliefs that: (1) all things and all events are intimately interconnected, as if by a seamless web, on all levels of reality; (2) objects that are perceptible to human senses are nothing more than local manifestations of larger energy patterns; (3) that which is imperceptible to human senses is just as important as that which is perceptible; (4) any event, anywhere, affects everything else, everywhere, as a result of vibrations transmitted throughout the web; and (5) everything, everywhere, is alive—that is, consciousness is all-pervasive; body, mind and spirit are all one; and the entire universe is sacred and has purpose and meaning. See text, Chapter 12. See also, "imaginal realm," "implicate order" and "shaman."

SOURCES

Page #   *Subject Matter:* **Source(s)**

Preface

xiv *"Transpersonal Experiences (TPEs)":* Grof, 1985;
Grof (Ed.), 1984; Grof & Grof (Eds.), 1989.

Chapter 1

22 *Key diagnostic criteria for Schizotypal Personality
Disorder:* American Psychiatric Association, 1994,
pp. 641-645

22 *"Perceptual and Motor Skills":* Brugger, et. al., 1993.

27 *Stanislav Grof's term "Transpersonal Experiences":*
Grof, 1985; Grof (Ed.), 1984; Grof & Grof (Eds.), 1989.

31 *Three studies with non-clinical populations:* Richards,
1991.

Chapter 2

36 *Study of high creativity and high I.Q. students:* Getzels &
Jackson, 1967.

37 *Testing revealed that eccentrics score high on scales
of ...:* Weeks & James, 1995.

39 *Belief in reincarnation was proclaimed anathema:* Weiss,
1988, p. 35.

39 *Explosion of super-nova in 1054 A.D.:* Hoagland, 1987,
p.91.

39 *Arrest of Gallileo Galilei:* McDaniel, 1993, p. 169.

40 *Last major organized group of Gnostics eliminated:*
Baigent, et. al., 1982, p. 57.

40 *The Left-Hander Syndrome:* Coren, 1992, pp. 1–2.

42(†)*Brookings Institute study:* McDaniel, 1993, pp. 167–169.

44 *Evidence supporting the veridicality of psi experiences:*
Dossey, 1993; Ostrander & Schroeder, 1997; Radin,
1997.

Page #   ***Subject Matter:* Source(s)**

71   *Many phenomena are strongly correlated with left-handedness:* Brugger, et. al., 1993; Coren, 1992; Coren & Searleman, 1987; Geschwind & Galaburda, 1985; Geschwind & Galaburda (Eds.), 1984; Hermann, 1989; Kunsendorf & Marsden, 1991; London, 1990; London & Butler; Obler & Fein (Eds.), 1988; Russell, 1979; Springer & Deutsch, 1981.

76   *Decreasing level of melatonin informs cell DNA ...:* Bock & Gayette, 1995; Pierpaoli & Regelson, 1995; Sahelian, 1995.

77   *Elevated levels of stress hormones are correlated with hypopigmentation:* Arcus, 1994.

77   *Stress hormones have been shown to be immuno-suppressive:* Achterberg, 1985; Arcus, 1994; Becker, 1990; Becker & Selden, 1995; Bock & Gayette, 1995; Dossey, 1993; Dossey, 1998; Korn & Johnson, 1983; Locke & Colligan, 1986; Ornstein & Sobel, 1987; Pelletier, 1977; Pierpaoli & Regelson, 1995; Shealey, 1999; Simonton, Simonton & Creighton, 1978; E. D. Wilson, 1991.

77   *Categories of stress:* Shealey, 1999, p. 156.

78   *Chromosomal abnormalities are correlated with left-handedness:* London & Butler.

78   *Interstital nuclei of the anterior hypothalamus:* Gorman, 1991.

Chapter 5

82   *Literature in the field of neurology:* Ardila, et. al., 1993; Geschwind & Galaburda, 1985; LaPlante, 1993; Persinger, 1987; Persinger, 1990; Teicher, et. al., 1993.

82   *Literature in the field of psychiatry:* Allison, 1980; Bliss, 1986; Braun (Ed.), 1986; Crabtree, 1985; Kluft, 1990; Kluft (Ed.), 1985; Putnam, 1989; Ross, 1989; Ross, 1995; Ross, 1997a; Ross, 1997b; van der Kolk, 1987.

82   *Literature in the field of transpersonal psychology:* Fiore, 1989; Grof & Grof (Eds.), 1989; Lucas, 1993; Persinger, 1974; Persinger, 1992; Reed, 1988; Richards, 1991; Ring, 1992; I. Wilson, 1989.

359

361

Page #   ***Subject Matter:*** **Source(s)**

Chapter 10

148 *Activities associated with the brain:* Bloom, et. al., 1985, p. 5.

148 *"The Origin of Consciousness in the Breakdown of the Bicameral Mind":* Jaynes, 1976.

151 *Primary diagnostic criterion for DID:* American Psychiatric Association, 1994, p. 484.

151(†)*"Mental Unity, Altered States of Consciousness and Dissociation":* Tinnen, 1990.

153 *Contemporary research with dolphins ...:* Coren, 2000; Grandin, 1995.

153 *Thinking in Pictures:* Grandin, 1995.

157*"Thin boundaries":* Hartmann, 1991.

157 *Brainwave frequency patterns of this [whole brain cognition] sort are associated with ...:* Arieti, 1976; Bentov, 1977; Csikszentmihalyi, 1996; Cytowic, 1993; Faraday, 1974; Gainer & Torem, 1994; Geschwind & Galaburda, 1985; Geschwind & Galaburda (Eds.), 1984; Green & Green, 1997; Hallowell & Ratey, 1994; Harmon & Rheingold, 1984; Hufford, 1982; Jamison, 1993; Kalweit, 1988; Korn & Johnson, 1983; LaPlante, 1993; Mahowald, et. al. (Eds.); Marvomates, 1987; Monroe, 1992; Ornstein & Sobel, 1987; Pelletier, 1977; Persinger, 1974; Persinger, 1987; Persinger, 1990; Ring, 1992; Rossi, 1986; Rossi & Cheek, 1988; Samuels & Samuels, 1975; Sanella, 1987; Simonton, et. al., 1978.

158 *Einstein's brain showed a highly coherent pattern of alpha brainwaves:* Zohar, 1993, p. 140.

158 *Scientific discoveries occurred in an Altered State of Consciousness:* Pearce, 1971, pp. 24–25.

159*"Perky Effect":* Baker, 1992, p. 142.

160 *Definition of the term "hallucinations":* Asaad, 1990, p. 4.

163 *Two different pathways by which ASCs can be accessed:* Hilgard, 1965; Hilgard, 1977.

164 *Dissociative pathologies and associative abilities:* Beahrs, 1982.

167*"Radar of the unconscious mind":* Wise, 1995.

362

363

364

Page #	**Subject Matter: Source(s)**

204   *Brains mathematically construct objective reality:*
Russell, 1979; Talbot, 1991.

204   *Capabilities of brain not explainable by neuroanatomical model:* Bohm, 1980; Russell, 1979, Talbot, 1986; Talbot, 1991; Zohar, 1983; Zohar, 1990.

206   *Projection from deeper order of reality —the "implicate order":* Bohm, 1980; Combs & Holland, 1990; Dossey, 1989; Grof, 1985; Grof (Ed.), 1984; Talbot, 1986; Talbot, 1991.

207   *Predominant brainwave frequencies of TPC:* Achterberg, 1985; Arieti, 1976; Combs & Holland, 1990; Green & Green, 1977; Harmon & Rheingold, 1984; Harner, 1980; Jamison, 1993; Kalweit, 1988; Korn & Johnson, 1983; LaPlante, 1993; Lucas, 1993; Marvomatis, 1987; Monroe, 1992; Persinger, 1974; Persinger, 1987; Persinger, 1990; Persinger, 1992; Persinger, et. al., 1980; Samuels & Samuels, 1975; Wise, 1995; Zohar, 1983; Zohar, 1990.

207   *Presence of strong flares of delta:* Lucas, 1993; Wise 1995.

207   *"Awakened mind":* Wise, 1995.

207   *"Schumann Resonance Frequency":* Becker & Selden, 1995; Bentov, 1977; Capra, 1991; Persinger, 1974.

208   *Similarities between mind processes and quantum mechanical processes:* Zohar, 1983, pp. 141–142.

208   *"Communication is unmediated …":* Dossey, 1989, p. 183.

211   *Evidence of mind on three levels:* Dossey, 1989, pp. 153–154.

212   *Existence of superimplicate order:* Bohm, 1980; Combs & Holland, 1990.

Chapter 12

230   *EEG biofeedback has shown promise in management of disorders:* Green & Green, 1977; Wise, 1995.

230   *Efficacy of EEG biofeedback in facilitating peak performance and experiences of psi:* Green & Green, 1977; Persinger, 1974; Wise, 1995; Zohar, 1983.

365

Selected

Bibliography

Achterberg, J. 1985. *Imagery in Healing—Shamanism and Modern Medicine.* Boston. New Science Library.

Allison, R. 1980. *Minds in Many Pieces.* New York. Rawson Wade.

American Psychiatric Association. 1994. *Diagnostic and Statistical Manual of Mental Disorders—Fourth Edition.* Washington, DC. American Psychiatric Association.

Arcus, D. "Biological Mechanisms and Personality: Evidence from Shy Children." In *Advances: The Journal of Mind-Body Health.*, Vol. 10, No. 4 (Fall, 1994).

Ardila, A., C. R. Nino, E. Pulido, D.B. Rivera and C.J. Vanega. "Episodic Psychic Symptoms in the General Population." In *Epilepsia,* Vol 34, No 1 (1993).

Arieti, S. 1976. *Creativity—The Magic Synthesis.* New York. Basic.

Aron, E. N. 1996. *The Highly Sensitive Person.* Secaucus, NJ. Carol.

Aron, E. N. and A. Aron. "Sensory Processing Sensitivity and its Relation to Introversion and Emotionality." In *Journal of Personality and Social Psychology.* 1998.

Asaad, G. 1990. *Hallucinations in Clinical Psychiatry.* New York. Brunner/Mazel.

Baigent, M., R. Leigh and H. Lincoln. 1982. *Holy Blood, Holy Grail.* New York. Dell.

Baker, R. A. 1990. *They Call It Hypnosis.* Buffalo, New York. Prometheus.

_____ 1992a. *Hidden Memories.* Buffalo, NY. Prometheus.

_____ 1992b. *Alien Abductions or Alien Productions.* Louisville, KY.

Baldwin, W. J. 1999. *CE-VI: Close Encounters of the Possession Kind.* Terra Alta, WV. Headline.

Bartholomew, R. E., K. Basterfield and G. Howard. "UFO Abductions and Contactees: Psychopathology or Fantasy Proneness?" In *Professional Psychology—Research and Practices,* Vol. 22, No. 3 (1991): 215-222.

Bates, B. 1983. *The Way of the Wyrd.* San Francisco. HarperCollins.

Beahrs, J. O. 1982. *Unity and Multiplicity.* New York. Brunner/Mazel.

Becker, R. O. 1990. *Cross Currents.* Los Angeles. Tarcher.

Becker, R. O. and G. Selden. 1995. *The Body Electric.* New York. Morrow.

Begich, N. and J. Manning. 1995. *Angels Don't Play This HAARP.* Anchorage, AK. Earthpulse.

Benson, H. 1975. *The Relaxation Response.* New York. Morrow.

Bentov, I. 1977. *Stalking the Wild Pendulum.* Rochester, VT. Destiny.

Blackmore, S. 1993. *Dying to Live.* Buffalo, NY. Prometheus.

Bliss, E. L. 1986. *Multiple Personality, Allied Disorders and Hypnosis.* New York. Oxford.

Bloom, F. E., A. Lazerson and L. Hostadter. 1985. *Brain, Mind and Behavior.* New York. Freeman.

Bock, S. J. and M. Gayette. 1995. *Stay Young the Melatonin Way.* New York. Dutton.

Bohm, D. 1980. *Wholeness and the Implicate Order.* London. Routledge & Kegan Paul.

Braun, B. G., (Ed.). 1986. *Treatment of Multiple Personality Disorder.* Washington, D.C. American Psychiatric Press.

Breggin, P. R. 1991. *Toxic Psychiatry.* New York. St. Martin's.

_____ 1998. *Talking Back to Ritalin.* Monroe ME. Common Courage.

Brown, B. B. 1980. *Supermind.* New York. Bantam.

Brugger, P., A. Gamma , R. Muri , M. Shafer and K. I. Taylor . "Correlates to Belief in the Paranormal: Functional Hemispheric Asymmetry and Belief in ESP - Toward a 'Neuropsychology of Belief.'" In *Perceptual and Motor Skills*, 77 (December, 1993): 1299-1308.

Budden, A. 1994. *Allergies and Aliens.* Trowbridge, Wiltshire, Great Britain. Redwood.

_____ 1995. *UFOs: Psychic Close Encounters*. London. Blandford.

_____ 1998. *Electric UFOs*. London. Blandford.

Capra, F. 1991. *The Tao of Physics.* Boston. Shambala.

Carlson, E. B. and F. W. Putnam. "Integrating Research on Dissociation and Hypnotizability." In *Dissociation,* Vol. II, No. 1 (March, 1989).

Collins, A. 1996. *From the Ashes of Angels.* London. Penguin.

Combs, A. and M. Holland. 1990. *Synchronicity.* New York. Random House.

Conway, F. and J. Siegelman. 1978. *Snapping.* New York. Dell.

Corbin, H. 1972. *Mundus Imaginalis or the Imaginal and the Imaginary.* Ipswich, England. Golgonooza Press.

Coren, S. 2000. *How to Speak Dog.* New York. Free Press.

_____ 1992. *The Left-Hander Syndrome.* New York. Free Press.

Coren, S. and A. Searleman. "Left Sidedness and Sleep Difficulty: The Alinormal Syndrome." In *Brain and Cognition,* 6 (1987): 184-192

Crabtree, A. 1985. *Multiple Man.* New York. Praeger.

Csikszentmihalyi, M. 1996. *Creativity.* New York. HarperCollins.

Cytowic, R. E.. 1993. *The Man Who Tasted Shapes.* Los Angeles. Tarcher.

Damgaard, J. A. "The Inner Self Helper." In *Noetic Sciences Review.* Sausalito, CA. Winter 1987.

Doore, G., (Ed.). 1988. *Shaman's Path.* Boston. Shambala.

Dossey, L. 1989. *Recovering the Soul.* New York. Bantam.

_____ 1991. *Meaning and Medicine.* New York. Bantam.

_____ 1993. *Healing Words.* New York. HarperCollins.

Drasin, D. "Zen ... and the Art of Debunkery." In P. D. Pursglove (Ed.). 1995. *Zen in the Art of Close Encounters.* Berkeley, CA. New Being Project.

Faraday, A. 1974. *The Dream Game.* New York. Harper & Row.

Fiore, E. 1978. *You Have Been Here Before.* New York. Doubleday.

_____ 1987. *The Unquiet Dead.* New York. Doubleday.

_____ 1989. *Encounters.* New York. Doubleday.

Frankel, F. H. 1976. *Hypnosis: Trance as a Coping Mechanism.* New York. Plenum.

Gainer, M. J. and M. S. Torem. "Sleep and Dissociation." In *ISSD News.* August 1994.

Gardner, H. 1983. *Frames of Mind.* New York. Basic.

Gardner, R. A. 1991. *Sex Abuse Hysteria.* Cresskill, NJ. Creative Therapeutics.

Gelernter, D. 1994. *The Muse in the Machine.* New York. Free Press.

Geschwind, N. and A. M. Galaburda. 1985. *Cerebral Lateralization.* Cambridge, MA. MIT Press.

Geschwind, N and A. M. Galaburda, (Eds.). 1984. *Cerebral Dominance.* Cambridge, MA. Harvard University Press.

Getzels, J. W. and P. W. Jackson. 1967. *Creativity and Intelligence.* New York. Wiley.

Goldberg, P. 1983. *The Intuitive Edge.* Los Angeles. Tarcher.

Goleman, D. "New Kind of Memory Found to Preserve Moments of Emotion." In *New York Times,* October 25, 1994.

Goldstein, E. 1992. *Confabulations.* Boca Raton, FL. SIRS Books.

Gorman, C. "Are Gay Men Born That Way?." In *Time,* September 9, 1991.

Graff, D. E. 1998. *Tracks in the Psychic Wilderness.* Boston. Element.

Grandin, T. 1995. *Thinking in Pictures.* New York. Vintage.

Green, E. and A. Green. 1977. *Beyond Biofeedback.* Ft. Wayne, IN. Knoll.

Greenwell, B. 1990. *Energies of Transformation—A Guide to the Kundalini Process.* Cupertino, CA. Transpersonal Learning Services.

Greer, S. M. 1999. *Extraterrestrial Contact.* Afton, VA. Crossing Point.

Grof, S. 1985. *Beyond the Brain.* Albany, NY. SUNY Press.

Grof, S., (Ed.). 1984. *Ancient Wisdom and Modern Science.* Albany, NY. SUNY Press.

Grof, S. and C. Grof, (Eds.). 1989. *Spiritual Emergency.* Los Angeles. Tarcher.

Halifax, J. 1979. *Shamanic Voices.* New York. Arkana.

Hallowell, E. M. and J. J. Ratey. 1994. *Driven to Distraction.* New York. Pantheon.

Harmon, W. and H. Rheingold. 1984. *Higher Creativity.* Los Angeles. Tarcher.

Harner, M. 1980. *The Way of the Shaman.* San Francisco. HarperSanFrancisco.

Harrison, R., E. Hartmann and J. Bevis. "The Hartmann Boundary Questionnaire—A Measure of Thick and Thin."

Hartmann, E. 1991. *Boundaries in the Mind.* New York. Basic.

Hassan, S. 1988. *Combatting Cult Mind Control.* Rochester, VT. Park Street .

Hermann, N. 1989. *The Creative Brain.* Lake Lure, N.C. Brain Books.

Herrenstein, R. J. and C. Murray. 1994. *The Bell Curve.* New York. Free Press.

Hilgard, E. R. 1965. *The Experience of Hypnosis.* San Diego, CA. Harcourt, Brace, Jovanovich.

_____ 1977. *Divided Consciousness.* New York. Wiley.

Hoagland, R. C. 1987. *The Monuments of Mars.* Berkeley, CA. North Atlantic.

Hopkins, B., D. M. Jacobs and R. Westrum. 1992. *Unusual Personal Experiences: Analysis of the Data from Three National Surveys Conducted by the Roper Organization.* Las Vegas, NV. Bigelow Holding Corporation.

Hufford, D. J. 1982. *The Terror That Comes in the Night.* Philadelphia. University of Pennsylvania Press.

Hughes, D. J. "Differences Between Trance Channeling and Multiple Personality Disorder on Structured Interview." In *Journal of Transpersonal Psychology,* Vol. 24, No. 2 (1992).

Jamison, K. R. 1993. *Touched With Fire.* New York. Free Press.

Jaynes, J. 1976. *The Origin of Consciousness in the Breakdown of the Bicameral Mind.* Boston. Houghton Mifflin.

Johnson, D. A. "Personality Characteristics of Persons Reporting Experienced Anomalous Trauma." In *Proceedings of the Third Conference on Treatment and Research of Experienced Anomalous Trauma.*

Kalweit, H. 1988. *Dreamtime and Inner Space.* Boston. Shambala.

Kiersey, D. and M. Bates. 1984. *Please Understand Me.* Del Mar, CA. Prometheus Nemesis.

Kluft, R. P. 1990. *Incest Related Syndromes of Adult Psychopathology.* Washington, D.C. American Psychiatric Press.

_____ (Ed.). 1985. *Childhood Antecedents of Multiple Personality.* Washington, D.C. American Psychiatric Press.

Korn, E. R. and K. Johnson. 1983. *Visualization—The Use of Imagery in the Health Professions.* Homewood, IL. Dow Jones - Irwin.

Kotulak, R. 1996. *Inside the Brain.* Kansas City, MO. Andrews McMeel.

Kramer, P. D. 1993. *Listening to Prozac.* New York. Viking.

Kunsendorf, R. B. and D. Marsden. "Dissociation in Ambidextrous Students." In *Perceptual and Motor Skills.* 72 (1991): 778.

LaPlante, E. 1993. *Seized.* New York. HarperCollins.

Larsen, G. E., D. L. Alderton, M. Neideffer and E. Underhill. "Psychological Factors in Differential Accident Rates for Right- and Left-Handers." A paper presented at the 101st annual convention of the American Psychological Association. August 22, 1993.

LeShan, L. 1966. *The Medium, The Mystic and The Physicist.* New York. Viking.

Locke, S. and D. Colligan. 1986. *The Healer Within.* New York. Dutton.

London, W. P. "Left-Handedness and Alcoholism." In S. Coren, (Ed.). 1990. *Left-Handedness: Behavioral Implications and Anomalies.* North Holland. Elsevier Science Publishers B.V.

London, W. P. and Butler, M.G. "Two Processes of Cerebral Lateralization and the Methylation of DNA." Unpublished.

Lucas, W. B. 1993. *Regression Therapy (Vol. I: Past Life Therapy).* Crest Park, CA. Deep Forest .

Lynn, S. J. and J. W. Rhue. "The Fantasy-Prone Person: Hypnosis, Imagination and Creativity." In *Journal of Personality and Social Psychology.* Vol. 51, No. 2 (1986): 404–408.

Lynn, S. J. and J. W. Rhue. "Fantasy Proneness." In *American Psychologist.* (January, 1988.)

Lynn, S. J. and J. W. Rhue, (Eds.). 1994. *Dissociation.* New York. Guilford.

Mahowald, M. W., C. H. Schenck and D. Gotlib, (Eds.). "Sleep/Wake State Dissociation." (A collection of articles from various sources).

373

Marvomatis, A. 1987. *Hypnagogia.* London. Routledge & Kegan Paul.

McDaniel, S. V. 1993. *The McDaniel Report.* Berkeley, CA. North Atlantic.

Mintz, E. E. 1983. *The Psychic Thread.* New York. Human Sciences.

Monroe, R. R. 1992. *Creative Brainstorms.* New York. Irvington.

Morse, M. with P. Perry. 1990. *Closer to the Light.* New York. Ivy.

Myers, I. B. with P. B. Myers. 1980. *Gifts Differing.* Palo Alto, CA. Counsulting Psychologists Press.

Myers, I. B. and M. H. McCaulley. 1985. *A Guide to the Development and Use of the Myers-Briggs Type Indicator.* Palo Alto, CA. Consulting Psychologists Press.

Naparstek, B. 1997. *Your Sixth Sense.* New York. HarperCollins.

Narby, J. 1998. *The Cosmic Serpent.* New York. Tarcher/Putnam.

Nickell, J. "A Study of Fantasy Proneness in the Thirteen Cases of Alleged Encounters in John Mack's *Abduction."* In *Skeptical Inquirer,* May/June, 1996.

Obler, L. K. and D. Fein, (Eds.). 1988. *The Exceptional Brain.* New York. Guilford.

Ornstein, R. 1993. *The Roots of the Self.* New York. HarperCollins.

Ornstein, R. and D. Sobel. 1987. *The Healing Brain.* New York. Simon & Schuster.

Ostrander, S. and L. Schroeder. 1997. *Psychic Discoveries.* New York. Marlowe.

Pearce, J. C. 1971. *The Crack in the Cosmic Egg.* New York. Julian.

Pelletier, K. R. 1977. *Mind as Healer, Mind as Slayer.* New York. Delta.

Persinger, M. A. 1974. *The Paranormal: Part II.* New York. MSS Information Corp.

_____ 1987. *Neuropsychological Bases of God Beliefs.* New York. Praeger.

_____ "Temporal Lobe Lability." In *Bulletin of Anomalous Experience.* Vol. 1, No. 6 (September 1990).

_____ "Neuropsychological Profiles of Adults Who Report 'Sudden Remembering' of Early Childhood Memories: Implications for Claims of Sex Abuse and Alien Visitation/Abduction Experiences." In *Perceptual and Motor Skills,* 75 (1992): 259-266.

Persinger, M. A., N. J. Carrey and L. A. Seuss. 1980. *TM and Cult Mania.* North Quincy, MA. Christopher.

Pierpaoli, W. and W. Regelson. 1995. *The Melatonin Miracle.* New York. Simon & Schuster.

Powers, S. M. "Fantasy Proneness, Amnesia and the UFO Abduction Phenomenon." In *Dissociation,* Vol. IV, No. 1 (March 1991).

Prince, M. 1975. *Psychotherapy and Multiple Personality.* Cambridge, MA. Harvard University Press.

374

Putnam, F. W. 1989. *Diagnosis and Treatment of Multiple Personality Disorder.* New York. Guilford.

Quail, R. A. 1993. *Prodigies: Extraterrestrial Telepathic Intelligence Phenomenon.* Atlanta, GA. ETIP.

Randles, J. 1994. *Star Children.* New York. Sterling.

Ratey, J. J. and C. Johnson. 1997. *Shadow Syndromes.* New York. Pantheon.

Radin, D. I. 1997. *The Conscious Universe.* New York. HarperCollins

Reed, G. 1988. *The Psychology of Anomalous Experience.* Buffalo, NY. Prometheus.

Restak, R. M. 1984. *The Brain.* New York. Bantam.

Restak, R. M. 1993. *Receptors.* New York. Bantam.

Richards, D. G. "A Study of the Correlation Between Subjective Psychic Experiences and Dissociative Experiences." In *Dissociation,* Vol. IV, No. 2 (June, 1991): 83–91.

Ring, K. 1982. *Life at Death.* New York. Quill.

_____ 1984. *Heading Toward Omega.* New York. Morrow.

_____ "Toward an Imaginal Interpretation of 'UFO Abductions.'" In *Revision,* Vol. 11, No. 4 (Spring, 1989).

_____ "Fantasy-Proneness and the Kitchen Sink." In the *Journal of UFO Studies*, Vol. 2 (1990): 186-187.

_____ 1992. *The Omega Project.* New York. Morrow.

Ritchey, D. "Of Lizards and Wizards." In *Bulletin of Anomalous Experience,* Vol. 4, No. 6 (December, 1993).

Rogo, D. S. 1986. *On the Track of the Poltergeist.* Englewood Cliffs, NJ. Prentice-Hall.

Ross, C. A. 1989. *Multiple Personality Disorder.* New York. Wiley.

_____ 1995. *Satanic Ritual Abuse.* Toronto. University of Toronto Press.

_____ 1997a. *Dissociative Identity Disorder.* New York. Wiley.

_____ "The CIA and Mind Control Research." On CKLN-FM (88.1), Toronto. *Mind Control Series.* March 16, 23, 30, 1997b.

Rossi, E. L. 1986. *The Psychobiology of Mind-Body Healing.* New York. Norton.

Rossi, E. L. and D. B. Cheek. 1988. *Mind-Body Therapy.* New York. Norton .

Russell, P. 1979. *The Brain Book.* New York. Dutton.

Sahelian, R. 1995. *Melatonin: Nature's Sleeping Pill.* Marina Del Ray, CA. Be Happier Press.

Samuels, M. and N. Samuels. 1975. *Seeing With the Mind's Eye.* New York. Random House.

Sanella, L. 1987. *The Kundalini Experience.* Lower Lake, CA. Integral.

Schnabel, J. 1994. *Dark White.* London. Hamish Hamilton.

Shallis, M. 1988. *The Electric Connection.* New York. New Amsterdam.

Shealey, N. 1999. *Sacred Healing.* Boston. Element.

Sheldrake, R. 1995. *A New Science of Life.* Inner Transitions.

Simonton, S. M., O. C. Simonton and J. L. Creighton. 1978. *Getting Well Again.* New York. Bantam.

Smith, C. W. and S. Best. 1989. *Electromagnetic Man.* New York. St. Martins.

Smith, S. L. 1991. *Succeeding Against the Odds.* Los Angeles. Tarcher.

Spencer, J. and A. Spencer. 1996. *The Poltergeist Phenomenon.* London. Headline.

Spiegel, H. and D. Spiegel. 1978. *Trance and Treatment.* New York. Basic.

Springer, S. P. and G. Deutsch. 1981. *Left Brain, Right Brain.* New York. Freeman.

Steiger, B. and S. H. Steiger. 1992. *Star Born.* New York. Berkley.

Strieber, W. 1995. *Breakthrough.* New York. HarperCollins.

Talbot, M. 1986. *Beyond the Quantum.* New York. Bantam.

_____ 1991. *The Holographic Universe.* New York. HarperCollins.

Targ, E. and M. Schlitz. 1998. "Psi Related Experiences: Research Directions and Clinical Experience."

Taylor, S. E. 1989. *Positive Illusions.* New York. Basic.

Teicher, M. H., C.A. Glod, J. Surrey and C. Swett. "Early Childhood Abuse and Limbic System Ratings in Adult Psychiatric Outpatients." In *Journal of Neuropsychiatry,* Vol. 5, No. 3 (Summer, 1993).

Tellegren, A. and G. Atkinson. "Openness to Absorbing and Self-Altering Experiences ('Absorption'), a Trait Related to Hypnotic Susceptibility." In Vol. 83, No. 3 (1974): 268–277.

Terr, L. 1990. *Too Scared to Cry.* New York. Harper & Row.

Terr, L. 1994. *Unchained Memories.* New York. Basic.

Tinnen, L. "Mental Unity, Altered States of Consciousness and Dissociation." In *Dissociation,* Vol. III, No. 3, (September 1990).

Vallee, J. 1979. *Messengers of Deception.* Berkeley, CA. And/Or Press.

_____ 1988. *Dimensions.* Chicago. Contemporary.

_____ 1990. *Confrontations.* New York. Ballantine

_____ 1991. *Revelations.* New York. Ballantine.

van der Kolk, B. H. 1987. *Psychological Trauma.* Washington, DC. American Psychiatric Press.

Walsh, R. 1990. *The Spirit of Shamanism.* Los Angeles. Tarcher.

Weiss, B. 1988. *Many Lives, Many Masters.* New York. Simon & Schuster.

Weeks, D. and J. James. 1995. *Eccentrics.* New York. Villard.

West, T. G. 1991. *In the Mind's Eye.* Buffalo, NY. Prometheus.

White, J. 1990. *The Meeting of Science and Spirit.* New York. Paragon.

Wilson, E. D. 1991. *Wilson's Syndrome.* Orlando, FL. Cornerstone.

Wilson, I. 1989. *Stigmata.* San Francisco. Harper & Row.

Wilson, S. C. and T. X. Barber. "The Fantasy-Prone Personality: Implications for Understanding Imagery, Hypnosis and Parapsychological Phenomena." In A. A. Sheikh, (Ed.). *Imagery: Current Theory, Research and Application.* 1983. New York. Wiley: 340–390.

Wise, A. 1995. *The High-Performance Mind.* New York. Tarcher.

Wolf, F. A. 1991. *The Eagle's Quest.* New York. Simon & Schuster.

Wonder, J. and P. Donovan. 1984. *Whole Brain Thinking.* New York. Ballantine.

Wright, L. 1994. *Remembering Satan.* New York. Knopf.

Yapko, M. 1994. *Suggestions of Abuse.* New York. Simon and Schuster.

Zohar, D. 1983. *Through the Time Barrier.* London. Paladin .

_____ 1990. *The Quantum Self.* New York. Quill.

Zukov, G. 1979. *The Dancing Wu Li Masters.* New York. Bantam.

Index

388

List of Tables

Page #	Title

LIST OF CHARTS

Notes

Notes

Notes

Notes

Notes

Notes

Notes

Notes

Notes

Notes